MRCGP
Applied Knowledge Test

1001 Questions and
Answers

Second edition

Rob Daniels

MA (Cantab), MRCGP
General Practitioner

Pastest

© 2016 Pastest Ltd
Egerton Court
Parkgate Estate
Knutsford
Cheshire
WA16 8DX

Telephone: 01565 752000

A percentage of the material in this book was previously published in *MRCGP Practice Questions: Applied Knowledge Test, Second Edition* (ISBN 9781905635665) and *nMRCGP Practice Papers: Applied Knowledge Test, Second Edition* (ISBN 9781905635597).

First Published 2013
Second Edition 2016

ISBN: 978 1 78414 003 8
eISBN: 978 1 78414 005 2 MobiPocket
          978 1 78414 004 5 ePUB

A catalogue record for this book is available from the British Library.

The information contained within this book was obtained by the author from reliable sources. However, while every effort has been made to ensure its accuracy, no responsibility for loss, damage or injury occasioned to any person acting or refraining from action as a result of information contained herein can be accepted by the publishers or author.

Pastest Online Revision, Books and Courses

Pastest provides online revision, books and courses to help medical students and doctors maximise their personal performance in critical exams and tests. Our in-depth understanding is based on over 40 years' experience and the feedback of recent exam candidates.

Resources are available for:
Medical school applicants and undergraduates, MRCP, MRCS, MRCPCH, DCH, GPST, MRCGP, FRCA, Dentistry, and USMLE Step 1.

For further details contact:
Tel: 01565 752000   Fax: 01565 650264
www.pastest.com   enquiries@pastest.com

Text prepared in the UK by Carnegie Book Production, Lancaster
Printed and bound in the UK by Bell & Bain Ltd, Glasgow

Contents

Acknowledgements

I would like to thank the patients of Townsend House Medical Centre, whose images appear in this book. I would also like to acknowledge, with thanks, the following people who have contributed additional clinical images:

Mr Peter Simcock, Consultant Ophthalmologist, Royal Devon & Exeter Hospital

Dr Chris Bower, Consultant Dermatologist, Royal Devon & Exeter Hospital

Mr Malcolm Hilton, Consultant Surgeon, Royal Devon & Exeter Hospital

Mr Ian Daniels, Consultant Surgeon, Royal Devon & Exeter Hospital

Dr Chris Cates, Senior Research Fellow, St George's University London

Thanks also to Lisa Daniels.

Contributors to the previous editions

Julius Bourke MBBS MRCPsych

Erika Damato MA (Cantab) MBBS MRCP

Alison Johnstone MBChB MRCGP DFFP

Priya Joshi MB ChB DRCOG MRCGP

Grant Neumegen MBChB (Otago) MRCGP

Seamus Phillips MA BM MRCS DOHNS MSc

Suzanne Renshaw BM DRCOG MRCGP

Andrew Rosewarne MBBS MRCS DFPP DCH MRCGP

Pinki Singh MBBS DGO DNB MRCOG

Ramanathan Visvanathan BM BCh, FRCS (Irel, Eng, Ed), ILTM

Amy Wilson MBChB MRCPCH

Kurt Wilson BSc MBChB MRCGP

Introduction

This book is intended predominantly to help candidates prepare for the Membership examination of The Royal College of General Practitioners. It is also hoped that this book will be useful for established GPs to identify learning needs as part of their appraisal process and perhaps prepare them for any future knowledge-based test introduced as part of revalidation.

About the exam

The MRCGP is the exit qualification for general practice training in the UK and consists of a written exam, a formal clinical skills assessment and workplace-based assessment. The written paper is a 200-question MCQ exam known as the Applied Knowledge Test (AKT). The subject matter is divided into critical appraisal and evidence-based clinical practice components (10% of total), health informatics and administrative questions (10%), and clinical medicine (80%).

The exam aims to test higher problem-solving at the level of an independent primary care physician, rather than simple fact recall, and questions are based on everyday clinical scenarios, practice issues and hot topics. There is no negative marking. Questions are in the following formats: single best answer, multiple best answer, extended matching questions, table/algorithm questions, picture format, drag-and-drop format, data interpretation, free text and drug calculations. Where calculations are required, an on-screen calculator will be available, but any arithmetic required will be simple and for most candidates a calculator will not be necessary.

The AKT takes place at the end of January, May and October each year, via computer terminals at 150 Pearson Vue professional testing centres around the UK. Candidates may take the exam in ST2 and ST3 stages of their general practice specialty training, but it is expected that most will do so during their third year of specialty training (ST3), when they will be working in primary care. The exam can be taken a maximum of four times. All questions will address important issues relating to general practice in the UK, and international applicants should note that the answers relate to standard clinical practice in the UK.

Preparing for the exam

The key to successful preparation is twofold. Similar to all medical exams good exam technique is vital. Two hundred questions have to be completed in 3 hours and 10 minutes at a rate of one question every 57 seconds. Practice is vital if questions can be answered at this rate. The second component of successful performance is an adequate knowledge base. The questions in this book are based on the GP curriculum, which is an excellent guide to planning your revision, ensuring that you cover less clinical areas of the curriculum such as practice management and information technology (see The Applied Knowledge Test Content Guide, August 2014, on the RCGP website – rcgp.org.uk).

In April 2016 the pass mark was 67.5% and the pass rate was 72.5%, although the cumulative pass rate after four attempts was approximately 95%. It is well worth reading recent examiners' reports describing areas of weak performance, which the examiners may concentrate on in future exams. Candidates usually perform well in clinical medicine, less well in critical appraisal and worst in administration questions. We have used these reports to update the questions for this second edition, but it is worth reading through them as they appear after each sitting.

The best way to prepare for clinical questions is to read up on problems that you see in general practice, ideally keeping a list of PUNs and DENs (patient's unmet needs and doctor's educational needs) encountered during each surgery. All of the examiners are practising GPs and questions are based on day-to-day practice.

Try to do as many practice multiple-choice questions as you can. PasTest also offer an online revision package specifically for the AKT, which gives instant progress feedback (www.pastest.co.uk). It should be possible to pick up on hot topics just through working in general practice and reading the *British Medical Journal* and *British Journal of General Practice*, but a 'hot topics' course just before the exam is usually money well spent. The RCGP's website suggests that candidates be familiar with the BNF, GMC's *Good Medical Practice*, RCGP's *Essential Knowledge Updates*, guidelines of the National Institute for Health and Care Excellence (NICE) and the Scottish Intercollegiate Guidelines Network (SIGN), Cochrane and the *Vaccine* update newsletter.

Information on management issues is best picked up by spending a session with your practice manager, attending practice meetings, reviewing the curriculum and doing multiple-choice questions to identify specific learning needs. Practising critical appraisal with a group from your GP training scheme is a useful way of learning this skill, and there are regular specimen questions on the *InnovAiT* website of SAGE Journals (http://ino.sagepub.com). I have included several statistics questions to illustrate various concepts, but all the data and graphs are made up, so please do not take the results too seriously.

Summary

In my experience the three best techniques to pass the exam are:

1. Practice, practice, practice: do as many MCQs as you can.
2. Don't leave any blanks: there is no negative marking.
3. Ensure that you cover the whole GP curriculum.

I have done my best to ensure that all the questions and answers are accurate and current. If you find any discrepancies or have any other comments please let me know and I will make the necessary changes.

Good luck!

Rob Daniels

Abbreviations

A&E	accident and emergency
ABPI	ankle–brachial pressure index
ACE	angiotensin-converting enzyme
ACL	anterior cruciate ligament
ACTH	adrenocorticotrophic hormone
ADH	antidiuretic hormone
ADHD	attention deficit hyperactivity disorder
AF	atrial fibrillation
AG	anion gap
AIDS	acquired immune deficiency syndrome
ALL	acute lymphoblastic leukaemia
ALP	alkaline phosphatase
ALT	alanine transaminase
AML	acute myeloid leukaemia
APTT	activated partial thromboplastin time
ARB	angiotension receptor antagonist
ARDS	acute respiratory distress syndrome
ARI	absolute risk increase
ARMD	age-related macular degeneration
ARR	absolute risk reduction
AST	aspartate transaminase
AV	atrioventricular
BCC	basal cell carcinoma
BCG	bacille Calmette–Guérin
βhCG	β-human chorionic gonadotrophin
BIPP	bismuth iodoform paraffin paste
BMI	body mass index
BNP	brain natriuretic peptide
BP	blood pressure
BTS	British Thoracic Society
CBT	cognitive-behavioural therapy
CC	case-control (study)
CER	control event rate
CF	cystic fibrosis
CHADS$_2$	CCF, hypertension, age >75, diabetes and stroke
CHD	coronary heart disease
CI	confidence interval
CIN	cervical intraepithelial neoplasia
CK	creatine kinase
CKD	chronic kidney disease
CLL	chronic lymphoblastic leukaemia
CML	chronic myeloid leukaemia
CMV	cytomegalovirus

CNS	central nervous system
COC(P)	combined oral contraceptive (pill)
COPD	chronic obstructive pulmonary disease
COX	cyclooxygenase
CPAP	continuous positive airway pressure
CPN	community psychiatric nurse
CPR	cardiopulmonary resuscitation
CREST	calcinosis, Raynaud's disease, (o)esophageal dysmotility, sclerodactyly and telangiectasia
CRP	C-reactive protein
CSF	cerebrospinal fluid
CT	computed tomography
CTG	cardiotocography
CVD	cardiovascular disease
CVS	chorionic villous sampling
DCIS	ductal carcinoma *in situ*
DES	direct enhanced service
DIC	disseminated intravascular coagulation/coagulopathy
DIP	distal interphalangeal
DKA	diabetic ketoacidosis
DMARD	disease-modifying anti-rheumatic drug
DNA	deoxyribonucleic acid
DSM-IV	*Diagnostic and Statistical Manual of Mental Disorders*, 4th edition
DVLA	Driver and Vehicle Licensing Agency
DVT	deep vein thrombosis
DXA	dual-energy X-ray absorptiometry
EBV	Epstein–Barr virus
ECG	electrocardiogram
EEG	electroencephalogram
EER	experimental event rate
eGFR	estimated glomerular filtration rate
ENT	ear, nose and throat
EPA	enduring power of attorney
ERCP	endoscopic retrograde cholangiopancreatography
ESR	erythrocyte sedimentation rate
FBC	full blood count
FEV1	forced expiratory volume in 1 second
FFP	fresh frozen plasma
FGM	female genital mutilation
FRC	functional residual capacity
FSH	follicle-stimulating hormone
FT_4	free thyroxine
FVC	forced vital capacity
G6PDH	glucose-6-phosphate dehydrogenase
GFR	glomerular filtration rate
GGT	γ-glutamyltransferase
GI	gastrointestinal
GLP	glucagon-like peptide
GMS	General Medical Services
GnRH	gonadotrophin-releasing hormone
GPPAQ	General Practice Physical Activity Questionnaire

GPwSI	general practitioner with a special interest
GTN	glyceryl trinitrate
GUM	genitourinary medicine
HbA1c	glycated haemoglobin
HDL	high-density lipoprotein
HELLP	haemolysis, elevated liver enzymes, low platelets
HIV	human immunodeficiency virus
HPV	human papillomavirus
HR	heart rate
HRT	hormone replacement therapy
HSP	Henoch–Schönlein purpura
IBS	irritable bowel syndrome
ICD-10	*International Classification of Disease*, 10th revision
ICP	intracranial pressure
ICU	intensive care unit
IMCA	independent mental capacity advocate
INR	international normalised ratio
IOP	intraocular pressure
IQ	intelligence quotient
IUCD	intrauterine contraceptive device
KUB	kidneys, ureters and bladder
LDH	lactate dehydrogenase
LDL	low-density lipoprotein
LES	local enhanced service
LFTs	liver function tests
LH	luteinising hormone
LHRH	luteinising hormone-releasing hormone
LMWH	low-molecular-weight heparin
LPA	lasting power of attorney
LRTI	lower respiratory tract infection
LTOT	long-term oxygen therapy
LVF	left ventricular failure
MALT	mucosa-associated lymphoid tissue
MAOI	monoamine oxidase inhibitor
MCH	mean corpuscular haemoglobin
MCV	mean corpuscular volume
MI	myocardial infarction
MMR	measles, mumps and rubella
MRI	magnetic resonance imaging
MRSA	methicillin-resistant *Staphylococcus aureus*
MSU	midstream urine
NCAA	National Clinical Assessment Authority
NICE	National Institute for Health and Care Excellence
NNH	number needed to harm
NNT	number needed to treat
NSAID	non-steroidal anti-inflammatory drug
NSTEMI	non-ST-elevation myocardial infarction
NYHA	New York Heart Association
OCD	obsessive–compulsive disorder
OSA	obstructive sleep apnoea
PCL	posterior cruciate ligament

PCOS	polycystic ovarian syndrome
PCR	polymerase chain reaction
PCT	primary care trust
PE	pulmonary embolus
PEFR	peak expiratory flow rate
PICA	posterior inferior cerebellar artery
PID	pelvic inflammatory disease
PIP	proximal interphalangeal
PMR	polymyalgia rheumatica
POP	progestogen-only pill
PPI	proton pump inhibitor
PSA	prostate-specific antigen
PT	prothrombin time
PTH	parathyroid hormone
PUVA	psoralen + UVA
QALY	quality-adjusted life-year
QOF	Quality and Outcomes Framework
RA	rheumatoid arthritis
RCT	randomised controlled trial
RICE	rest, ice, compression and elevation
RR	relative risk
RSV	respiratory syncytial virus
SCC	squamous cell carcinoma
SIGN	Scottish Intercollegiate Guidelines Network
SIR	standardised incidence ratio
SLE	systemic lupus erythematosus
SNRI	serotonin and noradrenaline reuptake inhibitor
SSRI	selective serotonin release inhibitor
STEMI	ST-elevation myocardial infarction
STI	sexually transmitted infection
SVC	superior vena cava
T_3	triiodothyronine
T_4	thyroxine
TB	tuberculosis
TED	thromboembolic deterrent
TFT	thyroid function test
TIA	transient ischaemic attack
TNF	tumour necrosis factor
TSH	thyroid-stimulating hormone
U&Es	urea and electrolytes
UTI	urinary tract infection
UTRI	upper respiratory tract infection
UVA	long-wavelength ultraviolet (light)
UVPP	uvulopalatoplasty
VEGF	vascular endothelial growth factor
VIN	vulval intraepithelial neoplasia
VRE	vancomycin-resistant enterococci
WCC	white cell count
WOMAC	Western Ontario and McMaster Universities Index of Osteoarthritis

Section 1
Clinical Medicine

Chapter 1
Cardiovascular problems

Single best answer questions

1.1   Blood pressure
        At a routine blood pressure check your practice nurse discovers a 20
        mmHg difference in systolic blood pressure between the right and left
        arms of a patient. She asks him to return and see you and, when he does,
        you note the same findings. What would be the SINGLE MOST appropriate
        next step in his management? Select ONE option only.

○   A   Ambulatory blood pressure monitoring

○   B   Ankle–brachial pressure measurement

○   C   Chest X-ray

○   D   Refer for tilt-table tests

○   E   Urinary catecholamines

1.2   Cholesterol
        A 29-year-old man asks for a cholesterol test. His father, aged 53, has just
        had a heart attack, although he was a heavy smoker. On checking his blood
        pressure you notice pale nodules on the tendons of his wrists. He tells you
        that he also has them on the back of his ankles, and that these are a family
        trait. His cholesterol is 7.8 mmol/l and his blood pressure is 134/80 mmHg.
        Which ONE of the following would be the SINGLE MOST appropriate
        management for this patient?

○   A   Advise on a low-fat diet and repeat his blood test in 6 months

○   B   Calculate his Framingham risk score and treat him with statins if his
         10-year risk is >20%

○   C   Start atorvastatin 10 mg once daily

○   D   Start simvastatin 20 mg once daily

○   E   Start simvastatin 80 mg once daily

1.3 **Fainting**
A 21-year-old student rower who is training for national trials complains that he has had a few episodes of palpitations and fainted during a heavy training session. On examination he is in sinus rhythm with a resting pulse of 54, his heart sounds reveal a soft systolic murmur and his blood pressure is 112/66. An ECG shows slightly enlarged R waves. Which ONE of the following is the SINGLE MOST likely diagnosis?

○ A Hypertrophic obstructive cardiomyopathy

○ B Overexertion

○ C Paroxysmal atrial fibrillation

○ D Recurrent supraventricular tachycardia

○ E Wolff–Parkinson–White syndrome

1.4 **Leg pain**
A 72-year-old man who underwent coronary artery bypass surgery 5 years ago presents with intermittent cramp-like pain in the buttock, thigh and calf. The symptoms are worse on walking and relieved by rest. On examination, both legs are of normal colour, but the pedal pulses are difficult to palpate. Sensation is mildly reduced in the left foot. Which of the following is the SINGLE MOST appropriate action?

○ A Advise him to reduce walking distance to prevent pain

○ B Doppler ultrasound

○ C Measure ankle–brachial systolic pressure index

○ D Magnetic resonance imaging (MRI) of the lumbar spine

○ E Referral for angiography

1.5 **Cholesterol**
The following results show the fasting lipid profile of a 35-year-old man who underwent routine testing as part of a general health check: total cholesterol 7.9 mmol/l, low-density lipoprotein (LDL) 4.9 mmol/l, high-density lipoprotein (HDL) 0.83 mmol/l and triglyceride 5.2 mmol/l. His father died of myocardial infarction (MI) at the age of 52. Which ONE of the following would be the most appropriate initial management? Select ONE option only.

○ A Initiate dietary modification and monitor response by re-testing in 3 months

○ B Initiate treatment with a fibrate

○ C Initiate treatment with simvastatin 10 mg once daily

○ D Initiate treatment with simvastatin 80 mg once daily; further testing is not required

○ E Refer for specialist opinion

1.6   Driving after myocardial infarction

A 65-year-old man has recently been discharged from hospital having suffered an ST-elevation MI. Coronary artery stenting was performed and he is now pain free. He enquires whether he can drive his own car. Which ONE of the following is the SINGLE MOST appropriate advice? Select ONE option only.

- ○ A   After an MI patients should not drive until they have undergone exercise or functional testing
- ○ B   Driving must cease for 6 months
- ○ C   Driving must cease for at least 4 weeks
- ○ D   The patient must notify the DVLA
- ○ E   The patient should be informed that the GP is obliged to inform the DVLA of this event

1.7   Antibiotic prophylaxis

A 64-year-old man who underwent mitral valve replacement 5 years ago has forgotten the advice that he was given regarding the use of prophylactic antibiotics to prevent endocarditis when he undergoes dental treatment or other procedures. Which one of the following is the most appropriate advice? Select ONE option only.

- ○ A   Antibiotic prophylaxis is not recommended for routine procedures, but he should be advised about the importance of maintaining good oral health
- ○ B   He should receive antibiotic prophylaxis for any future dental or surgical procedures
- ○ C   He should receive antibiotic prophylaxis for any procedures on the gastrointestinal or genitourinary tracts
- ○ D   He should receive antibiotic prophylaxis for dental procedures only
- ○ E   He should use chlorhexidine mouthwash before dental treatment

1.8   Hypertension

A 42-year-old man of Asian origin attends for a general health check. He is a non-smoker, drinks 21 units of alcohol per week, is physically well and active, and enjoys regular moderate exercise and a healthy diet. His body mass index (BMI) is 27.2 kg/m^2: His BP, measured on three occasions, was 162/100, 165/100 and 168/102 mmHg. Which one of the following would be the most appropriate initial management? Select ONE option only.

- ○ A   Advise about lifestyle modification and review in 6 months
- ○ B   Refer for investigation of a secondary cause of hypertension
- ○ C   Start a calcium-channel blocker
- ○ D   Start a thiazide diuretic
- ○ E   Start an ACE inhibitor

1.9   Calf pain
A 42-year-old woman has varicose veins that are normally asymptomatic. She presents with a 3-day history of moderately severe pain and erythema surrounding a superficial vein, below and medial to the right knee. On palpation, the varicose vein is hardened and tender; the rest of the calf is unremarkable. Which ONE of the following is the most appropriate management? Select ONE option only.

O   A   Refer for surgical assessment

O   B   Request a Doppler ultrasound scan of the leg

O   C   Start oral flucloxacillin

O   D   Treat with an NSAID and crepe bandage

O   E   Treat with topical corticosteroid

1.10   Collapse
A 21-year-old female student with no significant medical history consults you 24 hours after collapsing in a shop. The event was witnessed by a friend, who reports that she suddenly became pale and clammy, lost consciousness and fell to the floor. There was a short episode of twitching of all four limbs. She regained consciousness after less than 1 minute, rapidly became oriented and has felt well since the event. Neurological and cardiovascular examinations are normal, with a heart rate (HR) of 76/min and BP of 120/65 mmHg. Which ONE of the following is the SINGLE MOST likely diagnosis?

O   A   Epilepsy

O   B   Hyperglycaemia

O   C   Neurocardiogenic syncope

O   D   Paroxysmal arrhythmia

O   E   Pseudoseizure

1.11   Syncope
A 78-year-old man with a history of atrial fibrillation treated with sotalol complains of recurrent syncopal episodes. Examination reveals atrial fibrillation with a rate of 84/min and normal blood pressure. You ask your practice nurse to do an electrocardiogram (ECG) and while this is taking place he has another syncopal episode. A rhythm strip is obtained, which is shown below.

What would be the SINGLE MOST appropriate action in this situation?

O   A   Admit for pacemaker

O   B   Check bloods to exclude myocardial infarction

O   C   Give intravenous adrenaline and commence cardiopulmonary resuscitation (CPR)

O   D   Start amiodarone

O   E   Stop his β blocker

1.12 ECG abnormalities

A 35-year-old man presents with chest pain. The ECG below is carried out. Select the ONE feature from A to E shown that is most consistent with a diagnosis of pericarditis.

1.13   Raised blood pressure
A 56-year-old woman who looks after her daughter's three young children attends for a flu jab and is found to have raised blood pressure by the nurse. You see her and find that her blood pressure is elevated, but not as much as when the nurse saw her. There is no difference between her arms. You arrange a 24-hour blood pressure recording, the results of which are shown below.

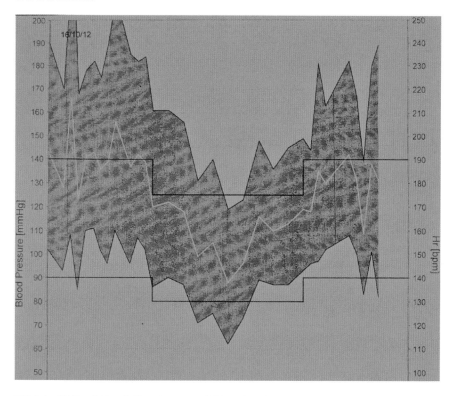

Which ONE of the following would be the SINGLE MOST appropriate management in this situation?

O   A   Advice her about healthy lifestyle and review in 3 months

O   B   Ask her to purchase her own blood pressure monitor and keep a diary of regular recordings for 2 weeks

O   C   Encourage her to attend relaxation classes

O   D   Reassure her that she has white coat hypertension and no treatment is needed

O   E   Start antihypertensives

1.14   Shortness of breath
A 79-year-old man presents with a 1-month history of mild shortness of breath on exertion. On examination, his pulse is irregular with a rate of 90 beats/min at rest. A systolic murmur is heard on auscultation. His ECG is shown below.

Which ONE of the following would be the SINGLE MOST appropriate in his management?

O   A   Amiodarone 200 mg once daily

O   B   Aspirin 300 mg once daily

O   C   Bendroflumethiazide 2.5 mg once daily

O   D   Diltiazem hydrochloride 60 mg twice daily

O   E   Furosemide 40 mg once daily

1.15   **Management of essential hypertension in patients under 55 years of age**

Select the rank order of the options (1–4) that best fulfils the requirements given in the question.

The following is a list of treatments for essential hypertension for white people aged <55:

1   ACE inhibitor or β blocker
2   α Blocker
3   Calcium-channel blocker
4   Thiazide diuretic

The responses (A–E) rank the treatments for essential hypertension in various orders. Select the response that places the options (1–4) in the order of **initial** treatment first to **final** step last. Select ONE rank order only.

○   A: 1, 3, 2, 4

○   B: 1, 3, 4, 2

○   C: 1, 4, 3, 2

○   D: 3, 1, 4, 2

○   E: 4, 3, 1, 2

Extended matching questions

ECG interpretation

1.16–1.19

Options

A   Atrial fibrillation
B   Atrial flutter
C   Sinus bradycardia
D   Sinus tachycardia
E   Ventricular extrasystoles
F   Wenckeback's phenomenon
G   Wolff–Parkinson–White syndrome

For each ECG rhythm strip shown below, select the SINGLE MOST likely diagnosis from the list above.

1.16

1.17

1.18

1.19

Heart failure

1.20–1.23

Options

A   Amlodipine
B   Atenolol
C   Carvedilol
D   Digoxin
E   Diltiazem
F   Furosemide
G   Ramipril
H   Spironolactone
I   Valsartan
J   None of the above

For each of the scenarios below, select the SINGLE MOST appropriate option from the list above. Each option may be used once, more than once or not at all.

1.20   A 67-year-old man had a heart attack last year. An echocardiogram 6 months after the heart attack showed left ventricular dysfunction for which he was started on an ACE inhibitor. He is still symptomatic and on examination he has a sinus tachycardia with a rate of 100. His previous medical history includes hypertension and hypercholesterolaemia, and he is taking aspirin, simvastatin and ramipril.

1.21   An 86-year-old man with heart failure has been started on lisinopril 8 weeks ago but complains of a persistent cough. His previous medical history includes chronic obstructive pulmonary disease for which he takes tiotropium and salmeterol.

1.22   A 73-year-old woman with left ventricular dysfunction after a myocardial infarction is taking valsartan and nebivolol at maximum doses. She was previously treated with ramipril but developed a cough. She is keen to improve her exercise capacity so that she can play with her grandchildren.

1.23   A 92-year-old woman who has been treated for many years for heart failure is taking digoxin for atrial fibrillation, ramipril and spironolactone. She has previously tried β blockers but developed cold feet. She is particularly bothered by her oedematous legs which make it very hard to find shoes that fit.

Treatment of hypertension

1.24–1.28

Options

A   Amlodipine
B   Atenolol
C   Bendroflumethiazide
D   Candesartan
E   Doxazosin
F   Furosemide
G   Hydralazine
H   No change indicated
I   Ramipril
J   Specialist referral

Select from the options above the SINGLE MOST appropriate treatment for each of the following scenarios. Each option can be used once, more than once or not at all.

1.24   A white 49-year-old man takes ramipril and amlodipine at their maximum doses for essential hypertension. His BP over the last 3 months has persistently been found to be between 148/92 and 154/96 mmHg.

1.25   A 56-year-old man of African–Caribbean origin takes bendroflumethiazide 2.5 mg once daily. His BP is persistently found to lie between 148/94 and 156/96 mmHg. He has a healthy diet and takes regular exercise. He is intolerant of calcium channel blockers.

1.26   A white 69-year-old man, who is otherwise well, takes atenolol and bendroflumethiazide for essential hypertension. His BP is 136/88 mmHg.

1.27   A 39-year-old businessman complains of daily headaches and stress at work. His BP is 186/116 mmHg and his urine is positive for protein on dipstick testing.

1.28   A previously well 42-year-old man has recently started taking an ACE inhibitor for essential hypertension. He complains of a dry cough, and has decided to stop his medication. On examination, his BP is 148/98 mmHg and auscultation of the chest is normal.

Angina

1.29–1.32

Options

A   Amlodipine
B   Anticoagulation
C   Atenolol
D   Clopidogrel
E   Emergency hospital admission
F   Glyceryl trinitrate (GTN)
G   Isosorbide mononitrate
H   Lisinopril
I   Nicorandil

For each of the scenarios below, select the SINGLE MOST appropriate treatment from the list above. Each option can be used once, more than once or not at all.

1.29   A 48-year-old man is seen at the end of the morning surgery, having experienced four episodes of chest pain that morning. Each episode lasted for 15–20 minutes and radiated to the left arm. He smokes 20 cigarettes a day and has a family history of MI. He takes no regular medication. He is now pain free, with a BP of 155/95 mmHg. Examination of the chest is normal.

1.30   A 72-year-old woman with angina experiences chest pain three to four times a week. Episodes usually occur on exertion and are relieved by sublingual GTN. She takes no other medication.

1.31   A 79-year-old man with known left ventricular dysfunction requires further control of his angina despite the use of a long-acting nitrate. He takes no other medication.

1.32   A 59-year-old man with angina, for whom standard treatment with calcium antagonists, β blockers and long-acting nitrates has been unsuccessful.

Pharmacological treatment of symptomatic heart failure due to left ventricular systolic dysfunction

1.33–1.38

Options

A	ACE inhibitor
B	Angiotensin II receptor antagonist
C	β Blocker
D	Digoxin
E	Diuretic therapy
F	Spironolactone

Complete the following algorithm, selecting options from the list above. Each option can be used once, more than once or not at all.

Free-text questions

1.39   Cholesterol treatment in diabetes
According to the 2014 NICE guidance, at what level of risk on the QRISK2 assessment tool should a statin be initiated in a patient with type 2 diabetes? Write the answer, as a percentage, in the box below.

┌─────────────┐
│   │
│   │
│   │
└─────────────┘

1.40   Shortness of breath
A 32-year-old woman with no previous medical history is seen 3 weeks after an uneventful delivery of her second baby. She complains that she has swollen ankles, is short of breath and has been waking up at night unable to breathe. Examination confirms pitting oedema of the ankles, a resting tachycardia of 120, with a regular heartbeat and bilateral basal crepitations on auscultation. In the box below, write the most likely diagnosis in this case.

┌──┐
│   │
│   │
│   │
│   │
└──┘

1.1   B: Ankle–brachial pressure measurement

A difference in systolic blood pressure between the arms of >10 mmHg is a risk factor for cardiovascular disease; systematic reviews suggest that a 15 mmHg difference is associated with a 70% increase in risk of occult peripheral arterial disease. Sustained differences should prompt ankle–brachial pressure index (ABPI) testing, particularly in patients with other cardiovascular risk factors. Ambulatory blood pressure monitoring should be used in patients with suspected white coat hypertension, whereas urinary catecholamines are used to exclude phaeochromocytoma in patients with fluctuating resistant hypertension.

1.2   E: Start simvastatin 80 mg once daily

Tendon xanthomas are diagnostic of familial hypercholesterolaemia. He is at very high risk of ischaemic heart disease and should be treated with simvastatin 80 mg once daily or equivalent regardless of his Framingham score. Diagnostic criteria for familial hypercholesterolaemia are a total cholesterol >7.5 with tendon xanthomas. Prevalence in the UK is 1:500 but it is higher in certain ethnic groups such as Afrikaners. Familial hypercholesterolaemia accounts for 10% of cases of heart disease in the under 60 group.

1.3   A: Hypertrophic obstructive cardiomyopathy

HOCM has a prevalence of 1:500 and is a common cause of sudden cardiac death in young people. Early symptoms include angina, dyspnoea and syncope. ECG changes include left ventricular hypertrophy and examination may show a systolic murmur, which characteristically diminishes on squatting and increases on Valsalva's manoeuvre. Echocardiography is the examination of choice.

1.4   C: Measure ankle–brachial systolic pressure index

These symptoms are typical of intermittent claudication. The history and an ABPI of <0.9 support the diagnosis. Walking distance can be improved by exercise and patients should be encouraged to continue walking beyond the distance at which pain occurs. Referral to a vascular surgeon is indicated if symptoms are lifestyle limiting. If there are bilateral symptoms, spinal stenosis should be considered.

1.5   A: Initiate dietary modification and monitor response by re-testing in 3 months

The premature death (at 52 years) of this patient's father and his abnormal lipid profile suggest a diagnosis of familial hyperlipidaemia, of which there are several types. Combined elevation of cholesterol and triglycerides suggests familial combined hyperlipidaemia, which affects 0.5–1% of the population and approximately 15% of patients who have an MI before the age of 60. In the absence of other risk factors (smoking, diabetes, hypertension) he can safely be managed by diet and, if there is no response, with statins. Should other risk factors be present, these should also be addressed.

1.6   C: Driving must cease for at least 4 weeks

DVLA medical standards of fitness to drive state that driving of a private car (a group 1 vehicle) must cease for 4 weeks after an ST-elevation MI. All acute coronary syndromes, including MI, result in disqualification from driving group 2 vehicles (eg a heavy goods vehicle or bus) for 6 months before re-licensing.

1.7   A: Antibiotic prophylaxis is not recommended for routine procedures, but he should be advised about the importance of maintaining good oral health

The use of prophylactic antibiotics to prevent endocarditis for patients with structural cardiac abnormalities and replacement valves has been longstanding, accepted medical practice, but there is little evidence of its effectiveness. Recommendations have been changed, based on the best available published evidence and multidisciplinary and expert consensus (NICE, March 2008).

1.8   E: Start an ACE inhibitor

This patient has a diagnosis of hypertension. With a BP >160/100 mmHg, he should be offered drug therapy. An ACE inhibitor is recommended as first-line treatment for patients aged <55 years. Patients aged >55, and black patients of any age, should initially be treated with a calcium-channel blocker or a thiazide diuretic.

1.9   D: Treat with an NSAID and crepe bandage

These features are typical of superficial thrombophlebitis, which can usually be adequately treated with NSAIDs. A crepe bandage will compress the vein and help prevent propagation of the thrombus. If phlebitis extends upwards in the medial thigh, towards the saphenofemoral junction, refer for Doppler ultrasound because there is potential for extension into the femoral vein.

1.10   C: Neurocardiogenic syncope

These features are typical of neurocardiogenic (vasovagal) syncope. The condition is benign and can be triggered by the following factors: emotion, pain, fear and anxiety, micturition, defecation, dehydration, a warm environment and prolonged standing. Advice to patients should include avoidance of precipitating factors. Other methods of prevention include compression hosiery or voluntary forceful contraction of the limb muscles at the onset of symptoms.

1.11   A: Admit for pacemaker

This ECG shows a 12-second episode of asystole. Atropine can be used if the episode is prolonged but a permanent pacemaker is needed. Amiodarone is used for atrial fibrillation, whereas adrenaline would be used in an arrest situation. If the patient collapses, basic life support should be instituted until he reaches hospital. Where pacing is not available, short-term treatment with isoprenaline might be helpful until definitive treatment is possible.

1.12   B

B indicates a saddle wave typical of acute pericarditis. This condition may cause ST elevation and also initially depression between the P wave and the start of the QRS complex. In later stages T-wave inversion may be seen.

1.13   E: Start antihypertensives

This graph shows that she has sustained hypertension with systolic readings consistently >140 mmHg. There are peaks, suggesting a stress response, but her average readings will be well above treatment targets. She should have lifestyle advice, start treatment and be assessed for end-organ damage and causes of hypertension, as well as having her 10-year cardiovascular risk calculated.

1.14   D: Diltiazem hydrochloride 60 mg twice daily

The ECG reveals AF with a rapid ventricular response. NICE clinical guidance on AF (2006) recommends that the most appropriate management strategy for this patient would be rate control with a rate-limiting calcium antagonist (or β blocker). Stroke risk stratification and anticoagulation are important, and it is likely that this patient would be a candidate for warfarin therapy (aged >75 with clinical evidence of valve disease).

1.15   B: 1 3 4 2

1 ACE inhibitor or β blocker; 3 Calcium-channel blocker; 4 Thiazide diuretic; 2 α Blocker

NICE guidance for the management of essential hypertension in adults aged >55 is to start with an ACE/ARB or if this is contraindicated with a β blocker. Poor control should prompt addition of a calcium-channel blocker. If control is still not gained a thiazide diuretic should be tried next. Spironolactone, although unlicensed for this indication, is recommended at stage 4 in the BNF. Failure to respond should prompt either an α blocker or specialist referral. Those aged >55 or of African–Caribbean origin should start with a calcium-channel blocker at stage 1.

ECG interpretation

1.16   B: Atrial flutter

This ECG shows atrial flutter with a 4:1 block. Atrial flutter is a supraventricular tachycardia with an atrial rate usually around 300, and either 2:1, 3:1 or 4:1 AV block, typically giving ventricular rates of 150, 100 or 75. The ECG shows characteristic saw-tooth flutter waves.

1.17   E: Ventricular extrasystoles

This ECG shows frequent broad complex ventricular extrasystoles, with a run of five consecutive complexes, usually followed by a compensatory pause. In healthy patients normally no investigation is required, but in patients with ischaemic heart disease investigation could trigger ventricular tachycardia.

1.18   F: Wenckeback's phenomenon

This ECG shows a lengthening P–R interval followed by a non-conducted P wave. Asymptomatic patients do not require treatment, and there is a low risk of progression to third-degree AV block, so pacing is rarely required.

1.19   G: Wolff–Parkinson–White syndrome

This ECG shows the characteristic delta waves (slurred slow rise of the initial portion of QRS) of Wolff–Parkinson–White syndrome. This is due to congenital accessory pathways causing episodes of tachyarrhythmia and a small risk of sudden cardiac death.

Heart failure

1.20   C: Carvedilol

First-line treatment for heart failure with left ventricular dysfunction consists of ACE inhibitor and a cardioselective β blocker such as carvedilol, bisoprolol or atenolol.

1.21   I: Valsartan

If ACE inhibitors are not tolerated, patients should be treated with an angiotensin receptor blocker. An alternative would be a β blocker, but in this patient there is COPD with reversibility, so caution should be exercised with β blockers.

1.22   H: Spironolactone

Patients symptomatic despite a β blocker and ACE inhibitor/ARB should be considered for an aldosterone antagonist.

1.23   F: Furosemide

Diuretics are useful for symptom relief but do not affect prognosis. They can cause postural hypotension so should be used with caution.

Treatment of hypertension

1.24	C:	Bendroflumethiazide
1.25	I:	Ramipril
1.26	H:	No change indicated
1.27	J:	Specialist referral
1.28	D:	Candesartan

The guidance produced by NICE suggests a stepwise protocol for the treatment of hypertension, as follows:

Step	Patients aged <55 years	Patients aged ≥55 years or black patients of any age
1	A	C or D
2	A + C or D	C or D + A
3	A+ C + D	A + C + D

A = ACE inhibitor (AIIRA if intolerant), C = calcium-channel blocker, D = thiazide diuretic.

Drug therapy should be offered to the following patients:

- Those with a persistent high blood pressure of ≥160/100 mmHg
- Those with a 10-year risk of CVD of >20%, and persistent high blood pressure of ≥140/90 mmHg.

Patients should be referred immediately if there are signs of accelerated hypertension or if phaeochromocytoma is suspected.

Angina

1.29	E:	Emergency hospital admission
1.30	C:	Atenolol
1.31	A:	Amlodipine
1.32	I:	Nicorandil

For patients with mild angina with fewer than two attacks per week, 'as required' treatment with GTN is appropriate. Introduction of further treatments should be stepwise in the following order: (1) β blocker, (2) long-acting dihydropyridine calcium-channel blocker (eg amlodipine) and (3) long-acting nitrate.

In the presence of left ventricular dysfunction, long-acting nitrates are used first line, with the addition of a long-acting dihydropyridine calcium-channel blocker if necessary. Nicorandil is recommended if standard treatment is unsuccessful but is contraindicated in left ventricular failure (LVF) and hypotension.

Pharmacological treatment of symptomatic heart failure due to left ventricular systolic dysfunction

1.33	A:	ACE inhibitor
1.34	B:	Angiotensin II receptor antagonist
1.35	C:	β Blocker
1.36	F:	Spironolactone
1.37	E:	Diuretic therapy
1.38	D:	Digoxin

Based on NICE clinical guidance, *Management of adults in chronic heart failure in primary and secondary care*, July 2003.

1.39   10%

NICE (July 2014), 'Lipid modification: cardiovascular risk assessment and the modification of blood lipids for the primary and secondary prevention of cardiovascular disease', states that, for primary prevention for people with type 1 diabetes, statin treatment should be considered for all adults who are over 40, or have had diabetes for 10 years or more, have nephropathy or other CVD risk factors. For patients with type 2 diabetes a statin should be initiated in patients with a 10% or higher 10-year risk as calculated on QRISK2. For both groups, atorvastatin 20 mg once daily is recommended as the drug of choice.

1.40   Peripartum cardiomyopathy

Peripartum cardiomyopathy occurs in the final 4 weeks of pregnancy or the first 6 months of delivery, and is characterised by impaired LVF. Most patients are managed medically but cardiac transplantation may be needed. The mortality rate is 20–50% although 30–50% recover without long-term complications. Recurrence rates are high and patients should be counselled about future pregnancies.

Chapter 2
Digestive problems, including nutrition

Single best answer questions

2.1 **Epigastric pain**
You are called to visit a 46-year-old man who complains of acute onset of severe upper abdominal pain, radiating to his back. He feels sweaty and nauseous and also reports pain in his shoulder. When you arrive he is sitting up, leaning over the back of a chair, and examination reveals marked epigastric tenderness. What is the SINGLE MOST likely diagnosis? Select ONE option only.

  ○   A   Acute cholecystitis

  ○   B   Acute pancreatitis

  ○   C   Oesophageal varices

  ○   D   Pancreatic cancer

  ○   E   Perforated duodenal ulcer

2.2 **Diarrhoea**
A 67-year-old man has been discharged from hospital after being treated for pneumonia. He has now developed a profuse watery diarrhoea, but has had no vomiting. There is no blood in the stool but he is febrile, tachycardic and hypotensive. What is the SINGLE MOST likely cause? Select ONE option only.

  ○   A   *Campylobacter* sp.

  ○   B   *Clostridium difficile*

  ○   C   *Escherichia coli*

  ○   D   Norovirus

  ○   E   Rotavirus

2.3   Hepatitis B serology
        For each pattern of hepatitis serological results in the table below, MATCH
        the MOST LIKELY disease status from the list below. All must be correctly
        matched to score ONE mark.

        A   Acute infection
        B   Immune due to previous infection
        C   Immune due to previous vaccination
        D   Susceptible

HBsAg	IgG anti-HBc	IgG anti-HBs	IgM anti-HBc	Hepatitis status
Negative	Negative	Negative	Negative	
Negative	Positive	Positive	Negative	
Negative	Negative	Positive	Negative	
Positive	Positive	Negative	Positive	

anti-HBc, antibodies to hepatitis core antigen; anti-HBs, antibodies to hepatitis
surface antigen; HBsAg, hepatitis B surface antigen.

2.4   Abdominal pain
        An 85-year-old woman with a previous history of peripheral vascular
        disease and hypertension presents with acute severe abdominal pain
        and loose bowels. The pain is colicky but examination findings are
        unremarkable apart from some tenderness in her abdomen, and an
        irregular pulse that has not been noted before. A rectal examination
        reveals blood-stained mucus. Which ONE of the following statements is
        correct with regard to this presentation? Select ONE option only.

        O   A   Blood-stained mucus is likely to be due to haemorrhoids

        O   B   Mesenteric ischaemia should be considered

        O   C   The absence of any significant examination findings suggests that
                   serious disease is unlikely

        O   D   The most likely diagnosis is diverticulitis

        O   E   The most likely diagnosis is irritable bowel syndrome (IBS) and the
                   patient should be given mebeverine

2.5 Coeliac disease
One of your patients has been diagnosed with coeliac disease. Which ONE of the following can she eat normally?

 ○ A Barley

 ○ B Porridge oats

 ○ C Rice

 ○ D Rye

 ○ E Wheat

2.6 Crohn's disease
Which of the following statements about Crohn's disease is true? Select ONE option only.

 ○ A Active disease should be treated initially with mesalazine

 ○ B Anti-mycobacterial therapies are an effective treatment if used early

 ○ C Anti-TNFα therapy is associated with remission rates of 80%

 ○ D Crohn's disease affects only the colon

 ○ E Patients should be referred early for surgery

2.7 Ulcerative colitis
Which ONE of the following statements about ulcerative colitis is true? Select ONE option only.

 ○ A Ulcerative colitis is always associated with perianal fistulas

 ○ B Mesalazine should always be prescribed generically

 ○ C Oral steroids are the mainstay of maintenance therapy

 ○ D Patients with ulcerative colitis should have regular colonoscopic follow-up to identify malignant change

 ○ E Ulcerative colitis can affect any part of the gastrointestinal tract

2.8 Abdominal pain
A 9-year-old child gives a 2-day history of intermittent abdominal pain that shifts to the right lower quadrant, preceded by nausea. She is mildly pyrexial with a tachycardia. Select the SINGLE MOST likely diagnosis from the list below. Select ONE option only.

 ○ A Appendicitis

 ○ B Incarcerated hernia

 ○ C Intussusception

 ○ D Malrotation

 ○ E Mesenteric thrombosis

2.9   Abdominal pain
A 35-year-old woman presents with a 3-day history of upper abdominal
pain that radiates to the right side, associated with nausea and bloating.
She is febrile and has upper abdominal tenderness and guarding. Select
the SINGLE MOST likely diagnosis from the list below.

○ A   Appendicitis

○ B   Cholecystitis

○ C   Ectopic pregnancy

○ D   Mesenteric thrombosis

○ E   Visceral perforation

2.10   Abdominal pain
A 74-year-old woman on long-term diclofenac for rheumatoid arthritis
presents with abdominal pain. She is hypotensive with a rapid pulse and
epigastric tenderness. Select the SINGLE MOST likely diagnosis from the
list below.

○ A   Acute pancreatitis

○ B   Appendicitis

○ C   Cholecystitis

○ D   Intussusception

○ E   Perforated ulcer

2.11   Abdominal rash
A 33-year-old woman has a violent coughing fit and shortly afterwards
notices an unusual rash over her lower abdomen. Her abdomen is shown
below:

Which ONE of the following is the SINGLE MOST likely underlying
diagnosis?

O   A   Disseminated intravascular coagulation (DIC)

O   B   Haemophilia

O   C   Psoas abscess

O   D   Rectus sheath haematoma

O   E   Von Willebrand's disease

2.12   Bowel cancer trial

A new test has been developed to pick up asymptomatic bowel cancer. This involves patients sending specimens of stool for analysis for dyskaryotic epithelial cells. It is reported by its inventors to be non-invasive and therefore safe and accurate. Initial trial data are shown below:

Total number of samples submitted	1000
Number suitable for analysis	500
Number of samples that tested positive	50
Number of true positives (confirmed by colonoscopy)	25
Total number of diagnoses in patients who submitted suitable sample	30
Number of false negatives	5
Number of diagnoses in all patients participating in trial	60

Which ONE of the following statements is true with regard to this data? Select ONE option only.

○   A   For patients submitting a suitable sample, the sensitivity of the test is 25/30, ie 83%

○   B   For patients submitting a suitable sample, the sensitivity of the test is 25/50, ie 50%

○   C   For patients submitting a suitable sample, the sensitivity of the test is 50/500, ie 10%

○   D   For patients submitting a suitable sample, the specificity of the test is 25/30, ie 83%

○   E   The data suggest that this test will make a significant impact on early diagnosis of bowel cancer

Extended matching questions

Complications of alcohol abuse

2.13–2.16

Options

A   Cirrhosis
B   Impotence
C   Korsakoff's psychosis
D   Oesophageal varices
E   Oesophagitis
F   Pancreatitis
G   Pellagra
H   Portal hypertension
I   Wernicke's encephalopathy

For each description below, select the SINGLE MOST likely diagnosis from the list above.

2.13   Characterised by retrograde amnesia, confabulation and an inability to memorise new information
2.14   The presence of caput medusa and splenomegaly strongly suggests this condition
2.15   Causes acute confusion, ophthalmoplegia and ataxia
2.16   May cause gynaecomastia, bruising and lethargy

Acute abdomen

2.17–2.21

Options

A	Appendicitis
B	Cholecystitis
C	Incarcerated hernia
D	Intussusception
E	Malrotation
F	Meconium ileus
G	Mesenteric thrombosis
H	Ruptured ectopic pregnancy
I	Septic abortion
J	Urinary tract infection
K	Visceral perforation

For each of the descriptions below, select the SINGLE MOST appropriate diagnosis from the list of options above. Each option may be used once, more than once or not at all.

2.17   A 6-year-old girl complains of 24 hours of generalised abdominal pain. On examination she is diffusely tender with some guarding. Urine dipstick testing is positive for nitrites.

2.18   A 28-year-old woman is admitted with a 14-hour history of sudden onset of severe lower abdominal pain with nausea and retching. Her last normal period was 10 weeks ago. Her pulse is 120 beats/min and her BP is 90/70 mmHg.

2.19   A 4-year-old boy is seen with an 8-hour history of colicky central abdominal pain and vomiting. He presents with an irreducible lump in the left groin, extending into the scrotum.

2.20   An 18-month-old toddler who has been on a weaning diet becomes fretful, clutches his abdomen and cries out. He refuses feeds and passes loose motions containing blood-stained mucus.

2.21   A 7-day-old male neonate has not opened his bowels since birth. Symptoms of bowel obstruction develop, with bile-stained vomiting. Respiratory investigations suggest cystic fibrosis.

Management of constipation in children

2.22–2.28

Options

A	High-dose osmotic laxative
B	Impaction not present
C	Impaction present
D	Maintenance-dose osmotic laxative
E	No red flags
F	Routine referral
G	Red flags present
H	Urgent referral

Complete the algorithm below describing the management of childhood constipation. Each option may be used once, more than once or not at all.

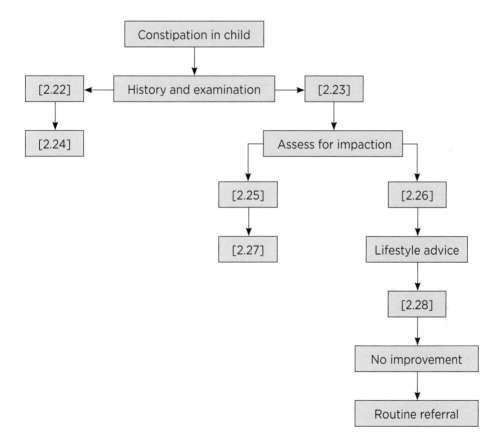

2.1   B: Acute pancreatitis

This is a typical presentation of acute pancreatitis. He should be admitted for investigation and management. Raised amylase will usually confirm the diagnosis. Oesophageal varices tend to cause haematemesis, whereas a perforated duodenal ulcer, although causing similar symptoms, is not usually relieved by sitting leaning forward.

2.2   B: *Clostridium difficile*

Watery diarrhoea starting after recent antibiotic therapy is usually caused by *Clostridium difficile*. The most common implicated antibiotics are amoxicillin, ampicillin, clindamycin and cephalosporins. Treatment consists of stopping the offending antibiotics, metronidazole or oral vancomycin, fluid replacement and barrier nursing. Toxic megacolon can occur and this should be managed surgically. *Campylobacter* sp. causes a diarrhoeal illness that is usually associated with eating chicken, whereas norovirus causes a transient diarrhoeal and vomiting illness. Rotavirus usually affects children.

2.3   Hepatitis B serology

HBsAg	IgG anti-HBc	IgG anti-HBs	IgM anti-HBc	Hepatitis status
Negative	Negative	Negative	Negative	Susceptible
Negative	Positive	Positive	Negative	Immune due to previous infection
Negative	Negative	Positive	Negative	Immune due to previous vaccination
Positive	Positive	Negative	Positive	Acute infection

Hepatitis B surface antigen (HBsAg) is the earliest indicator of acute hepatitis B infection and is seen in acute and chronic infection. Hepatitis B vaccination does not result in a positive HBsAg test. Hepatitis B core antigen (HBcAg) is not present in the vaccination and indicates past or present infection. IgM antibodies are produced only early in the course of the infection and IgG later, so IgM indicates acute infection, whereas IgG without IgM indicates previous exposure to the vaccine or the virus. The presence of anti-HBsAg without HBsAg indicates recovery from acute infection, absence of infectivity and immunity from future infection.

2.4   B: Mesenteric ischaemia should be considered

The presentation of acute severe abdominal pain in someone with arteriopathy, out of keeping with clinical findings, should suggest the possibility of ischaemic bowel. Initially there are few signs but, later on, blood-stained mucus, signs of bowel obstruction and shock are common. The prognosis is poor due to late diagnosis. Diverticulitis generally causes milder pain with more of a change in bowel habit whereas IBS would not normally cause severe pain.

2.5   C: Rice

Patients with coeliac disease should avoid wheat, rye and barley, but can eat rice and maize. Some coeliac disease patients are sensitive to pure oats but many patients can take these without any problem, although commercially available oats such as porridge oats are usually contaminated with wheat during the milling process, so patients should try to obtain pure oats.

2.6   C: Anti-TNFα therapy is associated with remission rates of 80%

Mesalazine is no better than placebo in the management of active disease. Its main use is in prevention of relapse after surgery. Infliximab is an effective anti-TNFα therapy in up to 80% of cases, but only 24% are steroid free. Surgery should be reserved for patients who do not respond to steroids, methotrexate or infliximab. Antibiotics should be used only for septic complications and perianal disease. Crohn's disease can affect any part of the gastrointestinal tract from the mouth to the anus.

2.7   D: Patients with ulcerative colitis should have regular colonoscopic follow-up to identify malignant change

Ulcerative colitis affects only the large bowel, whereas Crohn's disease can affect any part of the gastrointestinal tract. Mesalazine should be prescribed by brand. Ulcerative colitis is associated with bowel cancer and so patients should be regularly screened with colonoscopy. In most patients the disease can be controlled with mesalazine and where steroids are needed topical steroids such as Predfoam enemas should be used to reduce systemic effects. Perianal fistulas are associated with Crohn's disease.

2.8   A: Appendicitis

Acute appendicitis in children must be distinguished from acute mesenteric adenitis caused by systemic viral infections and urinary tract infections. In adolescent girls, mid-cycle pain, twisted ovarian cysts or ruptured ovarian follicles can mimic acute appendicitis.

2.9   B: Cholecystitis

Tenderness in the gallbladder area, a tender, palpable gallbladder and a positive Murphy's sign are all suggestive of acute calculous cholecystitis. An ultrasound scan would exclude empyema of the gallbladder, confirm stones in the gallbladder, and exclude duct stones and pancreatitis.

2.10   E: Perforated ulcer

Peptic perforation is a complication of peptic ulcer disease and is associated with anti-ulcer therapy non-compliance, alcohol abuse, long-term steroids and NSAIDs. A rare cause is gastrinoma (an islet-cell tumour), which stimulates gastric hypersecretion, causing multiple ulcers.

2.11   D: Rectus sheath haematoma

This is the typical appearance of a rectus sheath haematoma, which usually occurs spontaneously after coughing or vomiting. It is usually caused by blood leaking from the inferior epigastric artery, and commonly settles spontaneously.

2.12   A: For patients submitting a suitable sample, the sensitivity of the test is 25/30, ie 83%

Sensitivity = 100 × true positive/(true positive + false negative)

Specificity = 100 × true negative/(true negative + false positive)

The fact that half of all samples were unsuitable suggests that this test is unlikely to be useful on a population basis, because this resulted in 30 diagnoses being missed.

Complications of alcohol abuse

2.13   C: Korsakoff's psychosis

Usually seen in people with alcohol problems due to loss of nerve cells in the thalamic and mammillary bodies as a result of thiamine deficiency.

2.14   H: Portal hypertension

Worldwide the most common cause of this condition is schistosomiasis, but in the developed world liver cirrhosis is the most common cause. It results in splenomegaly, portosystemic shunting (eg caput medusa) and oedema, and 50% of patients have oesophageal varices, with 30% also having rectal varices.

2.15   I: Wernicke's encephalopathy

This is associated with alcoholism or other causes of acquired thiamine deficiency. Peripheral neuropathy is common, and untreated patients often develop Korsakoff's psychosis.

2.16   A: Cirrhosis

Characterised by fibrosis of the entire liver and formation of nodules, cirrhosis is irreversible. Of cases 60–80% are due to alcohol abuse, although only 10–20% of heavy drinkers develop cirrhosis.

Acute abdomen

2.17   A: Appendicitis

Appendicitis typically starts with vague abdominal pain that tends to localise to the right iliac fossa over 12–24 hours. Nitrites have low specificity for urinary tract infection. A pelvic appendix can mimic a urinary tract infection.

2.18   H: Ruptured ectopic pregnancy

Sudden onset of severe, persistent abdominal pain with hypotension and peritonism in a woman of childbearing age strongly suggests a ruptured ectopic pregnancy. A pelvic ultrasound scan will confirm the diagnosis.

2.19   C: Incarcerated hernia

Inguinal hernia in early childhood is caused by the virtual apposition of the internal and external rings during the development of the inguinal canal. The processus vaginalis is also patent, providing access of abdominal contents to the scrotum.

2.20   D: Intussusception

Intussusception in childhood is usually caused by hyperplasia of submucosal lymphoid tissue due to changes in bowel flora during weaning. The intussusception is initially intermittent but bowel obstruction rapidly supervenes which leads to ischaemia of the intussuscepted loop.

2.21   F: Meconium ileus

Meconium ileus is caused by inspissated meconium impacting in the terminal ileum and results from changes in bowel mucus associated with cystic fibrosis. If colonic washouts fail to restore patency, surgical evacuation is required.

Management of constipation in children

2.22   G: Red flags present

2.23   E: No red flags

2.24   H: Urgent referral

2.25   C: Impaction present

2.26   B: Impaction not present

2.27   A: High-dose osmotic laxative

2.28   D: Maintenance-dose osmotic laxative

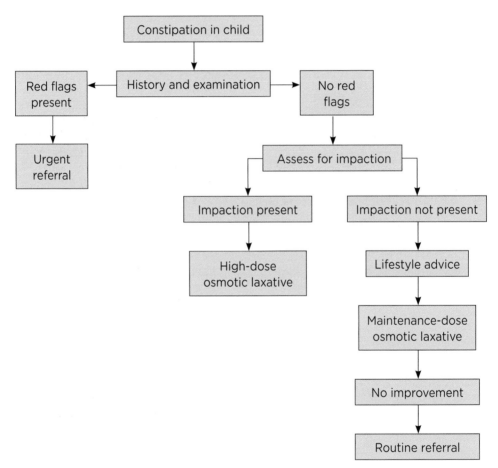

Chapter 3

Ear, nose and throat, and facial problems

Single best answer questions

3.1 **Reduced hearing**
A 67-year-old woman complains of 3 weeks of reduced hearing in one ear after an upper respiratory tract infection. She says that her head feels as if it is in a bucket. On examination she has no evidence of acute infection in her middle or outer ear but does have clinical evidence of a middle-ear effusion. She is otherwise well, and 2 months before this she had a full ENT assessment for reduced smell, which was normal. Which ONE of the following management strategies is effective in this situation?

○ A Nasal steroids

○ B Oral decongestant

○ C Otovent device

○ D Reassurance that her symptoms should resolve within 1–2 weeks

○ E Refer for grommets

3.2 **Sore throat**
A 19-year-old student is diagnosed with tonsillitis and starts antibiotic therapy. Twenty-four hours later she presents to the out-of-hours service with fever, ear pain, dysphagia and trismus. On examination her uvula is displaced away from the midline and her tonsils appear asymmetrically enlarged. What is the SINGLE MOST likely diagnosis?

○ A Epiglottitis

○ B Glandular fever

○ C Lemierre syndrome

○ D Quinsy

○ E Tonsillar lymphoma

3.3   Sore throat
A 16-year-old schoolboy complains of flu-like symptoms, sore throat and enlarged glands in his neck. On examination he has a temperature of 38.5°C, significantly enlarged lymph nodes in his neck, enlarged tonsils with white exudate and a yellowish tinge to his skin. Abdominal examination reveals some tenderness in the right upper quadrant. What is the SINGLE MOST likely diagnosis?

- ○   A   Epstein–Barr virus infection
- ○   B   Hepatitis A
- ○   C   Quinsy
- ○   D   Streptococcal tonsillitis
- ○   E   Viral sore throat

3.4   Enlarged tonsils
Persistent asymmetrical tonsillar enlargement in a 40-year-old man is best treated with which ONE of the following options?

- ○   A   Antifungals
- ○   B   Antibiotics
- ○   C   Referral for biopsy
- ○   D   Steroids
- ○   E   Watch and wait

3.5   Neck swelling
A child presents with a 3-cm swelling to the left of the midline in the lower part of the anterior triangle of the neck. It moves with swallowing and tongue protrusion. What is it MOST likely to be?

- ○   A   Branchial cyst
- ○   B   Lymph node
- ○   C   Thyroglossal cyst
- ○   D   Thyroid cyst
- ○   E   Sebaceous cyst

3.6   **Snoring**
A 54-year-old man with a BMI of 22 kg/m² complains of snoring and
waking up at night. He is tired during the daytime, and his partner says
that he seems to stop breathing for up to a minute every night. What is the
SINGLE MOST appropriate first-line treatment?

-    A   Advice on lifestyle changes and weight loss
-    B   Advise the use of earplugs
-    C   Refer for a sleep study
-    D   Refer for surgery
-    E   Refer to a dentist for a mandibular advancement device

3.7   **Hearing loss**
A 6-year-old girl has a 1-year history of 30 dB conductive hearing loss, flat
tympanograms and poor school performance. What is the SINGLE MOST
appropriate next-stage treatment?

-    A   Adenoidectomy
-    B   Bilateral grommet insertion
-    C   Conservative treatment
-    D   Nasal decongestants
-    E   Tonsillectomy

3.8   Facial swelling

An 86-year-old man is seen for a new patient check. While talking to him you notice a swelling in front of and inferior to the right ear. He tells you that this has been slowly growing for 10 years. On examination the swelling is firm but non-tender and mobile. He has no other findings of note. The swelling is shown below.

What is the SINGLE MOST likely diagnosis?

O   A   Acute bacterial parotitis

O   B   Adenocarcinoma

O   C   Lymphoma

O   D   Mumps

O   E   Parotid adenoma

3.9   Earache
        A 10-year-old girl complains of earache and a discharge from her ear and
        she has a fever. On examination you note the appearance below.

What is the SINGLE MOST likely diagnosis?

O   A   Acute otitis externa

O   B   Acute tympanic membrane perforation

O   C   Chronic otitis externa

O   D   Chronic tympanic membrane perforation

O   E   Glue ear

3.10 Itchy ears

A 27-year-old man with itchy ears has had several courses of eardrops over the last 3 months. He now complains of recurrent itchiness. On examination you note the appearance below.

What is the SINGLE MOST appropriate medical treatment?

○ A   Betnesol drops

○ B   Ciprofloxacin drops

○ C   Clotrimazole drops

○ D   Locorten-Vioform drops

○ E   Sofradex eardrops

3.11   Painful ear
        A 21-year-old girl has just returned from a holiday in Greece, where she
        developed a very painful ear. She has been taking regular ibuprofen,
        paracetamol and codeine from a local pharmacy, but to no effect. On
        examination her ear has the appearance shown below.

What is the ONE single diagnosis?

○   A   Acute otitis externa

○   B   Chronic suppurative otitis media

○   C   Fungal otitis externa

○   D   Otitis media with effusion

○   E   Otitis media with perforation

3.12 Loss of hearing

This picture shows the right tympanic membrane of a patient who presented with reduced hearing and discharge 2 days after the onset of earache and fever. The patient reports that the pain has eased somewhat since the onset of the discharge.

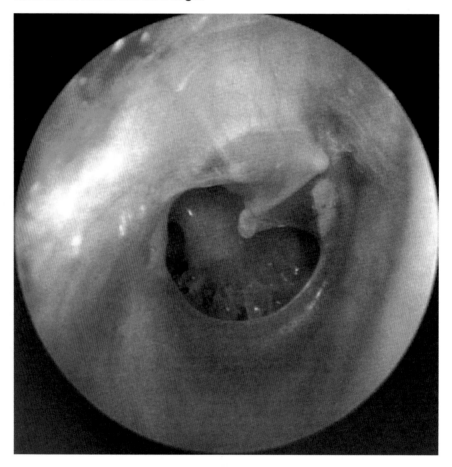

What is the SINGLE MOST likely diagnosis?

O   A   Cholesteatoma

O   B   Otitis externa

O   C   Otitis media

O   D   Otosclerosis

O   E   Tympanosclerosis

3.13   Audiograms
A patient with hearing problems has an audiogram carried out. Which
ONE of the options A-E would be MOST likely to be seen in a patient with
presbyacusis?

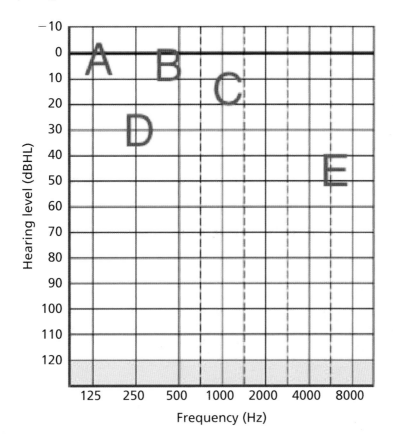

3.14   Ear discharge
A 45-year-old man presents with left ear discharge after swimming. The swab from this discharge shows the following results:

Organism: *Pseudomonas aeruginosa*

Sensitivity:

- Penicillin – resistant
- Neomycin – resistant
- Framycetin – resistant
- Metronidazole – resistant
- Ciprofloxacin – sensitive

What is the ONE SINGLE MOST appropriate treatment?

- O   A   Intravenous co-amoxiclav
- O   B   Oral ciprofloxacin
- O   C   Oral co-amoxiclav
- O   D   Topical aluminium acetate eardrops
- O   E   Topical ciprofloxacin eyedrops used as eardrops

3.15   Management of glue ear

A   4 weeks
B   6 weeks
C   3 months
D   6 months
E   12 months

Your local audiology department have produced a flowchart for the management of suspected glue ear in children. Complete the algorithm from the list of options above.

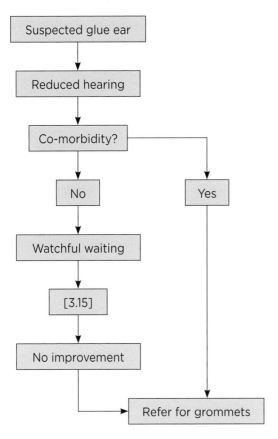

3.16 Medical management of chronic rhinosinusitis

Select the rank order of the options (1–4) that best fulfils the requirements given in the question.

The following is a list of treatment options for chronic rhinosinusitis:

1   1–2 weeks of oral antibiotics
2   4–6 weeks of oral antibiotics
3   Nasal steroid drops
4   Nasal steroid spray

The responses (A–E) rank the treatment options in various orders. Select the response that places the treatment options (1–4) in the order in which they should be used, with the **initial treatment** first to the **maximal medical therapy** last.

Select ONE rank order only.

○   A: 4, 2, 3, 1

○   B: 4, 3, 2, 1

○   C: 1, 3, 4, 2

○   D: 4, 1, 3, 2

○   E: 3, 4, 1, 2

Extended matching questions

Drug management of ENT disease

3.17–3.20

Options

A   Amoxicillin
B   Betnesol
C   Ciprofloxacin drops
D   Doxycycline
E   Erythromycin
F   Mometasone nasal spray
G   Montelukast
H   Phenoxymethylpenicillin
I   Sofradex
J   Sterimar

For each of the scenarios described below, select the most appropriate treatment option from the list above. Each option may be used once, more than once or not at all.

3.17   A 4-year-old boy complains of earache on one side. Examination shows a red, dull, bulging eardrum on that side. He has a temperature of 39.2°C and looks unwell.

3.18   A 24-year-old woman with long-standing perennial rhinitis not helped by antihistamines.

3.19   A 19-year-old man with a history of a chronically discharging ear. A swab is sent which shows *Pseudomonas* species.

3.20   A 51-year-old woman who is on a long-term nasal steroid spray complains of a blocked nose, and reduced smell and taste. Examination reveals bilateral nasal polyps.

Data interpretation question

3.21 **Tuning fork tests**

A 51-year-old woman complains of hearing loss in her right ear, which she thinks started after a recent flight to Spain. You conduct tuning fork tests.

MATCH EACH of the following diagnoses to the MOST LIKELY tuning fork results. All options must be correctly matched to score ONE mark.

A Left-sided conductive hearing loss
B Left-sided sensorineural hearing loss
C Normal
D Right-sided conductive hearing loss
E Right-sided sensorineural hearing loss

Right ear	Left ear	Weber's test	Diagnosis
BC > AC	AC > BC	Localises to right	
AC > BC	AC > BC	Localises to centre	
AC > BC	AC > BC	Localises to left	

AC, air conduction; BC, bone conduction.

Free-text question

3.22 Mouth pain

A 57-year-old woman complains of burning pain in her mouth for several months. She is otherwise well and takes no regular medication. Her buccal mucosa is shown below.

Write the SINGLE MOST likely diagnosis in the box below.

3.1   C: Otovent device

Middle-ear effusions are often seen on a background of acute upper respiratory tract infection and are typically unilateral. They can take several months to clear, but this can be improved with an Otovent device. Grommets might be necessary for refractory cases. Nasal decongestants and steroids are ineffective. Patients presenting with acute middle-ear effusions in adulthood should have nasendoscopy performed to exclude postnasal space lesions.

3.2   D: Quinsy

This presentation is typical of quinsy, or peritonsillar abscess. Treatment usually involves intravenous antibiotics and fluids, and incision of the abscess if it does not settle. Interval tonsillectomy is offered in most centres. Epiglottitis affects the epiglottis rather than the uvula and a lymphoma would not normally present over such a short period. Glandular fever does not usually cause significant asymmetry, whereas Lemierre syndrome causes more widespread disease throughout the mediastinum and patients are usually much more unwell.

3.3   A: Epstein–Barr virus infection

Epstein–Barr virus causes glandular fever. Most patients develop a sore throat, fever, malaise and cervical lymphadenopathy. Hepatosplenomegaly is not uncommon and most patients develop transient abnormalities of liver function. Treatment is supportive and most patients make a full recovery. Complications include cranial nerve palsies, encephalitis and splenic rupture, but these are rare. The symptoms usually last 2–4 weeks but up to 50% of patients report ongoing fatigue, which can take months to resolve.

3.4   C: Referral for biopsy

Asymmetrical tonsil enlargement in adults is suspicious of neoplasia, and biopsy is needed, as well as imaging of the head and neck.

3.5   C: Thyroglossal cyst

The thyroglossal cyst is a remnant of the thyroglossal duct, which descends from the tongue via the hyoid and neck to the thyroid during development. There can be a connection to the hyoid bone which explains its pattern of movement. Treatment is with surgical excision via Sistrunk's procedure.

3.6   C: Refer for a sleep study

Surgery for snoring is controversial, and evidence on its effectiveness is conflicting – some surgery might provide short-term help with snoring, but problems tend to recur. Any surgery should be carefully targeted at the source of the snoring. Lifestyle changes and earplugs will be ineffective with this patient. A mandibular advancement device might help, depending on the site of snoring, but, with a clear history of daytime somnolence and apnoea, a sleep study should be performed first – night-time continuous positive airway pressure (CPAP) might be all that is necessary to improve the patient's quality of life.

3.7   B: Bilateral grommet insertion

Typically, glue ear produces a 20–40 dB conductive loss with flat tympanograms – it is most common in children aged between about 3 years and 8 years, and tends to improve with time, although if it starts to affect development intervention is indicated. For cases of recurrent glue ear adenoidectomy has been shown, in the TARGET trial, to reduce the rate of recurrence.

3.8   E: Parotid adenoma

The most likely diagnosis in this case is a parotid adenoma. Parotid adenomas account for 90% of benign parotid tumours and are typically in the lower pole of the parotid. They are benign but can cause local damage to the facial nerve. They grow slowly and elderly patients might not require treatment. The diagnosis should be confirmed by fine-needle aspiration. Malignant tumours of the parotid tend to present more acutely due to rapid growth. Lymphomas tend to be more aggressive and often have a rubbery feel.

3.9   B: Acute tympanic membrane perforation

The history of fever and otalgia followed by otorrhoea suggests an acute otitis media followed by perforation. The discharge is thin and mucoid, which suggests middle-ear involvement rather than otitis externa, which causes a much thicker discharge which seldom runs from the ear. Chronic perforations can behave in this way but usually follow water exposure or coryza rather than an acute febrile illness. The tympanic membrane usually heals in 4–6 weeks.

3.10   C: Clotrimazole drops

This is a fungal otitis externa. Treatment is with 2 weeks of antifungal therapy and management of underlying risk factors, such as diabetes and excessive use of antibiotic or steroid preparations. Microsuction might be necessary where there is a lot of exudate.

3.11   A: Acute otitis externa

The presence of pain, particularly when moving the tragus, with creamy, thick exudate and meatal oedema is typical of otitis externa. The discharge in a tympanic membrane perforation tends to be more mucoid whereas in otitis media with effusion there is no exudate in the canal. Fungal otitis externa shows typical spores and hyphae.

3.12   C: Otitis media

This patient has most probably suffered from an acute middle-ear infection, resulting in a perforation and discharge, and later resolution of symptoms. Cholesteatoma usually causes a painless perforation that tends to be peripheral. Otitis externa rarely causes a perforation. Otosclerosis is a disease of the ossicles and causes a slowly progressive conductive hearing loss, and tympanosclerosis causes a conductive loss that is usually stable.

3.13 E

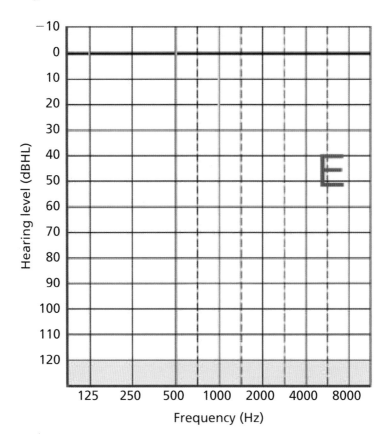

Presbyacusis is characterised by high frequency sensorineural hearing loss. Low-frequency loss is usually seen in Ménière's disease or conductive loss, whereas mid-frequency loss is often congenital. Severe hearing loss of any aetiology may affect any frequency.

3.14 E: Topical ciprofloxacin eyedrops used as eardrops

The presence of discharge after swimming suggests otitis externa. This is best treated with topical drops. Ciprofloxacin eye drops used topically in the ear, although off license, are effective in this situation. The patient should also be asked to keep his ears dry, and oral ciprofloxacin can be considered as a second-line treatment.

3.15 C: 3 months

Of cases of glue ear 90% settle within 3 months, so intervention before this period is indicated only if there is significant co-morbidity, eg blindness or Down syndrome.

3.16   **D: 4, 1, 3, 2**

Rank ordering: 4 Nasal steroid spray; 1 1–2 weeks of oral antibiotics; 3 Nasal steroid drops; 2 4–6 weeks of oral antibiotics

Initial management of chronic rhinosinusitis should be saline douching, which has a good evidence base for maintenance treatment of chronic rhinosinusitis. If this is not tolerated or is ineffective a nasal steroid spray is indicated. Failure to improve with regular nasal spray in the presence of signs of infection should prompt oral antibiotics. If there is still no improvement, 2–4 weeks of nasal steroid drops may prove effective. Continuing purulent discharge despite this is an indication for a 4- to 6-week course of antibiotics.

Drug management of ENT disease

3.17   **A: Amoxicillin**

Acute otitis media in a child who is unwell should be treated with antibiotics. If the child is not unwell a symptomatic approach might be appropriate, with the option of returning for antibiotics should the patient worsen.

3.18   **F: Mometasone nasal spray**

Second-line treatment in patients with rhinitis who have tried oral antihistamines is a nasal steroid. This can also help with ocular symptoms.

3.19   **C: Ciprofloxacin drops**

Pseudomonas sp. is often seen in patients with discharging ears and topical ciprofloxacin will often cure this. An alternative is Sofradex, but there are theoretical arguments against using this in patients without an intact tympanic membrane.

3.20   **B: Betnesol**

A short course of nasal steroid drops will often shrink nasal polyps, affording symptomatic relief in patients who are not fit for or who do not wish to have surgery. Mometasone nasal spray is licensed for the treatment of nasal polyps and is often effective in patients with smaller polyps and useful for preventing recurrence.

3.21   **Tuning fork tests**

Right ear	Left ear	Weber's test	Diagnosis
BC > AC	AC > BC	Localises to right	D
AC > BC	AC > BC	Localises to centre	C
AC > BC	AC > BC	Localises to left	E

AC, air conduction; BC, bone conduction.

Rinne's test involves placing a tuning fork in front of the ear and then on the mastoid. In a normal ear, air conduction is greater than bone conduction, which is described as Rinne positive. A Rinne-negative test is seen when air conduction is less than bone conduction, and is seen when there is a conductive hearing loss of 20 dB. Hence when AC > BC in the right ear, but BC > AC in the left ear, this signifies a left-sided conductive hearing loss.

Weber's test will determine if there is a unilateral sensorineural hearing loss. A tuning fork is placed in the midline. In the presence of a unilateral sensorineural hearing loss, it is heard louder on the unaffected side. Where hearing is normal it is heard on the midline. Where there is a unilateral conductive hearing loss with normal bone conduction in each ear, it is heard loudest on the affected side.

3.22   Lichen planus

Lichen planus is characterised by fine white streaking of the buccal mucosa. It affects all age groups but onset typically occurs in the fifth or sixth decade. It is most commonly seen on the posterior buccal mucosa, but may also affect the tongue, gums and lower lip. It may be asymptomatic, cause itching or burning, and may be bullous or erosive, both of which are associated with pain. At diagnosis patients should be referred for biopsy to exclude oral squamous cell carcinoma. Treatment may not be necessary if asymptomatic, but if pain is a feature oral steroids as a mouthwash, pellets or systemic treatment, may help. In refractory cases DMARDs may be necessary. The main differential diagnoses in buccal lichen planus are leukoplakia, candidiasis and secondary syphilis.

Chapter 4
Eye problems

Single best answer questions

4.1 Loss of vision

A 70-year-old woman complains of several weeks of generalised aches and pains and difficulty getting out of a chair. Over the last 24 hours she has become aware of loss of vision in her left eye, with pain in her jaw on chewing. On examination, she has a visual acuity of 6/60 and a left relative afferent pupillary defect. Her left disc appears pale and swollen. The SINGLE best option in the management of this patient is:

- ○ A   A 7-day course of 15 mg prednisolone and then review
- ○ B   Conservative management as the vision has already been lost
- ○ C   Refer to neurology with an MR scan
- ○ D   Start 80 mg prednisolone daily and arrange same-day assessment by ophthalmology
- ○ E   Urgent temporal artery biopsy

Select ONE option only.

4.2 Double vision

An 80-year-old man complains of sudden-onset double vision. He is otherwise well and not known to have high BP or high cholesterol, but he does smoke. On examination, he appears to have restricted lateral gaze in the left eye. His double vision is horizontal and worse on looking to the left and into the distance. His pupils react normally and there is no headache or ptosis. Which ONE of the following statements about his management is correct? Select ONE option only.

- ○ A   Advise him to attend his optometrist, who will prescribe glasses with prisms
- ○ B   Do nothing – it is likely that this will resolve in a few weeks
- ○ C   Start aspirin and investigate for cardiovascular risk
- ○ D   Start aspirin, investigate for cardiovascular risk and refer to ophthalmology
- ○ E   Urgent referral to neurosurgery

4.3   Painful red eye
A 68-year-old man complains of a painful red eye. He had cataract surgery
2 days ago and, aside from some mild grittiness, his eye was comfortable.
Since then his eye has become very red and painful, and he is no longer
able to see properly. The SINGLE MOST likely diagnosis is:

- O   A   Acute angle-closure glaucoma due to the drops used to dilate the
pupil before the surgery

- O   B   Endophthalmitis

- O   C   Postoperative iritis

- O   D   Severe allergic reaction to the anaesthetic injection

- O   E   Severe conjunctivitis

4.4   Visual problems
A myopic man complains of seeing flashing lights and floaters. The
appearance of his fundus is shown below:

Which ONE of the following statements about this patient is correct?
Select ONE option only.

- O   A   Being short-sighted usually reduces the risk of this condition

- O   B   He has a retinal tear that can be treated with laser in the outpatient
department

○   C   He has already lost vision and therefore surgery is not urgent

○   D   He will need an urgent operation to prevent irreversible visual loss

○   E   He will need surgery within 1 week

4.5   **Visual deterioration**

A 70-year-old woman complains of a gradual deterioration in vision in both eyes. Her visual acuity is 6/9 and 6/12. She has been told by her optician that she has macular degeneration and has heard of new treatments available for this condition. She would like your advice about treatment. Examination findings are shown below:

Which ONE of the following statements is correct with regard to this clinical situation? Select ONE option only.

○   A   She has evidence of diabetic maculopathy and needs to have her diabetes managed

○   B   She requires an urgent referral to ophthalmology for intravitreal Lucentis

○   C   She would be a suitable candidate for laser treatment

○   D   She would be a suitable candidate for photodynamic therapy

○   E   You should advise her to stop smoking and ensure a diet high in fresh fruit and vegetables

4.6 Diabetic eye problems

You see a young diabetic patient in your clinic. He is in his early 20s and has very poorly controlled type 1 diabetes. He doesn't like taking his insulin and he drinks and smokes to excess. His BP is slightly elevated. Fundoscopic findings are shown below:

Which ONE of the following statements is true with regard to his visual prognosis? Select ONE option only.

O A   After laser treatment his vision should remain stable

O B   He is at risk of visual loss due to retinal detachment

O C   He needs surgery to maintain his vision

O D   Regardless of the amount of laser treatment given, he is likely to be registered blind in 5 years

O E   With adequate laser and optimisation of diabetic control and risk factors, his vision can be maintained

4.7   Eye conditions
Which area of the eye would you expect to see a pterygium develop?
Select the SINGLE MOST appropriate option from A to E on the photo
below.

4.8 and 4.9   Loss of vision
A 73-year-old man with a history of essential hypertension complains of
sudden, painless loss of vision in his right eye. On examination his pupil
does not react to light and he cannot read any line on a Snellen chart. His
retina looks rather pale compared with the contralateral eye.

Part A
Which ONE of the following is the most likely diagnosis? Select ONE
option only.

A   Central retinal artery occlusion
B   Central retinal vein occlusion
C   Giant cell arteritis
D   Migraine
E   Retinal detachment

Part B
Which ONE of the following is the most appropriate treatment in this
situation? Select ONE option only.

A   Check the ESR and CRP
B   Emergency admission under stroke team
C   Emergency admission under ophthalmology
D   Prescribe oral prednisolone 60 mg once daily
E   Refer to rapid access stroke clinic

Extended matching questions

Eye problems

4.10–4.13

Options

A   Acute conjunctivitis
B   Blepharitis
C   Ectropion
D   Entropion
E   Pinguecula
F   Pterygium
G   Subconjunctival haemorrhage
H   None of the above

For each of the conditions below, select the SINGLE MOST likely diagnosis from the list above. Each option may be used once, more than once or not at all.

[4.10]

[4.11]

[4.12]

[4.13]

Visual fields

4.14–4.18

Options

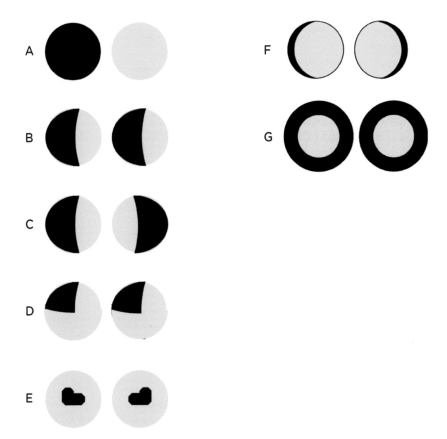

For each of the following patients, select the most likely visual field defect from the options above. Each option can be used once, more than once or not at all.

4.14   An elderly woman who has had a stroke
4.15   A person who is homeless, abuses alcohol and smokes
4.16   A man with acromegaly
4.17   A diabetic individual who has had panretinal photocoagulation
4.18   A patient with glaucoma

Management of eyelid problems

4.19–4.21

Options

A   Clean lid margin with cotton tip
B   Hot flannels applied for 10 minutes
C   Lubricants
D   Massage lump for 10 minutes
E   Oral antibiotics
F   Topical antibiotics

Complete the flowchart below describing the daily routine for self-management of chalazion and blepharitis from the list of options above. Each option may be used once, more than once or not at all.

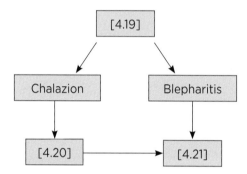

Free-text question

4.22   Interpretation of ophthalmological investigations
You receive a letter from a local optometrist regarding one of your patients. The results are summarised below:

Visual acuity right eye:	6/7
Visual acuity left eye:	6/6
Intraocular pressure right eye:	28
Intraocular pressure left eye:	27

In the box below write the most likely diagnosis based on these results.

4.1   **D:**   **Start 80 mg prednisolone daily and arrange same-day assessment by ophthalmology**

Giant-cell arteritis is an emergency. The patient has a high risk of blindness. In a patient such as the one in the question, the risk is to the other eye, which can rapidly become affected if the condition is not treated. Characteristically, patients have a prodrome of temporal artery tenderness, jaw claudication, malaise, weight loss and fatigue, and might have already been diagnosed with polymyalgia rheumatica. Classically, the ESR is very elevated, and is accompanied by a rise in the C-reactive protein (CRP). This is by no means always the case, however, and giant-cell arteritis can still occur in the absence of a very high ESR. Treatment comprises high-dose steroids, which are very slowly tapered down. To confirm the diagnosis, a temporal artery biopsy is performed by the ophthalmologist.

4.2   **D:**   **Start aspirin, investigate for cardiovascular risk and refer to ophthalmology**

The patient has developed a left VI nerve palsy. The most common reason for this to occur in a patient of this age is microvascular disease and cardiovascular risk factors should be addressed. Referral to ophthalmology is necessary to:

- confirm the diagnosis and exclude involvement of other cranial nerves (including the optic disc)

- obtain an orthoptic assessment in order to quantify the diplopia and prescribe the correct prisms

- arrange relevant investigations and follow-up.

It is also possible to develop cranial nerve palsies in association with giant-cell arteritis and so, if there is any suspicion of polymyalgia rheumatica, this diagnosis should be considered.

4.3   **B:**   **Endophthalmitis**

This is an emergency and the patient needs urgent referral to ophthalmology. This condition, where there is intraocular infection, can rapidly progress to irreversible blindness and retinal detachment. The classic presentation is one of a painful red eye developing a few days after surgery. There might be a hypopyon (pus in the anterior chamber) and slit-lamp examination will reveal significant intraocular inflammation. Deterioration to irreversible blindness or retinal detachment is rapid and prognosis is poor, even with prompt treatment. Management includes intravitreal sampling and injection of antibiotics. Vitrectomy might be necessary to clear debris. If retinal detachment occurs due to necrosis of the retina, further vitreoretinal surgery is indicated.

4.4   D: He will need an urgent operation to prevent irreversible visual loss

The photograph shows a large retinal tear and a peripheral retinal detachment. Small tears alone can be treated with laser in order to prevent retinal detachment but, once the retina has detached, surgery is necessary. The detachment is peripheral and the subretinal fluid has not reached the macula. This means that the patient's vision may be saved with urgent surgery to reattach the retina. Once the macula has detached, vision becomes poor – typically 6/60 or worse. Surgery can restore vision to some degree but not usually to previous levels. Myopic individuals are at higher risk of detachment because their eyes are relatively large.

4.5   E: You should advise her to stop smoking and ensure a diet high in fresh fruit and vegetables

The photo shows areas of drusen, pigment changes and atrophy consistent with dry macular degeneration. Dry macular degeneration is more common than wet macular degeneration and there is no treatment for this, with slowly progressive loss of central vision. Abstinence from smoking and a diet rich in fresh fruit and vegetables can help slow the progression of the disease. Wet macular degeneration is characterised by fluid leakage and subretinal oedema, resulting in visual distortion. Intravitreal Lucentis, an anti-VEGF drug, restores vision and prevents scarring. Photodynamic therapy destroys abnormal blood vessels near the macula. This treatment is aimed at preventing deterioration in vision, although the treatment itself causes significant scarring. It can be difficult to detect wet changes without a slit-lamp examination and therefore ophthalmology referral might be indicated. Most importantly, the patient should be aware that, if she starts to experience distortion of her vision, this could herald the development of wet changes and an urgent referral to ophthalmology would then be appropriate.

4.6   E: With adequate laser and optimisation of diabetic control and risk factors, his vision can be maintained

This photograph shows proliferative diabetic retinopathy with extensive neovascularisation at the optic disc. There are multiple dot-and-blot haemorrhages, microaneurysms and hard exudates. This patient is at high risk of visual loss due to vitreous haemorrhage and maculopathy. Urgent panretinal laser is indicated. It is likely that several sessions of laser will be needed to bring about regression and involution of the abnormal blood vessels. Management of the patient's risk factors is most important, including the psychological side of his condition. Surgery might be necessary if vitreous haemorrhage does not clear after several months, or if there is a progressive tractional retinal detachment. This type of detachment is different from that due to a retinal tear because it can remain stable for a long time, requiring monitoring only.

4.7   A

Pterygiums are benign overgrowths of the conjunctiva, usually seen at the medial canthus and growing laterally. They are thought to be due to exposure to heat, wind or dust. If they encroach on the cornea surgery may be indicated.

4.8 and 4.9   Loss of vision

Part A   A: Central retinal artery occlusion

Part B   C: Emergency admission under ophthalmology

This patient has symptoms of central retinal artery occlusion and should be admitted immediately to avoid permanent visual loss. Once treated, consideration should be given to screening for cardioembolism. Central retinal vein occlusion also causes sudden-onset, painless, unilateral visual loss, but the retinal veins look engorged and the disc swollen. Giant cell arteritis is usually painful, typically with jaw claudication and temporal artery tenderness. Migraine would be an unusual new presentation at this age and retinal detachment usually causes visual field loss rather than complete loss of vision.

Eye problems

4.10   A: Acute conjunctivitis

4.11   D: Entropion

4.12   G: Subconjunctival haemorrhage

4.13   H: None of the above

This is an allergic reaction to an insect bite.

Visual fields

4.14   B: Stroke usually causes a homonymous hemianopia.

4.15   E: Tobacco typically causes a caecocentral scotoma.

4.16   C: Optic chiasma compression (eg from a pituitary tumour) causes a bitemporal hemianopia.

4.17   G: Photocoagulation involves burning the peripheral visual field and results in constricted visual fields.

4.18   F: Glaucoma causes bilateral arcuate scotomas and delayed diagnosis can result in irreversible tunnel vision.

Management of eyelid problems

4.19   B: Hot flannels applied for 10 minutes

4.20   D: Massage lump for 10 minutes

4.21   A: Clean lid margin with cotton tip

This was described in the *British Medical Journal* (2010;**341**:c4044). Infected chalazia should be treated with oral antibiotics. Failure to resolve should prompt incision and drainage if affecting vision. Failure of blepharitis to improve should prompt oral doxycycline for 3 months.

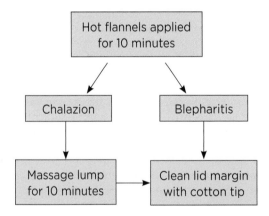

4.22   Glaucoma

Raised intraocular pressure is the hallmark of glaucoma. Visual acuity is preserved until late in the disease due to relative preservation of the macula. Field testing is much more sensitive in picking up early glaucoma, whereas slitlamp examination may show cupping of the optic disc.

Chapter 5
Genetics

Single best answer questions

5.1   Evidence-based practice
Which ONE of the following statements is correct with regard to the findings of the report *Familial cancer risk in people from ethnic minorities, 2012*? Select ONE option only.

○   A   Cultural influences are a significant barrier to effective healthcare in genetic disease

○   B   Risk assessment should not take into account ethnicity

○   C   Standardised referral and treatment pathways across the UK ensure equality of access to specialist services

○   D   The incidence of genetic disease is independent of ethnicity

○   E   The report recommended that counselling on cancer risk should be undertaken by specialist genetic counsellors only

5.2   Developmental concerns
You see the parents of a 30-month-old boy who are concerned about his development. He was born at term after a normal delivery and initially seemed to be developing normally, but they have now become concerned that he is not walking as well as he should. He falls frequently and when he stands he has to push himself up with his hands. Examination shows some wasting of his quadriceps and hypertrophy of his calves. What is the SINGLE MOST likely diagnosis?

○   A   Cerebral palsy

○   B   Down syndrome

○   C   Duchenne muscular dystrophy

○   D   Motor neurone disease

○   E   Myotonic muscular dystrophy

5.3 Causes of emphysema
A 49-year-old smoker has just been diagnosed with emphysema, and has been found to have α_1-antitrypsin deficiency. Which ONE of the following is a correct description of the aetiology of the emphysema? Select ONE option only.

- O A Environmental
- O B Multifactorial
- O C New mutation
- O D Single gene effect
- O E Sporadic

5.4 Cystic fibrosis
Which ONE of the following statements about cystic fibrosis is true? Select ONE option only.

- O A 98% of male patients are infertile
- O B It is transmitted as an X-linked recessive trait
- O C The disease is common in Asian and African–Caribbean individuals
- O D The incidence of cystic fibrosis in the UK is 1 in 10 000 live births
- O E The prevalence of carriers is 1 in 200 in the UK

5.5 Risk of Down syndrome
A 39-year-old woman with two children by her first marriage comes to see you to discuss pre-conception counselling now that she is to remarry. She is particularly concerned about the risk of Down syndrome. Which ONE of the following statements is true about this situation? Select ONE option only.

- O A All women with a risk >1 in 400 should be offered chorionic villous sampling (CVS)
- O B Nuchal translucency testing has 98% sensitivity and specificity for Down syndrome
- O C The risk at age 40 is 1 in 30
- O D The risk of Down syndrome is negligible below the age of 30
- O E The risk of having a baby with Down syndrome is significantly greater in parents who have already had a Down syndrome pregnancy

5.6   **Huntington's disease**
A 46-year-old man comes to see you to discuss his recent diagnosis of Huntington's disease. He was adopted and has no knowledge of his genetic family. He has two teenage sons and lost his wife 3 years ago to breast cancer. Which of the following statements is true about this situation? Select ONE option only.

- O   A   If his teenage sons show no signs of chorea, they can be reassured

- O   B   Testing the children to see if they will develop the condition is not possible

- O   C   The average life expectancy from diagnosis is 25 years

- O   D   The condition is inherited as an autosomal dominant trait and the risk of his sons developing the condition is 1 in 2

- O   E   This condition usually presents in the late teens

5.7   **Turner syndrome**
Which of the following statements is true about Turner syndrome? Select ONE option only.

- O   A   Affected individuals tend to be tall with hyperextensible joints

- O   B   Affected patients have the karyotype 47XXX

- O   C   The external genitalia are characteristically abnormal

- O   D   The incidence is 1:2500 live births

- O   E   Turner syndrome is invariably associated with learning disability

5.8   **Genetic counselling**
Which one of the following statements about genetic counselling in primary care is true? Select ONE option only.

- O   A   Family trees are not helpful in counselling families affected by Down syndrome

- O   B   Families with conditions with variable penetrance, eg tuberous sclerosis, can be successfully counselled in primary care

- O   C   Genetic counselling is a complex field and there is no place for genetic counselling in primary care

- O   D   Risk is best expressed as percentages (eg 0.1%), rather than as proportions (eg 1 in 1000)

- O   E   Two generations of a family tree are sufficient to identify a genetic predisposition

5.9 Phenylketonuria
A family who have recently joined your list come to see you to discuss phenylketonuria. The parents are unaffected but have had a son who has been diagnosed on the basis of a neonatal heel-prick test. They wish to discuss the risks relating to further pregnancies.

Which ONE of the following statements about this situation is true? Select ONE option only.

○ A   As the parents are unaffected, the affected son is the result of a new mutation and the recurrence risks are very rare

○ B   Phenylketonuria is an autosomal dominant trait so the lack of the disease in either parent suggests that the stated father is not the biological father

○ C   Phenylketonuria is an autosomal recessive trait, so both parents must be carriers

○ D   The risk of a future child being a carrier is 1 in 4

○ E   The risk of another child having phenylketonuria is 1 in 2

5.10 Skin lesions
A patient has had the lesions shown in the photograph below all over his body since childhood. He does not know anything about his family history because he was adopted at the age of 3 months. His wife is not affected. He is planning a family and consults you for advice as to whether their children are likely to be affected.

Which ONE of the following statements is true regarding the risk of passing the condition to any children? Select ONE option only.

○ A The condition is a spontaneous condition rather than genetic, so there is no risk of transmission to offspring

○ B The risk to affected offspring is 50%

○ C The risk to affected offspring is 100%

○ D The risk of children being carriers is 25%

○ E The risk of male children being carriers is 100%

5.11 **Genetic counselling**
A couple attend for pre-conception counselling after having two children affected by a genetic disease. They would like to have a third child but are concerned about the risk of recurrence. Their family pedigree is shown below:

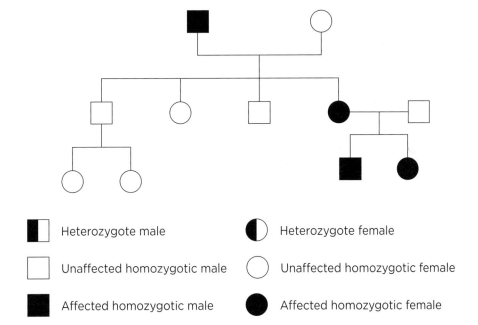

	Heterozygote male		Heterozygote female
	Unaffected homozygotic male		Unaffected homozygotic female
	Affected homozygotic male		Affected homozygotic female

Which ONE of the following statements about the pattern of inheritance is true? Select ONE option only.

○ A The condition is inherited as an autosomal dominant trait

○ B The condition is inherited as an autosomal recessive trait

○ C The condition is inherited as an X-linked recessive trait

○ D The condition is inherited as a Y-linked trait

○ E The condition is sporadic rather than an inherited trait

5.12 Causes of learning disability

Select the rank order of the options (1–4) that best fulfil the requirements given in the question.

The following is a list of genetic syndromes causing learning disabilities:

1 Down syndrome
2 Fragile X syndrome
3 Klinefelter syndrome
4 Turner syndrome

The responses (A–E) rank the genetic syndromes causing learning disabilities in various orders. Select the response that places the options (1–4) in the order of most common syndrome to **least** common.

Select ONE rank order only.

○   A: 1, 3, 4, 2

○   B: 1, 3, 2, 4

○   C: 3, 1, 2, 4

○   D: 3, 1, 4, 2

○   E: 3, 4, 1, 2

Extended matching questions

Prevalence of genetic disease

5.13–5.18

Options

A   0.05 per 1000 births
B   0.1 per 1000 births
C   0.5 per 1000 births
D   2 per 1000 births
E   5 per 1000 births
F   None of the above

For each of the diseases listed below, select the option from this list above that reflects most accurately the prevalence of the condition in the UK. Each option may be used once, more than once or not at all.

5.13   Familial combined hyperlipidaemia
5.14   β-Thalassaemia
5.15   Cystic fibrosis
5.16   Haemophilia A
5.17   Sickle cell anaemia
5.18   Neurofibromatosis

Modes of inheritance

5.19–5.22

Options

A Autosomal dominant
B Autosomal recessive
C Chromosomal translocation
D Non-dysjunction
E X-linked dominant
F X-linked recessive

For each of the conditions below, select the SINGLE MOST appropriate inheritance pattern from the list above. Each option may be used once, more than once or not at all.

5.19 Cystic fibrosis
5.20 Duchenne muscular dystrophy
5.21 Klinefelter syndrome
5.22 Huntington's disease

Diagnostic tests in genetics

5.23–5.27

Options

A Amniocentesis
B Carrier testing
C Chorionic villous sampling (CVS)
D Fetoscopy
E Fluorescent *in situ* hybridisation
F Guthrie test
G Heel-prick test
H Karyotyping
I Triple test
J Ultrasound

For each of the conditions affecting babies described below, select the SINGLE MOST appropriate diagnostic or screening test from the list above. Each option can be used once, more than once or not at all.

5.23 Hypothyroidism
5.24 Tay–Sachs disease
5.25 Phenylketonuria
5.26 Congenital cardiac disease
5.27 Thalassaemia major

Cancer genetics

5.28–5.32

Options

A	Acoustic neuroma
B	Acute lymphoblastic leukaemia
C	Colonic cancer
D	Gastrointestinal MALToma
E	Glioma
F	Kaposi's sarcoma
G	Meningioma
H	Non-Hodgkin's lymphoma
I	Oesophageal cancer
J	Retinoblastoma
K	Small-cell lung cancer
L	Thyroid cancer

For each of the genetic conditions described below, select the tumour that is MOST commonly associated with that condition from the list above. Each option can be used once, more than once or not at all.

5.28	**Neurofibromatosis**
5.29	**Tuberous sclerosis**
5.30	**Down syndrome**
5.31	**Familial adenomatous polyposis**
5.32	**Multiple endocrine neoplasia**

Antenatal testing

5.33–5.37

Options

A   0%
B   0.01%
C   0.25–0.5%
D   0.5–1%
E   5%
F   10–12 weeks
G   10–13 weeks
H   15–18 weeks
I   15–20 weeks
J   18–20 weeks
K   Diagnostic
L   Screening

The local midwives have constructed an information pack about antenatal testing to include in their booking information packs. Complete the table below from the list of options given. Each option may be used once, more than once or not at all.

	Nuchal translucency	Chorionic villous sampling	Amniocentesis	Combined test	Anomaly scan
Screening or diagnostic test?	5.33	5.34			
Gestational range for testing (weeks)			5.35		
Risk of adverse effects (%)		5.36		5.37	

Free-text question

5.38   **Genetic risk**
A couple have recently had a son diagnosed with cystic fibrosis. They are have been tested and both are heterozygous carriers of the *ΔF508* gene. What is the risk of their next born child having the disease? Write your answer in figures, as a percentage, in the box below.

5.1 A: Cultural influences are a significant barrier to effective healthcare in genetic disease

The report *Familial cancer risk in people from ethnic minorities* found that populations at increased risk of genetic disease face cultural and professional barriers to the delivery of effective treatment. Many patients favoured input from professionals from their own background, and the threshold for assessment should be tailored to both cultural beliefs and risk in that population.

5.2 C: Duchenne muscular dystrophy

Duchenne muscular dystrophy is an X-lined trait that usually manifests from 18 months of age but is typically not diagnosed until the age of 4–5 years. It causes progressive weakness, starting in the legs, and most patients are wheelchair bound by the age of 20. Myotonic dystrophy has an onset from late teens onwards and is characterised by hypogonadism, cataracts, weakening and wasting of sternocleidomastoid in particular. Motor neurone disease affects adults whereas cerebral palsy is non-progressive and usually present from birth.

5.3 B: Multifactorial

Patients with α_1-antitrypsin deficiency are at increased risk of heart and lung problems. The condition is inherited as a co-dominant trait, ie heterozygotes have 50% of normal enzyme activity, whereas homozygotes have only 10% normal activity. The development of emphysema depends on the enzyme activity and environmental insult, so development of pulmonary complications frequently occurs in the third and fourth decades in smokers, later in non-smokers. Homozygotes are also prone to cirrhosis and hepatocellular carcinoma. Treatment is aimed at avoiding smoking and in some centres recombinant α_1-antitrypsin is used.

5.4 A: 98% of male patients are infertile

Cystic fibrosis is the most common inherited condition in the UK and is transmitted as an autosomal recessive trait. The gene is carried by 1 in 25 people in the UK, but is rare in non-white individuals. The incidence is 1 in 2000 live births. Ninety-eight per cent of male patients are infertile and, now that the life expectancy is well into the 30s, fertility counselling plays an increasingly important role in the management of patients.

5.5 E: The risk of having a baby with Down syndrome is significantly greater in parents who have already had a Down syndrome pregnancy

Most cases of Down syndrome are due to non-dysjunction during meiosis, although some parents carry a balanced translocation, which puts them at high risk of recurrence. Karyotyping of parents should be considered after a Down syndrome pregnancy to exclude this risk. Nuchal translucency is a useful screening tool but is not specific for Down syndrome and can be a sign of Edwards' syndrome among others. It is therefore used as a screening test rather than a diagnostic test. In combination with serum screening as part of the 'integrated test', it is more sensitive and specific. Women with a risk of 1 in 200 or worse will usually be offered diagnostic tests such as CVS or amniocentesis. The risk of carrying a Down syndrome baby is 1 in 1400 at 25, 1 in 900 at 30, 1 in 400 at 35, 1 in 100 at 40 and 1 in 30 at 45. More babies are born with Down syndrome to women under 30 than to women over 40 due to the higher number of births in this age group.

5.6   D: The condition is inherited as an autosomal dominant trait and the risk of his sons developing the condition is 1 in 2

Huntington's disease usually manifests between 30 and 50 years of age and usually starts with chorea, with typical hemiballismus. Dementia develops later on, although there is often good insight, which leads to significant depression and suicide. The inheritance is autosomal dominant, giving offspring a 50% chance of developing the disease and their children a 25% chance of inheriting the disease, rising to 50% if their father develops the condition. The gene has been identified, so diagnosis is possible and although there is no cure this can be helpful in family planning.

5.7   D: The incidence is 1:2500 live births

Turner syndrome (45X) is seen in 1:2500 live births. Affected patients are often short, with wide-spaced nipples and a webbed neck. Coarctation of the aorta can occur and internal genitalia are abnormal, although the external genitalia and vagina are usually normal. This can present late as primary amenorrhoea. Oestrogen supplementation from puberty will encourage the development of normal secondary sexual characteristics. Learning disability is more commonly seen with Klinefelter syndrome in men. Many women with Turner syndrome live a normal life, albeit an infertile one.

5.8   A: Family trees are not helpful in counselling families affected by Down syndrome

Three generations of a family tree are needed, together with racial background, to identify genetic predisposition. Down syndrome arises in the parent as a balanced translocation (rare, <1% of cases) or spontaneously during meiosis, so family history is irrelevant. A basic working knowledge of genetics should be sufficient for GPs to advise on inheritance risks of different disorders, particularly with regard to pre-conception counselling. Conditions with variable penetrance or complex inheritance should be dealt with by the genetic counselling service because prediction of risk is complicated. Most people understand risk better as a proportion (eg 1 in 20 children would be affected and 19 in 20 would not be affected), rather than as a percentage (eg 5% are affected).

5.9   C: Phenylketonuria is an autosomal recessive trait, so both parents must be carriers

Phenylketonuria is an autosomal recessive disorder which affects 1 in 10 000 live births. The risk of recurrence of the condition is 1 in 4 and risk of future children being carriers is 1 in 2, whereas the risk of having a child free from the gene is 1 in 4. Screening at birth is important because early phenylalanine exclusion will lead to normal mental development. Where unusual patterns of inheritance are seen, the possibility of biological versus stated parenthood should be considered but there are many other causes, such as incomplete penetrance and new mutation, so this area is best broached by an expert rather than risk causing offence.

5.10   B: The risk of affected offspring is 50%

This picture shows café-au-lait patches and neurofibromas, so the patient has neurofibromatosis, which is inherited as an autosomal dominant trait. Offspring therefore have a 50% risk of being affected, but if they are not affected they will not be carriers. The condition is associated with brain tumours, including acoustic neuromas.

5.11   A: The condition is inherited as an autosomal dominant trait

The condition is expressed in three consecutive generations and is therefore most likely to be a dominant trait. It affects men and women and therefore is unlikely to be an X-linked trait, which tends to affect only males, whereas women are usually carriers or free of the trait. Affected males with X-linked traits cannot pass the condition to sons, whereas all daughters of affected males will be carriers. There are very few conditions associated with the Y chromosome and these would obviously affect only males.

5.12   D: 3, 1, 4, 2

> Ranking – 3: Klinefelter syndrome; 1: Down syndrome; 4: Turner syndrome; 2: fragile X syndrome

The incidence of Klinefelter syndrome is 1:500, Down syndrome 1:1000, Turner syndrome 1:2500, fragile X syndrome 1:4000.

Prevalence of genetic disease

An excellent resource for information on the frequency of genetic disease for patients and healthcare workers is available at www.geneticalliance.org.uk

5.13	E:	5 per 1000 births
5.14	A:	0.05 per 1000 births
5.15	C:	0.4 per 1000 births
5.16	B:	0.1 per 1000 births
5.17	B:	0.1 per 1000 births
5.18	C:	0.4 per 1000 births

Modes of inheritance

5.19   B: Autosomal recessive

Cystic fibrosis is inherited as an autosomal recessive with a 1 in 4 risk of two carriers having an affected child, a 2 in 4 risk of having a carrier child and a 1 in 4 risk of an unaffected child.

5.20   F: X-linked recessive

Duchenne muscular dystrophy is inherited as an X-linked recessive disorder. Women are very rarely affected (1 in 50 000 000) when both parents are carriers. Up to 30% of patients have the condition as a result of a new mutation.

5.21   D: Non-dysjunction

Non-dysjunction in meiosis causes the genotype 47XXY, the additional X chromosome coming from either parent. There is an association with increased maternal age.

5.22   A: Autosomal dominant

Huntington's disease is inherited as an autosomal dominant trait but does not usually present until middle age, by which time most patients have already had children. There is a 50% risk of children being affected.

Diagnostic tests in genetics

5.23   G: Heel-prick test

Shortly after birth a heel-prick blood sample is taken to test for TSH levels and a Guthrie test for phenylketonuria. In some areas, blood is also tested for immunoreactive trypsin, a marker for cystic fibrosis.

5.24   B: Carrier testing

Individuals of Ashkenazi Jewish extraction are tested for serum enzyme levels to detect carriers.

5.25   F: Guthrie test

Early diagnosis of phenylketonuria allows treatment of affected homozygotes, allowing normal neurological development.

5.26   J: Ultrasound

An anomaly scan at 18–20 weeks allows the prenatal diagnosis of congenital heart disease, allowing treatment in the immediate postnatal period or, in some cases, the prenatal period.

5.27   D: Fetoscopy

Fetoscopy allows cordocentesis for haemoglobinopathies at 16–20 weeks, as well as biopsies of skin and liver biopsy where relevant.

Cancer genetics

5.28   A: Acoustic neuroma

Neurofibromatosis is associated with acoustic neuromas, which usually present with sensorineural hearing loss or unilateral tinnitus.

5.29   E: Glioma

Tuberous sclerosis is an autosomal dominant inherited condition characterised by ash-leaf macules appearing on the skin in early childhood, followed by the development of red angiofibromatous papules on the face. The condition is also associated with seizures, interstitial lung disease and gliomas.

5.30   B: Acute lymphoblastic leukaemia

People with Down syndrome have an increased risk of acute lymphocytic leukaemia, whereas lymphoma is common in people with X-linked agammaglobulinaemia and ataxia telangiectasia.

5.31   C: Colonic cancer

Colonic cancer is seen at an early age (20s) in patients with the autosomal dominant condition, familial adenomatous polyposis, and these patients should all have regular colonoscopic screening from a young age.

5.32   L: Thyroid cancer

Multiple endocrine neoplasia is associated with pancreatic and pituitary tumours, peptic ulcer disease, phaeochromocytoma and medullary carcinoma of the thyroid. It has autosomal dominant inheritance and is inherited as a mutation in a tumour-suppressor gene, so patients are born as heterozygotes for that gene. Subsequent mutation of the other allele during the patient's lifetime then results in the development of cancer in that organ.

Antenatal testing

5.33	L:	Screening
5.34	K:	Diagnostic
5.35	H:	15–18 weeks
5.36	D:	0.5–1.0%
5.37	A:	0%

	Nuchal translucency	Chorionic villous sampling	Amniocentesis	Combined test	Anomaly scan
Screening or diagnostic test?	Screening	Diagnostic	Diagnostic	Screening	Screening
Gestational range for testing (weeks)	10-12	10-13	15-18	11-14	18-20
Risk of adverse effects (%)	0	0.5-1.0	0.25-0.50	0	0

5.38   25%

The *ΔF508* gene is carried by 1 in 30 white people, and when homozygous causes cystic fibrosis. When two parents are heterozygous carriers, they have a one in two risk of producing carriers, a one in four risk of an affected homozygote (ie disease sufferer) and a one in four risk of an unaffected homozygote, ie disease free.

Chapter 6
Haematology problems

Single best answer questions

6.1 **Sickle cell anaemia**
You are called to the minor injury unit see a 24-year-old woman suffering an acute painful sickle cell episode. She has already tried paracetamol, codeine and ibuprofen for the pain but still rates the pain as 9/10. Which one of the following would be the SINGLE MOST appropriate course of action in this situation? Select ONE option only.

   ○ A   Administer oxygen at 2 l/min

   ○ B   Give morphine as an intramuscular bolus

   ○ C   Give pethidine as an intramuscular bolus

   ○ D   Give rectal diclofenac 100 mg

   ○ E   Phone her surgery to check that she does have sickle cell anaemia and is not a drug seeker

6.2 **Leg pain**
A 76-year-old woman with a history of treated hypertension had a deep vein thrombosis 12 months ago after a flight from Miami. She complains that over the last few months she has a painful itchy leg. Examination reveals unilateral varicose veins with some hyperpigmentation and oedema. What is the SINGLE MOST likely underlying diagnosis? Select ONE option only.

   ○ A   Cellulitis

   ○ B   Peripheral arterial disease

   ○ C   Post-thrombotic syndrome

   ○ D   Recurrent deep vein thrombosis

   ○ E   Varicose eczema

6.3   Well's score

A 53-year-old woman with no previous history of note presents with a swollen left leg. She has no erythema but is tender posteriorly on the upper calf, and has no risk factors for deep vein thrombosis. You calculate her Well's score as 3. Which ONE of the following would be the SINGLE MOST appropriate action in this situation?

- O   A   Check her CRP levels

- O   B   Check her D-dimer levels and refer for imaging only if elevated

- O   C   Reassure her that a deep vein thrombosis is unlikely on the basis of her Well's score

- O   D   Refer for imaging

- O   E   Start anticoagulation as the diagnosis of deep vein thrombosis is confirmed by the Well's score

6.4   Thrombophillia

A 32-year-old woman suffered a deep vein thrombosis after breaking her leg skiing. She has been on warfarin for 6 months, but is concerned about the possibility of recurrence and asks you if you will test her for thrombophilia. She has no relevant family history, takes no regular medications and has no previous medical history of note. According to NICE guidance, which ONE of the following is an appropriate course of action in this situation? Select ONE option only.

- O   A   Do full thrombophilia screen before stopping warfarin

- O   B   Refer for pelvic ultrasound

- O   C   Refer her to haematology outpatients

- O   D   Stop warfarin and after 4 weeks carry out a full thrombophilia screen

- O   E   Stop warfarin and reassure her that no further testing is indicated at this time

6.5   Spherocytosis

A child has just registered with your practice because his family has moved to the area. He has recently been diagnosed with hereditary spherocytosis. Which ONE of the following statements about this condition is true?

- O   A   It is an X-linked recessive condition

- O   B   It is associated with aplastic crises

- O   C   It is usually diagnosed incidentally in adulthood on routine blood testing

- O   D   Patients should be treated with vitamin B_{12} supplementation

- O   E   There are usually no clinical signs

6.6 **Sickle cell anaemia**

You start a new job in a practice with a large African–Caribbean population, many of whom are affected by sickle cell anaemia. Which ONE of the following statements about this condition is true? Select ONE option only.

○ A   Infarction of the bone marrow causes severe pain

○ B   Osteomyelitis is rarely seen in patients with sickle cell disease

○ C   Sickle cell crises should usually be treated with paracetamol or nonsteroidal drugs rather than with opiates because of the risk of addiction

○ D   The condition is exclusively seen in African–Caribbean populations

○ E   The condition is inherited as an autosomal dominant trait

6.7 **Leukaemia**

A 19-year-old man comes to see you after being diagnosed by the haematology department with leukaemia. Which ONE of the following statements about acute leukaemia is true?

○ A   Of adults aged <50 with acute myeloid leukaemia (AML) 70% are treated successfully

○ B   Acute lymphoblastic leukaemia (ALL) is invariably associated with a white cell count (WCC) >20 × 10^9/l

○ C   ALL is usually diagnosed as an incidental finding on a routine full blood count (FBC)

○ D   AML is usually seen in children

○ E   Platelets are unaffected in acute leukaemia

6.8 **Back pain**

A 62-year-old man presents with a 6-month history of back pain and weight loss. He is a lifelong non-smoker and has no gastrointestinal symptoms. Examination is unremarkable, with no hepatosplenomegaly and no lymphadenopathy, but blood tests show an erythrocyte sedimentation rate (ESR) of 92 mm/h, raised calcium and creatinine levels, and a haemoglobin of 9.8 g/dl with normal white cells and platelets. The film has been reported as showing rouleaux. Which ONE of the following is the SINGLE MOST likely diagnosis?

○ A   Acute myeloid leukaemia (AML)

○ B   Chronic lymphocytic leukaemia (CLL)

○ C   Chronic myeloid leukaemia (CML)

○ D   Multiple myeloma

○ E   Myelodysplasia

6.9   Fatigue

A 78-year-old woman complains of several months of increasing fatigue and, more recently, bleeding gums. She has had no weight loss and no other symptoms. She takes no regular medication. Examination shows her to be pale, with no hepatosplenomegaly or lymphadenopathy. Blood tests show normal renal function and liver function and normal calcium and ESR, but an FBC shows: neutrophil count 0.4×10^9/l, platelets 18×10^9/l and reticulocyte count <1%. Which ONE of the following statements is true about this situation?

- ○ A   This woman has aplastic anaemia
- ○ B   This woman has chronic lymphocytic leukaemia
- ○ C   This woman has iron deficiency
- ○ D   This woman has myeloma
- ○ E   This presentation is typical of myelofibrosis

6.10   Mouth lesions

A 62-year-old man comes to see you 24 hours after being discharged from hospital where he had been admitted for a suspected myocardial infarction. He complains that shortly after discharge he started to get blood blisters in his mouth (shown below).

What is the SINGLE MOST likely diagnosis?

- ○ A   Aphthous ulceration
- ○ B   Behçet syndrome
- ○ C   Immune thrombocytopenia
- ○ D   Lichen planus
- ○ E   Trauma

Extended matching questions

Anaemia

6.11–6.15

Options

A   Alcoholism
B   Anaemia of chronic disease
C   Vitamin B_{12} deficiency
D   Folate deficiency
E   Glucose-6-phosphate dehydrogenase deficiency
F   Hereditary spherocytosis
G   Iron-deficiency anaemia
H   Sickle cell anaemia
I   Thalassaemia major
J   Thalassaemia trait

For each of the clinical scenarios below, select the SINGLE MOST appropriate diagnosis from the list above. Each option can be used once, more than once or not at all.

6.11   A 47-year-old, perimenopausal woman complains of fatigue and shortness of breath on exertion. On examination, she has glossitis and angular stomatitis, and she complains of brittle nails, which you find are spoon shaped.

6.12   A 36-year-old man with long-standing Crohn's disease complains of fatigue. A routine FBC shows a macrocytosis and a haemoglobin level of 10.5 g/dl. B_{12} levels are normal.

6.13   A 25-year-old woman from Iran is given nitrofurantoin for a urinary tract infection. Three weeks later she presents with fatigue and shortness of breath. Urine testing reveals haemoglobinuria and an FBC shows a haemoglobin level of 7.6 g/dl with reticulocytosis.

6.14   A 67-year-old woman with long-standing hypothyroidism and vitiligo has a routine FBC, which shows a macrocytic anaemia. Further blood tests are positive for parietal cell autoantibodies and intrinsic factor antibodies.

6.15   A 32-year-old woman has an FBC done as part of pre-conceptual counselling. She is noted to have a mild microcytic/hypochromic anaemia with normal ferritin levels.

Clotting disorders

6.16–6.20

Options

A   Antiphospholipid syndrome
B   Autoimmune thrombocytopenia
C   Disseminated intravascular coagulopathy
D   Factor V Leiden
E   Haemophilia
F   Idiopathic thrombocytopenia
G   Thrombocythaemia
H   Vitamin K deficiency
I   Von Willebrand's disease

For each scenario described below, select the SINGLE MOST appropriate diagnosis from the list above. Each option can be used once, more than once or not at all.

6.16   A 4-day-old breastfed baby whose mother has noticed bleeding from his umbilical stump.

6.17   A 36-year-old woman with recurrent miscarriages who has been treated by her GP for suspected rheumatoid arthritis for 10 years.

6.18   A 4-year-old girl is brought in by her parents with recurrent bruising. She has previously been fit and well and, apart from multiple bruises on her arms and legs, seems well.

6.19   A 14-year-old boy comes to see you after a traumatic dental extraction that resulted in a significant amount of bleeding. On reflection, his mother reports that he does seem to bruise more than his peers and also comments that his father and paternal uncle have had similar experiences at the dentist.

6.20   A 23-year-old girl experiences pain, swelling and erythema of her right calf after a flight to Hong Kong. Her only medication is the contraceptive pill and she does not smoke. On further questioning, she reports that her mother had a similar experience some years before.

Investigation of microcytic anaemia

6.21–6.25

Options

A α-Thalassaemia trait
B β-Thalassaemia trait
C Ferritin
D HbA$_2$
E Low
F No
G Normal
H Oral iron
I Raised
J Sickle cell trait
K Transfusion
L Yes

The following flow chart has been designed to simplify the investigation of microcytic anaemia (Hb = haemoglobin). From the list of options above, select the MOST appropriate choice for each numbered step in the flow chart. Each option can be used once, more than once or not at all.

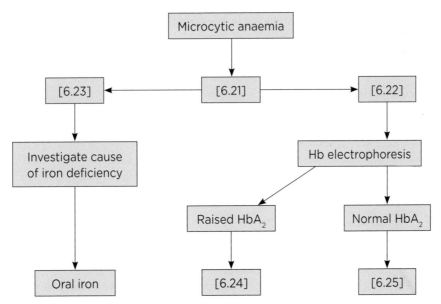

Data interpretation question

6.26 **Well man check**

A 53-year-old man with a history of treated hypertension has routine blood tests carried out as part of a 'well man' check. He smokes 10 cigarettes a day and drinks 10–15 units of alcohol a week. His blood results are shown below:

	Result (normal range)
Haemoglobin	20.7 g/dl (12.0-18.0 g/dl)
Platelets	196 × 10^9/l (150–450 × 10^9/l)
WCC	2.43 × 10^9/l (0.9-4.5 × 10^9/l)
Neutrophils	5.58 × 10^9/l (1.9-9.0 × 10^9/l)
Haematocrit	0.58 (0.4-0.5)
Mean corpuscular volume (MCV)	90 fl (80-99 fl)
Mean corpuscular haemoglobin (MCH)	31.7 pg (27-32 pg)

Which ONE of the following is the SINGLE MOST likely diagnosis?

O   A   Acute myeloid leukaemia

O   B   Vitamin B$_{12}$ deficiency

O   C   Chronic lymphocytic leukaemia

O   D   Essential thrombocythaemia

O   E   Polycythaemia rubra vera

Free-text question

6.27 **Anticoagulants in pregnancy**

A 27-year-old woman on warfarin for an artificial heart valve consults for family planning advice. She has been advised by her cardiologist that she should continue anticoagulation for life. What drug would be the most appropriate anticoagulant to use during pregnancy? Write the answer, in words, in the box below.

6.1   B: Give morphine as an intramuscular bolus

Patients with acute sickling crisis suffer extreme pain and should be treated accordingly. Although some drug addicts have used this condition as a way of obtaining drugs, patients should be given prompt adequate analgesia when presenting. Most patients manage their crises at home but where they present with severe pain not responding to oral medication parenteral opioids should be used. Supplementary oxygen helps, but the primary concern should be controlling pain. Pethidine should not be used due to a tendency to develop addiction.

6.2   C: Post-thrombotic syndrome

Post-thrombotic syndrome affects 25% of patients suffering a deep vein thrombosis within 12 months and is due to venous obstruction with secondary venous hypertension. Patients are at increased risk of venous ulcers. Compression hosiery has been shown to reduce the risk of this condition by 50% and should be started as soon as possible after diagnosis of a DVT.

6.3   D: Refer for imaging

A Well's score estimates the probability of a deep vein thrombosis using clinical markers, including swelling, tenderness and oedema, as well as risk factors in the history such as previous DVT or cancer. It is not a diagnostic test. A Well's score ≥2 should prompt imaging. Point of care testing of D-dimer together with use of Well's score have been estimated to reduce demand for imaging by up to 90% (*Br J Gen Pract* 2010:**60**;742).

6.4   E: Stop warfarin and reassure her that no further testing is indicated at this time

NICE guidance (*Venous thromboembolic diseases: the management of venous thromboembolic diseases and the role of thrombophilia testing*, 2012) suggests the following:

- Do not offer testing to patients who are continuing anticoagulation treatment
- Consider testing patients who have had unprovoked DVT or PE (pulmonary embolus) if it is planned to stop anticoagulation treatment
- Consider testing patients who have had unprovoked DVT or PE with a first-degree relative who has had DVT or PE if it is planned to stop anticoagulation treatment
- Do not offer testing to patients who have had provoked DVT or PE
- Do not routinely offer thrombophilia testing to first-degree relatives of people with a history of DVT or PE and thrombophilia.

In this patient her DVT was provoked, so no further investigation is necessary unless she has a further DVT or PE. If there is a suspicion of malignancy (eg smoker) consider screening for occult malignancy.

6.5 B: It is associated with aplastic crises

Hereditary spherocytosis is an autosomal recessive condition that affects 1 in 5000 live births. It usually presents in childhood as jaundice or with aplastic crises, often triggered by parvovirus infections. Most children receive folic acid supplementation. Splenomegaly is common. It is rarely diagnosed in adulthood.

6.6 A: Infarction of the bone marrow causes severe pain

Sickle cell anaemia affects 1 in 4 West African and 1 in 10 African–Caribbean individuals. It is inherited as an autosomal recessive trait and is also carried in Mediterranean and Middle Eastern populations. Homozygotes suffer from infarction of bone marrow and haemolysis during times of low oxygen levels (eg with infections), causing a haemolytic anaemia and extreme bone pain, often requiring opiates. Infection of infarcted bone marrow is common.

6.7 A: Of adults aged <50 with acute myeloid leukaemia (AML) 70% are treated successfully

In ALL, 50% of patients have a normal WCC but typically have blasts present on the film and a normocytic anaemia. AML is rarely seen in children, whereas ALL is usually seen in children and young adults. The prognosis in AML is better for the under-50s, those with a WCC <50 × 10^9/l and those without extramedullary disease at presentation. ALL usually presents with signs of marrow failure or bone pain. Platelets are usually reduced and a diagnosis of leukaemia should always be considered in children with apparent thrombocytopenia.

6.8 D: Multiple myeloma

Myeloma often presents with bone pain and there are usually few abnormal findings on clinical examination. At presentation, many patients will have biochemical evidence of nephropathy and bone destruction, and hyperviscosity is often seen, with a raised ESR and rouleaux formation. Bence Jones protein is characteristically raised. AML and ALL tend to present with signs of bone marrow failure and extramedullary infiltration (eg meningeal signs in AML). CLL presents as a routine finding on an FBC in most cases, whereas CML is usually associated with signs of bleeding and hepatosplenomegaly. Myelodysplasia generally presents with fatigue.

6.9 A: This woman has aplastic anaemia

Myelofibrosis typically presents over a longer period of time and is associated with hepatosplenomegaly due to extramedullary haematopoiesis. Aplastic anaemia is idiopathic in at least 70% of cases and has a poor prognosis, with <50% of patients surviving 6 months.

6.10 C: Immune thrombocytopenia

Immune thrombocytopenia is typically caused by heparin, sulfonamides, chloramphenicol, sulfasalazine, quinine and quinidine. It typically comes on 2–3 days after taking a drug that has been taken in the past, or 7 days after taking a new drug. It is reported to occur in up to 25% of patients on heparin. The platelet count typically rises 7–10 days after stopping the medication.

Anaemia

6.11   **G:**   **Iron-deficiency anaemia**

Iron deficiency can be caused by blood loss through heavy menstrual bleeding or parasitic infection, or by poor iron intake. An FBC will usually show a microcytosis.

6.12   **D:**   **Folate deficiency**

Folate deficiency can be due to poor intake or to malabsorption (eg coeliac disease, Crohn's disease). Bloods show a macrocytic anaemia and low folate levels. Treatment is with folate supplementation.

6.13   **E:**   **Glucose-6-phosphate dehydrogenase (G6PDH) deficiency**

G6PDH deficiency affects up to 25% of people from southern Africa and the Middle East. Haemolysis can follow infection, fava bean ingestion and drugs (eg dapsone, quinine, antibiotics). Hospital admission is required to avoid renal damage and correct the haemolysis.

6.14   **C:**   **Vitamin B_{12} deficiency**

Vitamin B_{12} is found in animal foods, including milk and eggs, but not in vegetables, so vegans are at risk of deficiency. Other causes of vitamin B_{12} deficiency include malabsorption (eg after gastrectomy) and autoimmune disease. There is a strong association with vitiligo and Hashimoto's thyroiditis. Treatment is with 3-monthly vitamin B_{12} injections.

6.15   **J:**   **Thalassaemia trait**

Thalassaemia trait is usually symptomless and is really of significance only if both partners in a relationship are affected.

Clotting disorders

6.16   **H:**   **Vitamin K deficiency**

Vitamin K deficiency in babies is seen in exclusively breastfed babies who have not received vitamin K and manifests as bleeding, usually between days 2 and 4 of life. The cause is a combination of low natural levels at birth coupled with lack of bacterial vitamin K synthesis in the gut and immature liver function. Breast milk is low in vitamin K, whereas formula milk has vitamin K added.

6.17   **A:**   **Antiphospholipid syndrome**

Antiphospholipid syndrome can be primary or secondary to connective tissue disease, most commonly SLE. It causes recurrent fetal loss, thrombocytopenia and recurrent ischaemic events. It is characterised by the presence of high titres of IgG antiphospholipid antibodies and is thought to be due to a coagulopathy rather than to a vasculitis.

6.18   F: Idiopathic thrombocytopenia

Idiopathic thrombocytopenia is the most likely diagnosis in children, although child abuse and leukaemia should be excluded. In adults taking medication, autoimmune thrombocytopenia is more likely.

6.19   I: Von Willebrand's disease

Von Willebrand's disease is inherited as an autosomal dominant trait and is characterised by excessive bleeding after dental extractions and prolonged bleeding time. The bleeding is usually much less severe than in haemophilia and can usually be controlled with tranexamic acid.

6.20   D: Factor V Leiden

Factor V Leiden is a variant of factor V that predisposes to venous thromboembolism. Patients with a suspicious family history should be tested before prescribing the combined oral contraceptive pill.

Investigation of microcytic anaemia

6.21   C: Ferritin

6.22   G: Normal

6.23   E: Low

6.24   B: β-Thalassaemia trait

6.25   A: α-Thalassaemia trait

HbA$_2$ is raised in β-thalassaemia trait, but is normal in α-thalassaemia trait.

6.26   E: Polycythaemia rubra vera

The raised haematocrit and haemoglobin, with normal MCH and MCV suggest that the diagnosis is polycythaemia. These results, with a normal plasma volume and raised red cell mass, suggest true polycythaemia, rather than dehydration. Secondary causes include hypoxia, smoking and chronic lung disease. Patients should have a bone marrow biopsy to exclude myeloproliferative disease. Treatment is usually regular venesection to keep the haematocrit <0.45.

6.27   Heparin

Warfarin crosses the placenta and is associated with significant risk to the fetus. Heparin does not, so is safe in pregnancy, but must be given by daily injection.

Chapter 7
Immunology problems

Single best answer questions

7.1 Vaccination in pregnancy

A woman in week 23 of her second pregnancy asks you if you would recommend her to have a flu vaccine this winter. Which ONE of the following statements is true with regard to this situation?

- ○ A   All influenza vaccines available in the UK are live vaccines

- ○ B   All vaccines are contraindicated in pregnancy

- ○ C   Immunity lasts up to 5 years so patients vaccinated before becoming pregnant do not need a booster during pregnancy

- ○ D   Pregnant women are considered an 'at risk' category for influenza vaccination in the UK

- ○ E   Vaccination of pregnant women with H1N1 vaccine is associated with a higher risk of miscarriage than H1N1 infection

7.2 Rabies vaccination

A 19-year-old man is due to leave for a gap year travelling around Asia and asks your advice about rabies vaccination. Which SINGLE ONE of the following statements is correct with regard to this vaccine?

- ○ A   Three doses of rabies vaccine provide lifelong protection against rabies

- ○ B   Patients attacked by animals in rabies endemic countries need treatment only if skin is broken

- ○ C   Patients receiving animal bites in the UK may be reassured that they do not need rabies vaccination

- ○ D   Patients receiving animal bites in endemic countries do not need further treatment if they have received a full vaccination course before exposure

- ○ E   Patients receiving animal bites in endemic countries should seek urgent medical attention for wound treatment, regardless of the extent of the injury

7.3   Immunotherapy
Which SINGLE ONE of the following statements about the use of immunotherapy in allergic conditions is true?

O   A   Grazax is effective in patients with allergic rhinitis due to house-dust mite only where RAST tests are positive

O   B   Sublingual immunotherapy can be used on an as-needed basis

O   C   Sublingual immunotherapy is effective in patients with allergic rhinitis only

O   D   Sublingual immunotherapy results in angioedema in 15% of patients

O   E   Use of sublingual grass allergen tablets results in a significant reduction in medication use

7.4   Pneumococcal vaccination
You are updating the protocols for pneumococcal vaccination in the practice. Which SINGLE ONE of the following patient groups needs a booster vaccination after routine primary immunisation?

O   A   Patients with asthma

O   B   Patients with chronic kidney disease

O   C   Patients with chronic obstructive pulmonary disease

O   D   Patients with diabetes

O   E   Patients with stable ischaemic heart disease

7.5   Allergic rhinitis
With regard to the drug management of allergic rhinitis, which SINGLE ONE of the following statements is true?

O   A   Anticholinergics are effective for rhinorrhoea

O   B   Antileukotrienes are effective for ocular but not nasal symptoms

O   C   Nasal steroids are effective for nasal symptoms, but not for ocular symptoms

O   D   Oral antihistamines are the most effective treatment for nasal symptoms

O   E   Treatment of asthma has no effect on allergic rhinitis

7.6 Interpretation of skin changes
Consider the picture below:

Which SINGLE ONE of the following statements about this situation is true?

○ A   This patient has experienced a fixed drug reaction

○ B   This patient has had patch testing performed

○ C   This patient has had skin-prick testing

○ D   This patient is suffering from bullous pemphigoid

○ E   This patient is suffering from erythema multiforme

Extended matching questions

Allergy testing

7.7–7.11

Options

A   Exclusion diet
B   IgE levels
C   None of these options
D   Patch testing
E   RAST
F   Skin-prick testing
G   Symptom diary

For each of the situations described below, select the SINGLE MOST appropriate investigation from the list above. Each option may be used once, more than once or not at all.

7.7	A 35-year-old marketing executive complains of abdominal bloating and cramps after eating certain foodstuffs.
7.8	A 48-year-old woman who complains of 5 years of fatigue and myalgia, which she feels are due to mercury in her dental fillings.
7.9	A 13-year-old boy complains of rhinitis and wheeze for most days of the year, which are worse when he visits his father's house and better when he goes on holiday.
7.10	A 36-year-old paramedic complains of recurrent dermatitis affecting his hands when he is at work, which rapidly improves on holiday.
7.11	A 28-year-old man requests testing for wasp sting allergy.

Vaccines

7.12–7.16

Options

A   Inactivated
B   Immunoglobulins
C   Live attenuated
D   Recombinant antigen
E   Toxoid

For each of the vaccine types given below, select the SINGLE MOST appropriate option to describe its mode of action from the list above. Each option may be used once, more than once or not at all.

7.12	Pertussis
7.13	Measles, mumps and rubella (MMR)
7.14	Tetanus
7.15	Hepatitis B
7.16	Salk polio vaccine

Allergy management in primary care

7.17–7.21

Options

A   Admit
B β_2 Agonist
C β Blockade
D   Depo-Medrone
E   Intramuscular adrenaline
F   Intravenous adrenaline
G   Oral antihistamine
H   Oral prednisolone

For each of the numbered gaps in the following allergy management flow chart, select the single most appropriate option from the list above. Each option can be used once, more than once or not at all.

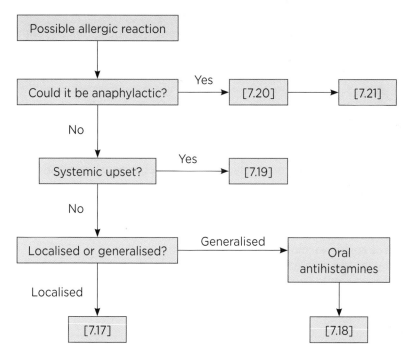

Data interpretation question

7.22   Chickenpox
A 24-year-old woman is 12 weeks pregnant. She works as a preschool teacher and one of the children has recently been diagnosed with suspected chickenpox. She feels as if she has a temperature but has no rash. She is not sure if she has had chickenpox in the past, and her mother cannot recall this either. Blood tests are carried out which show the following results:

Varicella IgG	Elevated
Varicella IgM	Normal
Measles IgG	Normal
Measles IgM	Normal

Which SINGLE ONE of the following statements about this patient's varicella status is correct?

O   A   She has been infected with varicella in the past and is now immune

O   B   She has not been exposed in the past to chickenpox

O   C   She has recently been infected with chickenpox

O   D   She is measles immune

O   E   The results are most likely to be due to childhood vaccination

Free-text question

7.23   Herpes zoster vaccination
A 77-year-old man enquires about having a vaccination against herpes zoster. He would like to know more about the risks involved and asks if it is a live or inactivated vaccine. Which of these is correct? Write the answer, in words, in the box below.

7.1   D: Pregnant women are considered an 'at risk' category for influenza vaccination in the UK

Patients developing influenza while pregnant are at increased risk of morbidity and mortality and therefore, since 2010, have been included in the clinical risk categories. Vaccination is safer than infection, and all but one of the vaccines available in the UK are inactivated. There is a theoretical risk from using live vaccines in pregnancy so they are usually avoided, unless risk outweighs benefits.

7.2   E: Patients receiving animal bites in endemic countries should seek urgent medical attention for wound treatment, regardless of the extent of the injury

Management of animal bites in rabies endemic countries involves urgent wound debridement and management to avoid increasing the risk of infection, together with assessment of risk. All cases should be discussed with a rabies specialist. Where mucous membranes have potentially been contaminated with saliva, even where there is no obvious wound, urgent irrigation is required to prevent infection through this route.

7.3   E: Use of sublingual grass allergen tablets results in a significant reduction in medication use

Grazax, a purified grass allergen extract in tablet form, is taken up to 16 weeks before the start of the allergy season in patients with proven IgE-mediated grass pollen sensitivity (through either RAST or skin-prick testing). It is well tolerated and results in a 30% reduction in symptoms and a 38% reduction in medication use. Serious side effects have not been reported in trials (*J Allergy Clin Immunol* 2006;**118**:434–40). Meta-analysis has shown that immunotherapy also reduces symptoms and medication use in children with asthma (*Chest* 2007;**133**:599–609).

7.4   B: Patients with chronic kidney disease

Patients with chronic kidney disease, hyposplenism or asplenia should have booster doses of pneumococcal vaccine and haemophilus vaccine every 5 years. Children vaccinated routinely should also have a booster dose at 13 months.

7.5   A: Anticholinergics are effective for rhinorrhoea

The ARIA (Allergic Rhinitis and its Impact on Asthma) guidelines for the treatment of allergic rhinitis suggest that oral antihistamines are effective for sneezing, rhinorrhoea and eye symptoms, but not for nasal obstruction. Intraocular antihistamines are effective only for eye symptoms. Corticosteroids are the most effective treatment for all symptoms, although they are not as effective for eye symptoms as intraocular antihistamines. Decongestants are effective only for nasal obstruction, whereas anticholinergics are effective only for rhinorrhoea. Antileukotriene antagonists are moderately effective for all symptoms except nasal itch. Treatment of asthma will often improve symptoms of allergic rhinitis and vice versa.

7.6   B: This patient has had patch testing performed

This patient has had patch testing, which is suitable for occupational allergies (eg contact dermatitis). Aeroallergens are better tested with skin-prick testing.

Allergy testing

7.7   A: Exclusion diet

Food intolerance is distinct from food allergy and can have a metabolic basis (eg lactase deficiency). Symptoms are distinct from food allergy, an IgE-mediated reaction characterised by nausea, vomiting, diarrhoea, urticaria and angioedema. Food intolerance can be diagnosed by exclusion diet but ideally this should be under the supervision of a dietician if there are multiple potential causes, to avoid malnutrition.

7.8   C: None of these options

These symptoms are not suggestive of allergy or intolerance. She should be questioned about other somatic symptoms and a diagnosis of depression considered. She would be best advised to seek dental advice regarding her fillings.

7.9   E: RAST

RAST will help to identify allergic reactions, which would allow some lifestyle modification, eg if cats or dogs are involved. If allergy to house-dust mite is detected this is often difficult to manage because of the prevalence of this allergen and the limited evidence for efficacy of house-dust mite elimination.

7.10   D: Patch testing

Patch testing will identify most T-cell-mediated delayed hypersensitivity contact allergens. Around 20–30 suspect allergens are tested as a batch and the responses used to identify which the culprits are. Appropriate precautions, eg hypoallergenic gloves or soaps, can then be taken.

7.11   F: Skin-prick testing

Skin-prick testing is suitable for insect stings. Where this is not available RAST may be used but may give a false negative if there has not been recent exposure.

Vaccines

7.12   A: Inactivated

The pertussis vaccine, either on its own or as part of a combination vaccine, contains inactivated *Bordetella pertussis*.

7.13   C: Live attenuated

MMR is a live attenuated vaccine.

7.14   E: Toxoid

Tetanus vaccine is a toxoid and is either given alone or in combination.

7.15   D: Recombinant antigen

Hepatitis B vaccine is a recombinant vaccine containing hepatitis B surface antigen (HBsAg) cultured from yeast cells.

7.16   A: Inactivated

Inactivated polio vaccines are now the norm, and oral live vaccine is no longer used routinely in the UK. The current vaccine in use contains three strains of poliovirus.

Allergy management in primary care

7.17   G: Oral antihistamine

7.18   H: Oral prednisolone

7.19   H: Oral prednisolone

7.20   E: Intramuscular adrenaline

7.21   A: Admit

7.22   A: She has been infected with varicella in the past and is now immune

IgM is the first antibody to be produced in infection; IgG is produced later. Recent infection therefore results in raised virus-specific IgM, whereas historical infection results in raised IgG with normal IgM.

7.23   Live

The herpes zoster vaccine is a live attenuated vaccine, and hence should not be used in immunocompromised patients, or those on steroids.

Chapter 8
Infectious diseases

Single best answer questions

8.1 **Sore throat**
A 13-year-old asylum seeker recently arrived from Georgia is brought to see you by her mother. She has had a sore throat for the last 48 hours but is now drowsy and restless, and cannot walk unaided. She has no previous history of note. On examination she is febrile and tachycardic, and has a thick white exudate over her tonsils. Which of the following is the SINGLE MOST likely diagnosis?

   ○ A   Diphtheria

   ○ B   Glandular fever

   ○ C   Poliomyelitis

   ○ D   Scarlet fever

   ○ E   Vincent's angina

8.2 **Unwell child**
A 13-year-old boy has been treated for chickenpox for the last 72 h.
His mother is concerned about his balance and asks for a home visit. On examination you note nystagmus, a tremor and difficulty walking heel to toe, and a bilateral tremor worse when trying to touch your finger. What is the SINGLE most likely diagnosis? Select ONE option only.

   ○ A   Encephalitis

   ○ B   Meningitis

   ○ C   Sepsis

   ○ D   Space-occupying lesion

   ○ E   Stroke

8.3   Jaundice
A 47-year-old man who works in a water treatment plant complains of flu-like symptoms of headache, myalgia and fever. He has been taking over-the-counter medication for this but after 6 days he becomes concerned because his skin looks yellow. On examination he has widespread lymphadenopathy and an enlarged liver, and is jaundiced. Reviewing his medical notes you see that he has been vaccinated against hepatitis A and hepatitis B and has no other risk factors. What is the SINGLE MOST likely diagnosis?

○   A   *Campylobacter* sp.

○   C   *Escherichia coli* O157

○   B   Epstein–Barr virus

○   D   Leptospirosis

○   E   Shigellosis

8.4   HPV vaccination
Your next patient is a 12-year-old girl who has come with her mother. The girl is due to have her human papillomavirus (HPV) vaccination at school soon. Her mother is very uneasy about this and asks your advice on whether it is worth having. Which ONE of the following statements is true with regard to this issue? Select ONE option only.

○   A   A single dose is given at age 13

○   B   The HPV vaccine will prevent her getting genital warts and cervical cancer

○   C   The vaccine is associated with potentially serious adverse reactions

○   D   Vaccination does not need to start until a girl becomes sexually active

○   E   Where three doses of vaccine are given it is >97% effective

8.5   Antimalarials in pregnancy
        According to current guidelines, what are the recommendations for
        antimalarial chemoprophylaxis for pregnant women travelling to malarial
        areas? Select ONE option only.

O   A   Doxycycline is safe in all trimesters of pregnancy

O   B   Mefloquine is thought to be safe in treatment doses in the second and
        third trimesters

O   C   Pregnant women are less at risk of developing malaria, so
        chemoprophylaxis should be avoided

O   D   Pregnant women taking chloroquine should receive supplementation
        with 5 mg folic acid daily

O   E   Women who have taken mefloquine before or during the first trimester
        should consider a termination

8.6   Dysuria
        A 19-year-old woman presents with a burning sensation when passing
        urine and a yellow, blood-stained vaginal discharge. She admits to having
        had unprotected sexual intercourse 4 days ago. What is the SINGLE MOST
        likely diagnosis?

O   A   Bacterial vaginosis

O   B   Chlamydia infection

O   C   Gonorrhoea

O   D   Syphilis

O   E   Trichomoniasis

8.7   Unwell child
        A 4-year-old girl is brought in by her mother with a 3-day history of cough,
        runny nose and watery eyes. Today, mum has noticed red spots with white
        centres inside the girl's cheeks. Which ONE of the following is the SINGLE
        MOST likely diagnosis?

O   A   Measles

O   B   Rhinovirus

O   C   Rubella

O   D   Scarlet fever

O   E   Varicella

8.8   Insects

A concerned mother comes to see you having found an insect in her daughter's sleeping bag after a school trip to the New Forest. She is concerned that her daughter may be at risk of disease and would like to know what action should be taken. Her daughter is asymptomatic and there are no abnormal findings on examination. The insect is shown below.

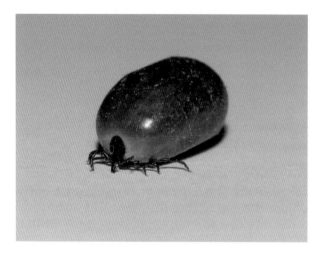

Which ONE of the following would be appropriate management in this situation? Select ONE option only.

○   A   Prescribe amoxicillin

○   B   Prescribe flucloxacillin

○   C   Prescribe topical mupirocin to use on any insect bites

○   D   Reassure the mother that in the absence of a rash or systemic symptoms no treatment is necessary

○   E   Take blood for Lyme serology from the patient

8.9   Skin lesion
This 38-year-old soldier returned from a tour of duty in the Middle East
6 weeks ago. He has developed a lesion on his skin that started as an
erythematous papule:

What is the SINGLE MOST likely diagnosis from the list below?

O   A   Cutaneous leishmaniasis

O   B   Cutaneous tuberculosis

O   C   Leprosy

O   D   Syphilis

O   E   Systemic lupus erythematosus

Extended matching questions

Antibiotics

8.10–8.13

Options

A   Admit for intravenous antibiotics
B   Amoxicillin
C   Co-amoxiclav
D   Flucloxacillin
E   Fusidic acid cream
F   Metronidazole
G   No treatment necessary
H   Trimethoprim for 3 days
I   Trimethoprim for 7 days
J   None of the above

For each of the following scenarios select the most appropriate antibiotic from the list of options. Each option can be used once, more than once or not at all.

8.10   A 4-year-old boy has had a yellow, crusted lesion on his chin for a few days and has now developed a similar one on his right arm.

8.11   A woman with dysuria and frequency is currently 32 weeks pregnant.

8.12   A 64-year-old man comes to consult after a cat scratch to his face. On examination, he is afebrile with cellulitis around the scratch.

8.13   High vaginal swab results for a 38-year-old woman show bacterial vaginosis.

Management of respiratory tract infections

8.14–8.17

Options

A   5 years
B   65 years
C   80 years
D   Facial pain
E   Postnasal drip
F   Symptoms persisting for more than 5 days
G   Significant co-morbidity
H   Systemically unwell

Complete the algorithm below identifying patients in need of antibiotics in respiratory tract infection using the options above. Each option may be used once, more than once or not at all.

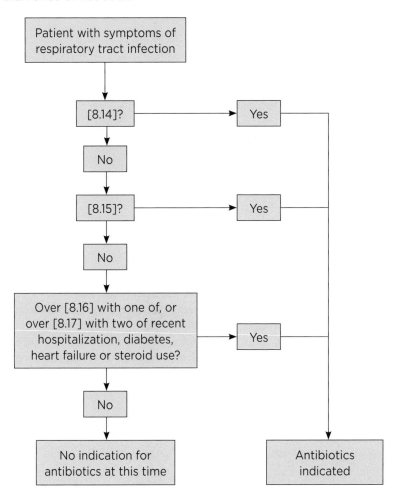

Data interpretation question

8.18   Unwell child
A 9-month-old girl presents with a fever and vomiting. A urine sample was sent to the laboratory and you receive the following result:

White cells	>100 cells/ml
Red blood cells	>100 cells/ml
Organisms	3+
Epithelial cells	1+
Culture	*Escherichia coli* >10^8

Which ONE of the following would be the SINGLE MOST appropriate initial management for this child? Select ONE option only.

○   A   Refer immediately for an urgent ultrasound scan of the kidneys

○   B   Repeat the urine sample to ensure that it is not a contaminated specimen

○   C   Start antibiotics, continue with a prophylactic dose and review in 2 months

○   D   Start antibiotics immediately and refer for urgent paediatric assessment

○   E   Start antibiotics immediately and repeat the urine sample in 7–10 days to confirm that the infection has cleared

Free-text questions

8.19   Dog bite
A 56-year-old woman with no previous medical history of note is bitten by her dog while breaking up a fight with another dog. She has a small puncture wound on her hand that is bleeding. She takes no regular medications and has no allergies. What would be the SINGLE MOST appropriate antibiotic, if any, to use in this situation? Write your answer in the box below.

8.20 and 8.21   Occupational health

According to current Department of Health guidance, risk of HIV infection in healthcare settings can be classified as high or low risk, depending on the type of exposure.

Part A

MATCH each exposure to the MOST APPROPRIATE column with regard to risk of infection following OCCUPATIONAL EXPOSURE. All six items must be correctly matched to score ONE mark.

A   Amniotic fluid
B   Blood
C   Faeces
D   Synovial fluid
E   Urine
F   Vomit

Low risk	High risk

Part B

What is the MINIMUM number of WEEKS after a needlestick injury that follow-up serology should take place? White your answer in the box below, in numbers.

8.1 A: Diphtheria

Diphtheria is uncommon in the UK but is prevalent in the former Soviet republics and South Africa. It is caused by a diphtheria toxin produced by the bacteria infecting the throat. It may be carried asymptomatically, cause a mild pharyngitis without the pharyngeal pseudomembrane, or cause systemic illness with myocarditis and cardiac failure. Treatment is with anti-toxin and macrolide or β-lactam antibiotics to clear the organism and prevent infection of others. Vaccination is effective to prevent the disease, but many of the UK population are not fully immunised.

8.2 A: Encephalitis

Chickenpox encephalitis usually presents with ataxia 3–4 days after the onset of the rash, often in the recovery phase of chickenpox, and usually affects the cerebellum. Where the cerebrum is affected, seizures are common. 80% of patients make a full recovery, although there may be permanent seizures and intellectual disability. Meningitis usually presents with meningism, altered mental status and headache. Patients with sepsis are usually unwell; stroke is uncommon in this age group and a space-occupying lesion would not normally present with acute onset of symptoms.

8.3 D: Leptospirosis

Leptospirosis can be spread by a number of different rodents but is usually associated with rats. People who work in environments with large numbers of rats are most at risk (eg sewage workers). Infection causes an initial flu-like illness, after which a proportion of patients go on to develop jaundice, renal failure and meningism. Most patients make an uneventful recovery. Diagnosis is by complement fixation of urine culture for *Leptospira* sp. Penicillin or tetracycline is usually effective treatment.

8.4 E: Where three doses of vaccine are given it is >97% effective

The HPV vaccination programme aims to prevent infection with the strains of HPV (16 and 18), which are associated with genital warts and cervical cancer in the UK. These vaccines are given in three doses from age 13 and provide 97–99% coverage. There have been no reports of serious adverse reactions. The vaccine covers some wart viruses but not all, so patients can still develop genital warts. There are currently two vaccines available in the UK, Gardasil and Cervarix. Gardasil also provides coverage against HPV6 and HPV11, so it is likely to provide additional cover against warts. Vaccination should start before sexual activity begins to ensure adequate protection before first exposure.

8.5   B: Mefloquine is thought to be safe in treatment doses in the second and third trimesters

There is no strong association between mefloquine in treatment doses and stillbirths or miscarriages in the second and third trimesters, although lack of data on its use in the first trimester has encouraged caution. Pregnant women have an increased risk of developing severe malaria and have a higher risk of fatality. Doxycycline is contraindicated in pregnancy and those taking proguanil should also take folic acid. Women who have taken mefloquine before or during the first trimester should be advised that this is not an indication to terminate the pregnancy.

8.6   C: Gonorrhoea

The early signs of gonorrhoea can be mild and are often missed, but symptoms in women can include a painful and burning sensation when passing urine and a yellow, blood-stained, vaginal discharge. Symptoms usually appear 2–10 days after becoming infected. Chlamydia infection usually presents 1–3 weeks after becoming infected. Symptoms include bleeding between periods, an unusual vaginal discharge and lower abdominal pain. Around 70% of women have no symptoms at all. The symptoms of syphilis are generally non-specific and it usually presents with a painless but infectious sore anywhere on the body, which resolves spontaneously in 2–6 weeks. Bacterial vaginosis presents with a typical grey–yellow, fishy, offensive discharge and it is not a sexually transmitted infection. Trichomoniasis presents with a typical yellow–green, frothy discharge and is less common than other sexually transmitted infections.

8.7   A: Measles

Tiny, bluish-white spots with surrounding erythema seen on the buccal mucosa of the cheek, known as 'Koplik's spots', are pathognomonic of early stage measles. The first symptoms of measles include cough, coryza, conjunctivitis, fever and malaise. A florid erythematous maculopapular rash, which starts at the head, appears 3–4 days later. Koplik's spots can appear 1–2 days before the rash.

8.8   D: Reassure the mother that in the absence of a rash or systemic symptoms no treatment is necessary

Ticks are frequently found in areas of long grass and woodland and prophylactic treatment in the absence of symptoms is not usually justified. Patients should be reassured and advised to report a rash or systemic symptoms. If these occur antibiotics should be used. Doxycycline, amoxicillin or cefuroxime is commonly used but advice from local microbiology services should be obtained before treatment.

8.9   A: Cutaneous leishmaniasis

Leishmaniasis is a parasitic disease spread by infected female sandflies and is mainly seen in the tropics and subtropics. It can be visceral, cutaneous or mucocutaneous. Visceral leishmaniasis is serious and can be fatal. Cutaneous leishmaniasis presents with one or more skin lesions that start as red papules and develop into ulcers. These can change in shape and appearance over time. There can be associated lymphadenopathy. With no treatment these ulcers will heal themselves, usually within 10 months, but can leave depigmented scars or go on to cause mucocutaneous leishmaniasis, which is very disfiguring. It is therefore advisable to treat after seeking advice from the local centre for disease control.

Antibiotics

8.10   D: Flucloxacillin

This is impetigo that has spread. As a result of increasing resistance, current advice is for topical treatment to be reserved for very localised lesions.

8.11   I: Trimethoprim for 7 days

Current guidelines for urinary tract infections in pregnancy suggest that trimethoprim is unlikely to cause problems in the fetus in the third trimester, so first-line antibiotics for urinary tract infections in pregnancy are trimethoprim and nitrofurantoin; second-line antibiotics are cefalexin and amoxicillin. All these antibiotics should be given for 7 days in pregnancy.

8.12   C: Co-amoxiclav

Co-amoxiclav is used for facial cellulitis, and is the drug of choice for animal scratches and bites. Flucloxacillin or erythromycin (if penicillin allergic) can be used for cellulitis elsewhere, unless the infection is due to an animal scratch or bite. A febrile or ill patient should be admitted for intravenous antibiotics.

8.13   F: Metronidazole

Bacterial vaginosis can be treated with oral or vaginal metronidazole or vaginal clindamycin cream.

Management of respiratory tract infections

8.14	H:	Systemically unwell
8.15	G:	Significant co-morbidity
8.16	C:	80 years
8.17	B:	65 years

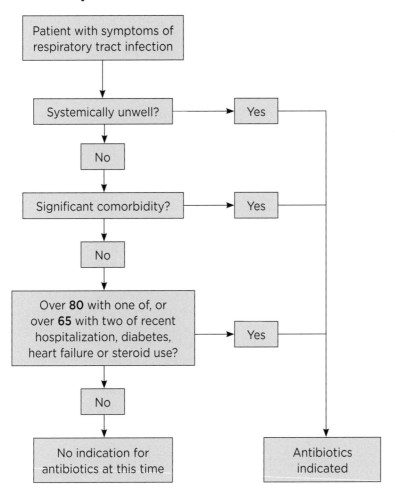

8.18   D: Start antibiotics immediately and refer for urgent paediatric assessment

This result indicates a genuine bacterial infection. The risks of ascending infection and renal damage are high from birth to 6 years of age. Infection at this age suggests a possible renal tract abnormality.

8.19   Co-amoxiclav

All animal bites should be treated with prophylactic antibiotics. Where patients are penicillin allergic, metronidazole or doxycyline is a suitable alternative.

8.20 and 8.21   Occupational health

Part A

Low risk	High risk
Faeces	Amniotic fluid
Urine	Blood
Vomit	Synovial fluid

Part B   12 weeks

Blood-stained fluid, or fluid from within a mucous membrane, may pose a risk of infection if significant occupational exposure occurs, ie percutaneous injury, exposure of broken skin or exposure of mucous membranes including the eye. Unless blood stained, exposure to urine, vomit, saliva or faeces is considered low risk and postexposure prophylaxis is not usually required. Where postexposure prophylaxis is used, this should be given as soon as possible, and follow-up serology should not be carried out until at least 12 weeks after exposure, due to the time taken to seroconvert. The risk of occupational infection from a needlestick injury is around 3 in 1000, but is higher in patients with a high viral load, eg in terminal AIDS. The risk from mucocutaneous exposure is less than 1 in 1000. Where zidovudine is used for postexposure prophylaxis, it reduces risk of seroconversion by 81%. Most regimens in the UK now use triple or quadruple drug regimens.

Chapter 9
Intellectual and learning disabilities

Single best answer questions

9.1   Learning difficulties
Which ONE of the following is the MOST APPROPRIATE definition of a learning disability? Select ONE option only.

  ○ A   Disability occurring at any age characterised by an inability to acquire new skills which is approximately two or more standard deviations (SDs) below the mean

  ○ B   Disability occurring before the age of 18 years old characterised by significantly below-average intellectual functioning and adaptive behaviour which is approximately two or more SDs below the mean

  ○ C   Disability originating during the developmental period characterised by significantly below-average intellectual functioning and adaptive behaviour which is approximately two or more SDs below the mean

  ○ D   Disability characterised by an age-specific IQ (intelligence quotient) score <50

  ○ E   Disability characterised by an age-specific IQ score <100

9.2   Epidemiology of learning disability
Which ONE of the following statements is true with regard to learning disability in the UK? Select ONE OPTION only.

  ○ A   Of the population 0.5% have an IQ <50

  ○ B   Of the population 10% have an IQ <70

  ○ C   Patients with an IQ between 50 and 70 have a significantly increased prevalence of psychiatric illness

  ○ D   Patients with an IQ <70 are invariably unable to live independently

  ○ E   The aetiology of learning disability is exclusively biological

9.3 Long-term health for patients with learning disability
Which ONE of the following statements is CORRECT with regard to long-term health in patients with learning disabilities? Select ONE option only.

- O A All-cause mortality rates in patients with moderate-to-severe learning disabilities are twice the rate in the general population

- O B Down syndrome is associated with a reduced risk of leukaemia

- O C One in twenty adults with learning disabilities rates their health as not good

- O D Patients with learning disability living in residential care have worse oral health than those living with their families.

- O E The prevalence of epilepsy in patients with learning disability is 20 times higher than in the general population

9.4 Consent and learning disability
An 18-year-old girl with Down syndrome attends with her boyfriend who also has Down syndrome. She would like to go on the pill. She lives with her parents, who are strict Catholics, and does not wish to discuss this issue with them. She understands and communicates to you that without contraception she is at risk of unplanned pregnancy, and that there are small risks with taking the pill. Which ONE of the following statements is CORRECT in this situation? Select ONE option only.

- O A An independent mental capacity advocate (IMCA) must be appointed to make a decision in this case

- O B Her mother is assumed to be her next of kin and must be consulted before treatment

- O C If she can demonstrate that she has capacity, there is no need to consult her parents before treatment

- O D If her parents disagree with her wishes, a referral to the court of protection must be made

- O E She is under 19 years old and therefore cannot consent to medical treatment without her parents' agreement

9.5 Childhood autism
Which ONE of the following statements about childhood autism is true?

- O A It involves a preference for consistency and routine
- O B It involves the normal early development of social interactions
- O C It is a subtype of psychosis
- O D It is associated with a reciprocal 'social smile'
- O E It is not associated with self-harm

Extended matching questions

Early signs of learning disability

9.6–9.9

Options

A   Attention deficit hyperactivity disorder
B   Auditory processing disorder
C   Autism
D   Dyscalculia
E   Dysgraphia
F   Dyslexia
G   Dyspraxia
H   Global developmental delay
I   Monochromatism
J   None of the above

For each of the descriptions below, select the SINGLE MOST LIKELY diagnosis from the list above. Each option may be used once, more than once or not at all.

9.6   A child was noted at preschool to not talk as much as his peers and often mispronounced words and struggled to remember the names of things

9.7   A child entering primary school is noted to have trouble grouping items by size, shape and colour. At home she struggles to sort cutlery into spoons, knives and forks

9.8   A child is noted by his parents to have trouble with join-the-dots puzzles, and often struggles to keep colouring within the lines of a drawing

9.9   A child won't play alone and needs a parent to direct play, has trouble finishing simple tasks, asks lots of questions but doesn't seem to follow the answers, and often gets angry with other children who disagree with him

Inheritance of learning disabilities

9.10-9.13

Options

A   Down syndrome
B   Edward syndrome
C   Fragile X syndrome
D   Prader–Willi syndrome
E   William syndrome

For each of the descriptions below, select the SINGLE MOST likely diagnosis from the list above. Each option may be used once, more than once or not at all.

9.10   A dominant X-linked gene with incomplete penetrance
9.11   The most common chromosomal disorder in the UK
9.12   Caused by trisomy with a weak association with maternal age
9.13   Most cases are due to chromosome deletion

Classification of learning disability

9.14-9.17

Options

A   Mild learning disability
B   Moderate learning disability
C   No learning disability
D   Profound learning disability
E   Severe learning disability
F   Suggestive of Down syndrome

For each of the IQ scores below, select the SINGLE MOST appropriate statement from the list above. Each option can be used once, more than once or not at all.

9.14   IQ: 100
9.15   IQ: 38
9.16   IQ: 63
9.17   IQ: 28

Assessing mental capacity

9.18–9.21

Options

A   Act accordingly
B   Court of Protection
C   Discuss best interests
D   IMCA referral

Using the list of options above, complete the flowchart below, to describe the process that must be followed under the Mental Capacity Act 2005, when an adult with learning difficulties is judged not to have capacity.

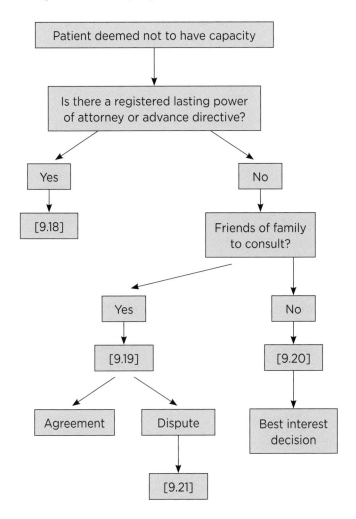

Data interpretation questions

9.22 and 9.23   Fatigue

A 37-year-old woman with Down syndrome is brought to see you by her carer, concerned that she is tired all the time, has no interest in group activities and often complains of joint pain. Examination is unremarkable, although you note that she has put on 1 kg in weight since last being seen. She takes no regular medication apart from the pill for menorrhagia.

You arrange blood tests, which show the following results:

Na$^+$	139 (132–144) mmol/l
K$^+$	5.1 (3.5–5.5) mmol/l
eGFR	84 ml/min
CRP	5 (<6) mg/l
HbA1c	48 mmol/mol
TSH	5.1 (0.4–4.5) mU/l
T$_4$	11 (10–24) pmol/l
Hb	9.9 (11.5–16.5) g/dl
WBC	17.3 (3.8–10.8) × 10^9/l
Platelets	134 (150–400) × 10^9/l
MCV	82 (77–95) fl

Part A

Which is the SINGLE MOST likely diagnosis? Select ONE option from A–E only.

- O   A   Acute lymphoblastic leukaemia
- O   B   Glandular fever
- O   C   Iron-deficient anaemia
- O   D   Subclinical hypothyroidism
- O   E   Type 2 diabetes mellitus

Part B

Which is the SINGLE MOST appropriate management at this stage? Select ONE option from F–J only.

- O   F   Prescribe levothyroxine and repeat blood tests in 3 months
- O   G   Prescribe oral iron and arrange to repeat blood tests in 6 weeks

O   H   Refer urgently to haematology

O   I   Repeat blood tests in 3 months

O   J   Trial of antidepressants

Free-text questions

9.24   Medication doses in attention deficit hyperactivity disorder
One of your patients has severe ADHD. His paediatrician has recommended methylphenidate in a twice-daily dose. Your patient weighs 30 kg. The BNF recommends a maximum daily dose of 2.1 mg/kg daily. The tablets come in strengths of 5 mg, 10 mg and 20 mg. They cannot be broken.

What is the maximum 12-hourly dose of methylphenidate that you could prescribe in tablets? Write the NUMBER OF MILLIGRAMS in FIGURES in the box below.

9.25   Statistics in learning disability
A survey of the IQ of residents in a residential unit for learning disabilities is carried out. The results are shown below.

IQ of residents

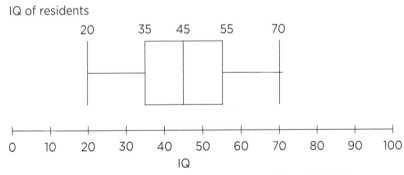

What statistical term is represented by the number 45? Write your answer in words in the box below.

9.1 C: Disability originating during the developmental period characterised by significantly below-average intellectual functioning and adaptive behaviour which is approximately two or more SDs below the mean

There are several different working definitions of learning disability but the key feature is that they arise during the developmental phase. Thus a patient who develops an inability to learn new tasks after a stroke does not have a learning disability. The latest version of the *International Classification of Diseases* (ICD-11) uses the definition above. Classification on the basis of IQ was previously used to describe levels of mental handicap but this is no longer considered useful. The UK Department of Health use the working definition of a significantly reduced ability to understand new or complex information and learn new skills, and a reduced ability to cope independently, which start before adulthood with lasting effects on development.

9.2 A: Of the population 0.5% have an IQ <50

Of the population 2.5% have an IQ <70, whereas 0.5% have an IQ <50. People with an IQ between 50 and 70 do not have an increased risk of psychiatric difficulties, but those with an IQ <35 have higher incidence of abnormal behaviour. At school entry 2.5–3.0% of children have a measured IQ <70, and social factors are as important as biological ones in the aetiology. It should be borne in mind that IQ compares individuals with age-matched peers.

9.3 E: The prevalence of epilepsy in patients with learning disability is 20 times higher than in the general population

All-cause mortality rates in patients with moderate-to-severe learning disabilities are three times higher than the rate in the general population. One in seven adults with learning disabilities rates their health as not good and the risk of carer-reported poor health in children with learning disability is 2.5–4.5 times greater than their peers. Down syndrome is associated with a particularly high risk of leukaemia. Epilepsy is very common in patients with learning disability, and seizures tend to be more resistant to treatment. Overall, cancer rates are lower but around 50% of cancer deaths are due to gastrointestinal cancers, compared with 25% in the general population. Carriage of *Helicobacter pylori* is very common in residential care facilities. Oral health tends to be poor, and is usually worse in patients living in the community.

9.4 C: If she can demonstrate that she has capacity, there is no need to consult her parents before treatment

Under the Mental Capacity Act she is assumed to have capacity regardless of any previous medical history. If she can communicate, understand, retain and balance the information given to her, she has capacity with regard to that decision. If she does not have capacity, her care should be discussed with friends and family. If agreement is not possible a referral to the Court of Protection should be made at that time. If she has no friends or family an IMCA should be consulted.

9.5   A: Involves a preference for consistency and routine

Autism is typified by abnormalities of language and social interaction, which are marked and early. There is a strong preference for routine, and alterations to routines already established will often be met with an abnormal behavioural response, which can include forms of self-injurious behaviour. Children with autism develop unusual preoccupations with objects and this will extend to toys, which will typically be played with in a way that suggests interest in function rather than fantasy. Compulsions are common and there can be poor speech comprehension. There is a lack of normal attachment behaviour, including reciprocal smiling (a 'social smile'), which is often deeply distressing for parents.

Early signs of learning disability

9.6   F: Dyslexia

Dyslexia is characterised by a child who speaks like a younger child (due to delayed language development), has trouble with names (due to central difficulty labelling objects and symbols), struggles with rhymes (due to trouble isolating and breaking words into individual sounds) and struggles with following multistep commands (due to failure to register all of the words).

9.7   D: Dyscalculia

Dyscalculia is characterised by trouble with counting, categorising and sorting. This may manifest as difficulties attaching a number to a group of items, sorting items in logical ways, a poor memory for numbers, eg home phone number, and difficulty sensing passage of time. As children get older difficulties with maths often become more obvious.

9.8   E: Dysgraphia

Dysgraphia causes trouble controlling and using small muscles in the hands. As a result children struggle with fine control, get tired easily, and struggle with tasks that require them to monitor how things look and connect, and find it particularly hard to copy text or drawings. They may be misdiagnosed as ADHD due to an apparent inability to write or draw for any sustained period.

9.9   A: Attention deficit hyperactivity disorder

In preschool children ADHD is characterised by difficulties with focus and planning, difficulty controlling impulses, difficulty regulating emotions and reacting appropriately to others, and the child often needs constant stimulation and movement.

Inheritance of learning disabilities

9.10   C: Fragile X syndrome

This is the second most common heritable cause of mental handicap. It results from a dominant X-linked gene with penetrance of 50% in females. Severity increases down the generations of affected families as the triple repeats expand and, of patients with the full mutation, 80% of males are mentally handicapped, 20% of males are normal and 30% of females are mildly affected.

9.11   A: Down syndrome

Down syndrome has an incidence of 1 in 700 in the UK and 95% are due to trisomy 21, whereas 5% result from mosaicism or translocation. Although being more common in older mothers, there is a risk at all ages and women aged <20 have a 1 in 1600 risk, and most children with Down syndrome are born to younger mothers.

9.12   B: Edward syndrome

Down syndrome is caused in most cases by trisomy 18 and affects 1 in 6000 live births with a male:female ratio of 1:2. There is only a weak association with maternal age and risk of recurrence is low. Of children with the syndrome <10% survive their first year.

9.13   D: Prader–Willi syndrome

Prader–Willi syndrome is characterised by neonatal hypotonia, behavioural disturbance and mild-to-moderate mental handicap. 60% of cases are due to deletion of a portion of the paternal chromosome 15. It affects 1 in 150 00 births.

Classification of learning disability

9.14   C: No learning disability

9.15   B: Moderate learning disability

9.16   A: Mild learning disability

9.17   E: Severe learning disability

The IQ ranges for the determination of the severity of learning disability are: mild 50–69, moderate 35–49, severe 20–34 and profound <20. Lower IQ has an association with lower social class of parents. With increasing severity there are an increasing number of organic causes associated with learning difficulty, the vast majority of which are detectable *in utero* or during the perinatal and postnatal period. The cause (eg Down syndrome) cannot be elucidated by IQ measurement, however.

Assessing mental capacity

9.18–9.21

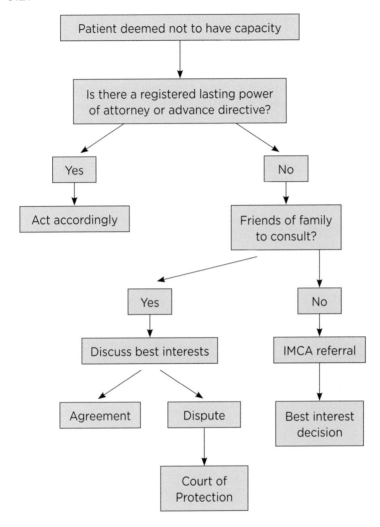

9.18   A: Act accordingly

9.19   C: Discuss best interests

9.20   D: IMCA referral

9.21   B: Court of Protection

The five principles of the Mental Capacity Act are that: capacity is assumed to be present, people should be helped to have capacity, people are entitled to make unwise decisions, decisions for people without capacity should be in their best interests and decisions for people should be as least restrictive as possible. To assess capacity a person must be able to communicate his or her decision, understand information given to him or her, and retain that information and balance it. If the person is deemed not to have capacity, the flowchart should be followed.

9.22 and 9.23   Fatigue

Part A   A: Acute lymphoblastic leukaemia

Part B   H: Refer urgently to haematology

ALL is 10–30 times more common in patients with Down syndrome than the general population, and patients with Down syndrome have a 1:150 chance of developing the condition. The condition may present with symptoms of bone marrow infiltration or bone marrow failure. Bloods tend to show anaemia, low neutrophils, low platelets, raised white cells and circulating blasts in most cases. Hypothyroidism is also more common in patients with Down syndrome, but this patient has a normal T_4. Although this may represent subclinical hypothyroidism, the presence of abnormal red cell indices suggests that this is not the prime diagnosis. Iron-deficient anaemia would usually be associated with a microcytic picture.

9.24   30 mg

The maximum daily dose is 2.1 × 30 kg = 63 mg. This equates to a maximum 12-hourly dose of 31.5 mg. The tablets come as 5, 10 and 20 mg, so the maximum dose that can be prescribed is therefore 1 × 10 mg tablet and 1 × 20 mg tablet every 12 h.

9.25   Median

Boxplots show the maximum (70 in this graph), minimum (20 in this graph), lower quartile (35 in this graph), median and upper quartile (55 in this graph). These are used to display information about the distribution of data within a population.

Chapter 10
Mental health problems

Single best answer questions

10.1 **Postnatal mental health**
One of your patients attempts suicide after suffering an acute postnatal psychotic illness. Which ONE of the following statements is correct with regard to this situation? Select ONE option only.

  ○ A   Education to A level or degree level is protective against severe postnatal depression

  ○ B   Most women suffering severe postnatal depression have a history of mental illness

  ○ C   Severe postnatal depression is more common in women under the age of 25 years

  ○ D   Severe postnatal depression is more common in woman without a current partner

  ○ E   Women suffering severe postnatal depression who attempt suicide tend to choose violent methods, eg hanging or jumping from a bridge

10.2 **Psychosis**
You see a 21-year-old patient who has recently been discharged from a mental health unit after a psychotic incident. His mother thinks that it has been caused by smoking cannabis. Which ONE of the following statements with regard to this association is correct? Select ONE option only.

  ○ A   Cannabis use moderates pre-existing psychotic symptoms

  ○ B   Patients with recent psychosis are twice as likely to have used cannabis as patients without psychosis

  ○ C   Skunk is associated with psychosis, but cannabis is not

  ○ D   There is no evidence of long-term harm from cannabis use

  ○ E   There is unequivocal proof that smoking cannabis causes psychosis

10.3 Schizophrenia
Which ONE of the following statements about the risk factors for schizophrenia is correct? Select ONE option only.

○ A Development of schizophrenia is not associated with physical health

○ B Genetic factors account for 90% of the risk of developing schizophrenia

○ C Patients with premorbid schizoid personality traits are more likely to develop schizophrenia

○ D Studies have failed to show any genetic factors in schizophrenia

○ E There are no known biochemical triggers for the development of schizophrenia

10.4 Physical health in mental illness
Which ONE of the following statements about physical health in mental illness is correct?

○ A Physical health improves during manic periods in patients with bipolar disorder

○ B Physical health is at risk in patients with mental health problems

○ C Physical health is significantly better in obsessive–compulsive disorder (OCD) when compared with the general population

○ D Physical health is unaffected by depression

○ E Physical health is unaffected by schizophrenia

10.5 Delirium
Which ONE of the following statements about delirium is correct?

○ A Delirium is best treated with antipsychotics

○ B Delirium is categorised as an organic disorder

○ C Delirium is typified by auditory hallucinations

○ D Delirium occurs only in elderly people

○ E Delirium occurs only in those with a pre-existing psychiatric diagnosis

10.6 Obsessive–compulsive disorder
Which ONE of the following statements about obsessive–compulsive disorder (OCD) is correct?

○ A OCD involves unpleasant thoughts that the individual does not recognise as being his or her own

○ B OCD is commonly associated with anxiety and depression

○ C OCD is commonly associated with mania

○ D OCD raises the risk of suicide in sufferers

○ E The onset of OCD tends to be earlier in men than in women

10.7 Suicide
Which ONE of the following statements about suicide is correct?

○ A Rates are highest over the Christmas and New Year holiday period

○ B Suicide by dangerous methods is more common in women

○ C Suicide is more common in men

○ D The incidence is 1/100 000 per year

○ E The risk of suicide is reduced in schizophrenia when accompanied by akathisia

10.8 Management of depression
According to the NICE guidance, *Management of depression in primary and secondary care*, which ONE of the following statements is the SINGLE MOST accurate?

○ A 'Doing nothing' is an appropriate course of action in an initial presentation of mild depression

○ B CBT is more effective than antidepressants in the treatment of an initial presentation of a severe depressive episode

○ C SSRIs are the first choice in the management of mild depressive episodes

○ D Tricyclic antidepressants are more effective than SSRIs

○ E Venlafaxine can be introduced in primary care for patients who have failed to respond to other agents

10.9 Treatments for depression

This is a Kaplan–Meier survival plot for the number of patients maintaining remission after a severe depressive episode treated with antidepressants compared with placebo.

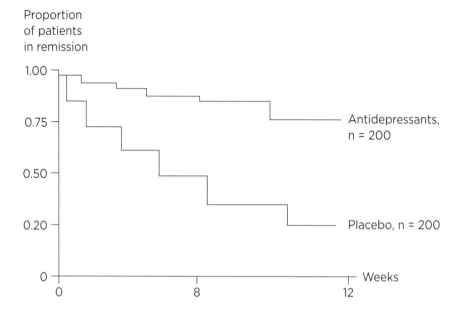

Which ONE of the following best describes the data as they are represented?

○ A   All patients taking antidepressants maintain their initial improvement after 12 weeks of treatment

○ B   Approximately 150 patients taking antidepressants remain in remission at the end of the treatment represented by the graph

○ C   Approximately 75% of patients in the placebo arm remain in remission at the end of the treatment represented by the graph

○ D   Patients taking placebo and patients taking antidepressants show a similar rate of relapse after 12 weeks of treatment

○ E   Placebo and antidepressants are ineffective for maintaining long-term remission

Extended matching questions

Side effects of antidepressants

10.10–10.14

Options

A   Amisulpiride
B   Citalopram
C   Fluoxetine
D   Lamotrigine
E   Mirtazepine
F   St John's wort
G   Tryptophan
H   Venlafaxine

For each of the descriptions of side effects below, select the most likely drug from the list above. Each option can be used once, more than once or not at all.

10.10   Sedation and weight gain are common side effects.
10.11   This antidepressant can cause a rise in anxiety levels during initial titration.
10.12   Blood pressure should be monitored during initiation of this antidepressant.
10.13   Gastrointestinal side effects often occur with this antidepressant.
10.14   Caution should be exercised when choosing an antidepressant in a patient who is self-medicating with this.

Mental Health Act assessment in the community

10.15–10.19

Options

A   1
B   2
C   3
D   4
E   135(2)
F   136
G   A clinical psychologist
H   A community psychiatric nurse
I   A consultant psychiatrist
J   A layperson
K   An approved social worker
L   Section 12

The following algorithm describes the process for detention under the Mental Health Act 1983. Using the list of options above, select the SINGLE MOST appropriate option for each stage in the flow chart. Each option can be used once, more than once or not at all.

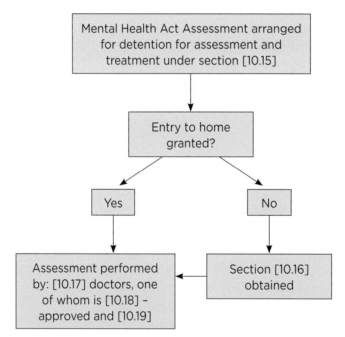

Data interpretation question

10.20-10.22 Eating disorders

You see a 25-year-old women with a long history of anorexia who has avoided medical help for some years. On examination you note the following:

BMI = 16.3 kg/m²

Sitting blood pressure = 94/48 mmHg

Standing blood pressure = 88/46 mmHg

Pulse = 44 beats/min

Haemoglobin = 9.2 g/dl

White cell count = 2.4 × 10⁹/l

Platelets = 131 × 10⁹/l

Sodium = 132 mmol/l

Potassium = 3.1 mmol/l

Glucose = 2.6 mmol/l

Part A

What practice procedure should be carried out at this point in your assessment? Write the answer in words in the box below.

Part B

Which TWO of the following are criteria for same-day medical admission? Select TWO options only.

A   Abnormal liver function tests
B   BMI <15 kg/m²
C   Glucose <3.0 mmol/l
D   Potassium <3.0 mmol/l
E   Pulse <40/min
F   Temperature <36.0°C

Free-text question

10.23 **Postnatal depression**

You see a new mother who has been referred by the health visitors over concerns that she has postnatal depression. After assessing her you agree with her request for antidepressants. She is breastfeeding and keen to continue doing so and has previously had side effects with tricyclic antidepressants, so you decide to use a selective serotonin reuptake inhibitor. Which one of these drugs would be the SINGLE MOST appropriate option in this situation? Write your answer in the box below.

10.1 **E:** **Women suffering severe postnatal depression who attempt suicide tend to choose violent methods, eg hanging or jumping from a bridge**

The Confidential Enquiry into Infant and Maternal Deaths has identified a significant number of deaths due to suicide in women with severe postnatal depression. The demographics of high-risk groups are different from other depressive or psychotic illness, however, and this group are more likely to choose violent suicide methods. They are typically aged >30, have supportive backgrounds, no history of mental illness and often well educated. A high index of suspicion and proactive screening for depression is recommended.

10.2 **B:** **Patients with recent psychosis are twice as likely to have used cannabis as patients without psychosis**

There is clear evidence of a link between cannabis use and psychosis, although it is not clear whether this is causal or represents self-medication of pre-existing low-grade symptoms. A prospective study of cannabis use in Swedish conscripts showed that regular cannabis use before the age of 18 was associated with a sevenfold increase in risk of developing psychosis in the next 15 years. Cannabis use has increased from 10% of people ever having used it in the late 1960s to 50% in the twenty-first century but the incidence of psychosis has not increased this much, suggesting that any influence is likely to be multifactorial. Stronger strains of cannabis such as skunk seem to be more likely to produce mental health problems, but these are seen with all types of cannabis.

10.3 **C:** **Patients with premorbid schizoid personality traits are more likely to develop schizophrenia**

There are numerous associations with the development of schizophrenia. Premorbid schizoid personality traits (fanaticism, hypochondriasis, excessive shyness, eccentricity) and a positive family history are both associated with increased risk of developing schizophrenia, as is drug use (both cannabis and LSD/amphetamines). Twin studies show a 10–15% concordance for dizygotic twins and 30–60% concordance for monozygotic twins. Life events such as bereavement or losing a job, or brain injury (eg after a head injury) can be associated with the onset of schizophrenia.

10.4 **B:** **Physical health is at risk in patients with mental health problems**

Physical health is often a significant concern in mental disorder, eg schizophrenia is associated with a lower life expectancy, and this is unrelated to the effects of antipsychotic medication. This is generally well known, but depression is also associated with significant co-morbidity and health risks, including a greater risk of myocardial infarction (MI). OCD does not protect physical health, but is the only mental disorder that is thought to protect against suicide.

10.5   B: Delirium is categorised as an organic disorder

Delirium is listed under 'Organic mental disorders' in ICD-10. It is also commonly referred to as an 'acute confusional state'. It is a non-specific syndrome characterised by concurrent disturbances of consciousness, perception, cognition, behaviour, emotion and the sleep–wake cycle. Although its frequency rises with age, it is not unique to elderly people. The highest frequency is seen in terminally ill patients (American Psychiatric Association, 1999). Disorientation in time and place is almost universal. Patients have a marked difficulty in sustaining concentration. These two points often make the assessment challenging. It is best treated by the management of the underlying cause, which can be as simple as a urinary tract infection or a recent change in medication. Low-dose antipsychotics and benzodiazepines can be used to treat the disorder symptomatically. Visual hallucinations are typical and the presence of these should always alert one to the possibility of an organic cause.

10.6   E: The onset of OCD tends to be earlier in men than in women

OCD comprises the experience of intrusive obsessional thoughts and the compulsion to do something in response. It is commonly associated with depression (30%), anxiety and depersonalisation. The obsessional thoughts experienced are recognised as being the individual's own, are unpleasant, and at least one must still be resisted in order for the diagnosis to be made. The mean age of onset is 20 years but it often occurs earlier in men, who can experience it in their early teens. The best treatment is through gradual exposure to environmental cues combined with response prevention, although in practice (serotoninergic) antidepressant therapy is also required.

10.7   C: Suicide is more common in men

Suicide has an incidence in the UK of approximately 1/10 000 per year. The risk is raised in all mental disorders with the exception of OCD, and in schizophrenia the risk is higher in those who experience akathisia as a side effect of antipsychotic medication. The rates are highest during the summer and the spring in both hemispheres. It is more common in men, who are also more likely to choose dangerous or violent methods such as shooting. Jumping from structures is more commonly a method used in young than in elderly people. Remember that an individual does not need to have a mental disorder to commit suicide and that sociopolitical solutions are often more important than psychiatric ones.

10.8   A: 'Doing nothing' is an appropriate course of action in an initial presentation of mild depression

'Watchful waiting' is often the most appropriate course of action in such a presentation. The natural history of low mood dictates that over the following 2 weeks it might resolve (in which case the diagnosis of an adjustment disorder might be considered), stay the same or worsen. SSRIs are as effective as tricyclic antidepressants with a more favourable side-effect profile, and should be considered as first-line therapy for moderate and severe episodes treated in primary care. Venlafaxine should be initiated only by specialist mental health medical practitioners, including GPs with a special interest in mental health. For those presenting with severe depression, a combination of cognitive–behavioural therapy (CBT) and an SSRI should be considered as this is considered more cost-effective. There is no evidence to suggest that CBT alone is a superior management strategy.

10.9   B: Approximately 150 patients taking antidepressants remain in remission at the end of the treatment represented by the graph

This graph shows the number of patients maintaining improvement on antidepressants compared with placebo after 12 weeks of initial treatment. It shows that after this 12-week treatment period only 25% maintain their improvement on placebo, whereas approximately 75% (ie 150 patients) of those on antidepressants maintain their treatment response.

Side effects of antidepressants

10.10   E: Mirtazepine

10.11   B: Citalopram

10.12   H: Venlafaxine

10.13   C: Fluoxetine

10.14   F: St John's wort

Mirtazepine's action at the histamine receptor is greater than at the noradrenergic receptor at the starting dose (15 mg). This is outweighed at higher doses so that the initial sedation experienced by most patients generally subsides. This can be usefully taken advantage of in patients with insomnia and a predominantly anxious presentation. Anxiety is a common side effect on starting citalopram, which might require symptomatic treatment, but patients should be advised that this is likely to pass after the first week or two. St John's wort is available over the counter. It is an enzyme inducer and possesses serotoninergic activity, which, when combined with selective serotonin reuptake inhibitors (SSRIs) or other serotoninergic drugs, can give rise to the serotonin syndrome. Fluoxetine frequently causes diarrhoea in the first 2–3 weeks but this usually settles in time.

Mental Health Act assessment in the community

10.15	C:	3
10.16	E:	135(2)
10.17	B:	2
10.18	L:	Section 12
10.19	K:	An approved social worker

The Mental Health Act is currently in the process of being revised to allow indefinite detention for people with personality disorders but for the time being the above rules apply.

10.20–10.22   Eating disorders

Part A   ECG

Patients who are bradycardic, especially where there is low potassium, should have an ECG carried out to measure the Q–T interval. In the long-term management of these patients an annual DXA scan should be carried out alongside regular blood tests.

Part B   D: Potassium <3.0 mmol/l

E: Pulse <40 beats/min

Other criteria for admission include temperature <34.5°C, BMI <12 kg/m^2, weight loss >1 kg/week, BP <80/60 mmHg or with a postural drop ≥20 mmHg, haemoglobin <9.0 g/dl, sodium <130 mmol/l, glucose <2.5 mmol/l or LFTs twice the normal upper limit.

10.23   Sertraline

SSRIs are not licensed for use when lactating but data suggest that sertraline is probably the safest. Fluoxetine has a license for use during pregnancy but excessive sleepiness has been reported in children whose mothers breastfeed while taking this drug. Paroxetine has a discontinuation effect of jitteriness and citalopram has been reported to cause problems with weight gain and sleepiness. Studies of 30 babies have shown no harm from sertraline, although all of these drugs would be used off-licence.

Chapter 11
Alcohol and substance misuse problems

Single best answer questions

11.1   Guidance on safe drinking levels
       Which ONE of the following statements reflects the latest Department
       of Health guidance (2016) on safe consumption of alcohol? Select ONE
       option only.

  O   A   Men and women should both drink no more than 14 units of alcohol a
          week

  O   B   Men should drink no more than 14 units a week, women 7 units a week

  O   C   Men should drink no more than 21 units of alcohol a week, women 14
          units a week

  O   D   Men should drink no more than 28 units of alcohol a week, women 21
          units a week

  O   E   Pregnant women should drink 7 units or less to avoid increased risk to
          the fetus

11.2   **Drug driving and the statutory medical defence**
Which ONE of the following statements is true with regard to drug driving?
Select ONE option only.

○   A   The 'statutory medical defence' can be used in all driving offences where the causative drug has been prescribed

○   B   The 'statutory medical defence' can be used to avoid prosecution when patients are charged with driving under the influence of cannabis, if the patient has been diagnosed with depression

○   C   The 'statutory medical defence' can be used to avoid prosecution when a patient taking opioids on prescription is charged with falling asleep at the wheel

○   D   The 'statutory medical defence' can be used to avoid prosecution when patients have a controlled drug blood level higher than statutory limits

○   E   Where a doctor is aware that a patient is driving while taking prescription opioids, they have a statutory duty to inform the Driver and Vehicle Licensing Authority (DVLA)

11.3   **The healthcare team in the management of drug abuse**
Which ONE of the following members of the healthcare team is responsible for prescribing maintenance methadone for shared care patients? Select ONE option only.

○   A   Community pharmacist

○   B   Community psychiatric nurse

○   C   Consultant psychiatrist

○   D   General practitioner

○   E   Social worker

11.4   **Treatment of drug addiction in pregnancy**
Which ONE of the following statements is true with regard to the management of drug addiction in pregnancy? Select ONE option only.

○   A   Methadone is the substitution treatment of choice in pregnancy

○   B   Neonatal withdrawal syndrome always presents within 24 hours of birth

○   C   Opioid use in pregnancy, whether illicit or prescribed, is associated with an increased risk of fetal abnormalities

○   D   Patients on substitution treatment who become pregnant should have their dose reduced at the earliest opportunity

○   E   Women who have a previous history of intravenous drug abuse should not breastfeed

11.5   Methadone prescribing
Which ONE of the following statements is correct with regard to primary care prescribing of methadone? Select ONE option only.

  ○ A   Instalment prescriptions must be issued daily

  ○ B   Instalment prescriptions should be written on an FP10, annotated to show that they should be dispensed in instalments

  ○ C   Methadone can be prescribed only for supervised daily consumption

  ○ D   Methadone prescriptions can be computer printed

  ○ E   Patients who fail to collect a dose on the specified day should receive two doses the following day to compensate

Multiple best answer questions

11.6 and 11.7   Risks of drug misuse

Which TWO of the following statements is correct with regard to the initial management of intravenous drug abusers? Select TWO options only.

  A   Patients should be offered hepatitis A vaccination

  B   Patients should be offered hepatitis B vaccination

  C   Patients should be offered hepatitis C vaccination

  D   Patients who do not inject drugs do not require HIV testing

  E   Patients who test positive for HIV should be offered BCG vaccination

11.8 and 11.9   Screening for harm caused by alcohol

Which TWO of the following blood results suggest harm from alcohol use? Select TWO options only.

  A   Hyeruricaemia

  B   Hypertriglyceridaemia

  C   Low g-glutamyltransferase (GGT)

  D   Low mean corpuscular volume (MCV)

  E   Raised vitamin B_{12} level

  F   Raised serum sodium

Extended matching questions

Drug treatment of alcohol abuse

11.10–11.13

Options

A   Acamprosate
B   Carbamazepine
C   Chlordiazepoxide
D   Chlorpromazine
E   Disulfiram
F   Haloperidol
G   Phenytoin
H   Thiamine
I   Vitamin B complex
J   Vitamin C
K   Vitamin E

For each of the descriptions below, select the SINGLE most appropriate choice from the list above.

11.10   The first-line choice for acute alcohol withdrawal
11.11   Recommended for acute hallucinations during detoxification
11.12   If large quantities of alcohol are consumed with this drug, cardiac arrhythmias may occur
11.13   Reduces the desire to drink

Management of drug abuse

11.14–11.20

Options

A   Abstinence
B   Detoxification
C   Maintenance
D   Harm prevention
E   Relapse
F   Structured treatment and rehabilitation
G   Vaccinations

The flowchart below describes the processes in managing drug misuse. From the list of options, COMPLETE the flowchart.

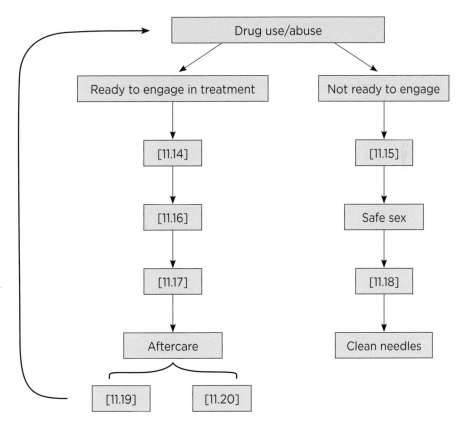

Data interpretation questions

11.21   Calculating alcohol consumption
When assessing alcohol consumption drinks are converted to units.

MATCH each drink to the MOST APPROPRIATE number of units. All four must be correctly matched to score one mark.

A   1 unit
B   1.5 units
C   2 units
D   3 units

Drink	Number of units
Large (175 ml) glass of wine	
One pint of strong lager	
One small sherry	
One Alcopop	

Free-text question

11.22   Heroin overdose
A patient is found collapsed in the car park of your surgery. He has pinpoint pupils and is unresponsive with a respiratory rate of 8 breaths/min. What drug is most appropriate to use in this situation?

Type your answer in the following text box.

11.1 A: **Men and women should both drink no more that 14 units of alcohol a week**

The 2016 guidance from the Department of Health is that men and women should both drink no more than 14 units a week, consumed over 3 days or more, and there should be several alcohol-free days a week. Drinking in pregnancy can lead to fetal harm, and the more alcohol consumed the greater the risk.

11.2 D: **The 'statutory medical defence' can be used to avoid prosecution when patients have a controlled drug blood level higher than statutory limits**

In 2013 an amendment was made to the Road Traffic Act 1988 that made it an offence to drive with specified controlled drugs in the body in excess of a specified limit. It allows for a 'statutory medical defence' where a prescription drug has been prescribed and is used in line with the prescriber's instructions and/or the patient information leaflet which will avoid prosecution if patients test above the statutory limit. Where driving is impaired, eg drowsiness or sleeping at the wheel, the statutory medical defence cannot be used.

11.3 D: **General practitioner**

Patients in shared care schemes are initially managed by a specialist team with specialist drug workers (often community psychiatric nurses or CPNs) working alongside psychiatrists specialising in addiction. Once stabilised, prescribing is taken over by GPs as long as they have received training, and prescriptions are dispensed by community pharmacists.

11.4 A: **Methadone is the substitution treatment of choice in pregnancy**

Drug use in pregnancy is best managed by a specialist multidisciplinary team, aiming to support the mother before, during and after birth. Methadone is the substitution drug of choice, because it has beneficial effects on fetal growth, survival and risk of prematurity. Stable consumption should be the goal, because attempts to reduce the dose may result in harmful illicit opioid use. Close support is needed in the first trimester when morning sickness may result in loss of methadone doses, and in the third trimester when haemodilution may reduce methadone effects. Breastfeeding should be encouraged unless HIV positive, and infants should be monitored for withdrawal symptoms for at least 5 days, because onset is often delayed with methadone use. Although the rate of stillbirths is higher, there is no increase in fetal abnormalities in opioid abusers.

11.5   D: Methadone prescriptions can be computer printed

Instalment prescribing should be done on an FP10 (MDA) form, which may be hand written or computer printed, and should specify the frequency of dispensing, although this does not have to be daily in established stable consumption. Pharmacists may supervise consumption or give supplies for patients to consume at home, but a high index of caution should be maintained to ensure that drugs are not diverted. Failure to pick up a prescription should result in forfeiture of that dose, and several days' failure suggests continuing use of illicit opioids.

11.6 and 11.7   Risks of drug misuse

> **A: Patients should be offered hepatitis A vaccination;**
> **B: Patients should be offered hepatitis B vaccination**

Patients who misuse drugs should be encouraged to be tested for HIV, HBV and HCV, and consideration should be given to testing for STIs including HIV in sex workers or TB if clinically indicated. Patients with HIV should not receive the BCG vaccination. Patients should be encouraged to practise safe sex and to encourage their partners to be tested. Vaccination against hepatitis A, hepatitis B and tetanus are recommended as routine in patients who inject drugs.

11.8 and 11.9   Screening for harm caused by alcohol

> **A: Hyeruricaemia;**
> **B: Hypertriglyceridaemia**

Blood results that suggest heavy alcohol consumption include raised uric acid levels, raised triglycerides, macrocytosis, raised GGT, alanine transaminase (ALT), aspartate transaminase (AST) and raised cholesterol. Vitamin B_{12} and folic acid levels are often low in chronic alcoholism, due to poor diet.

Drug treatment of alcohol abuse

11.10   C: Chlordiazepoxide

This is the drug of choice for acute alcohol withdrawal to prevent delirium tremens due to its long half-life and low risk of diversion to street use. Daily dispensing and family support are advised to ensure compliance, with a reducing dose over 7 days.

11.11   F: Haloperidol

This is the antipsychotic of choice for acute hallucinations not responding to benzodiazepines. It may increase the risk of seizures so patients at increased risk of seizure should be managed in secondary care.

11.12   E: Disulfiram

This blocks alcohol oxidation leading to accumulation of acetaldehyde, which causes abdominal pain, flushing, headache and vomiting. Large quantities of alcohol can cause arrhythmia. The intensity of the reaction is unpredictable.

11.13   A: Acamprosate

This acts on GABA/glutamate pathways to reduce the desire to drink. It does not interact with alcohol and is licensed for prevention of relapse; it should be used together with psychological treatment, and started as soon as possible after withdrawal.

Management of drug abuse

11.14	F:	Structured treatment and rehabilitation
11.15	D:	Harm prevention
11.16	B:	Detoxification
11.17	C:	Maintenance
11.18	G:	Vaccinations
11.19	E:	Relapse
11.20	A:	Abstinence

Patients who are unable to engage in structured treatment should receive treatment aimed at prevention of adverse consequences, such as overdose, blood-borne disease and safe sex. They should be regularly offered the opportunity to engage in treatment programmes.

11.21 Calculating alcohol consumption

Drink	Number of units
Large (175 ml) glass of wine	2 (**C**)
One pint of strong lager	3 (**D**)
One small sherry	1 (**A**)
One Alcopop	1.5 (**B**)

A unit of alcohol is 8 g of alcohol. It can be calculated from the formula below, or an online calculator can be used.

Units = volume of drink (ml) × ABV (%)/1000

Most bottled alcoholic drinks sold in the UK have the number of units printed on the label.

11.22 Naloxone

Naloxone is a specific antidote for opioid poisoning and should be used at a dose of 400 mcg intramuscularly, intravenously or subcutaneously if the patient is unconscious and bradypnoeic. It has a short half-life and repeated doses may be needed.

Chapter 12
Metabolic and endocrine problems

Single best answer questions

12.1   Breast symptoms
        A 52-year-old man complains of pain in the area of his nipples. He is
        otherwise fit and well, and his only medication is ranitidine for dyspepsia.
        Examination reveals tenderness in both breasts and slightly enlarged
        breast tissue. There is no lymphadenopathy. What is the SINGLE MOST
        likely cause of his symptoms? Select ONE option only.

   O   A   Breast cancer

   O   B   Hormonal changes with age

   O   C   Over-the-counter drug use

   O   D   Ranitidine

   O   E   Recreational drug use

12.2   Weight gain
        A 66-year-old woman who is being treated for polymyalgia rheumatica
        complains that she has gained 15 kg weight in the last 6 months. She is
        particularly bothered by weight gain in her face and says that she has
        developed a hump on her back. Her skin is thin and her face flushed. What
        is the SINGLE MOST likely diagnosis? Select ONE option only.

   O   A   Addison's disease

   O   B   Cushing's disease

   O   C   Cushing syndrome

   O   D   Diabetes mellitus

   O   E   Hypothyroidism

12.3 Infertility

A 32-year-old man attends with his partner for fertility advice. She has two children by a previous partner but they would like children of their own. On closer questioning he admits to poor sex drive and difficulty maintaining erections, and that he has always needed to shave less than his peers. He has no previous history of note and takes no regular medications. He is otherwise well. You check his bloods and these show a raised FSH level with a low testosterone and a normal prolactin level. What is the SINGLE MOST likely diagnosis? Select ONE option only.

O   A   Cushing's disease

O   B   Drug use

O   C   Primary hypogonadism

O   D   Prolactinoma

O   E   Secondary hypogonadism

12.4 Insulin

Insulin comes in different forms with different onsets of action. MATCH each insulin brand to the MOST APPROPRIATE DESCRIPTION with regard to speed of onset. All FOUR must be correctly matched to score ONE mark.

A   Actrapid
B   Humalog
C   Lantus
D   NovoMix

Speed of action	Insulin brand
Biphasic	
Long acting	
Short acting	
Very rapidly acting	

12.5   Bone health
You see a 57-year-old postmenopausal woman who has just had a DEXA scan carried out at a local private hospital as part of a well woman check. The results show that she has a T score of –1.8. She has a normal diet, normal BMI, exercises most days and does not smoke. You review her medical records and these show that she has no major previous medical history. Routine blood tests are carried out, which are normal. She would like to be treated. Which ONE of the following is the SINGLE MOST appropriate management?

○   A   Calcium and vitamin D supplements

○   B   No treatment required

○   C   Oral bisphosphonate

○   D   Teriparatide

○   E   Three-monthly intravenous bisphosphonate

12.6   Erectile dysfunction
A 46-year-old man complains of problems with erections. He has been through a divorce after a long and unhappy marriage and has now started a new relationship. His new partner is frustrated by his erectile problems and would like him to try Viagra. His previous medical history is unremarkable, he takes no regular medications and he has no children. He is a new patient so you undertake a physical examination, which is normal. Which ONE of the following would be the SINGLE MOST appropriate next step in his management?

○   A   Check FSH and testosterone levels

○   B   Prescribe sildenafil at 25 mg initially and review in 2 weeks

○   C   Prescribe testosterone supplements

○   D   Refer for psychosexual counselling

○   E   Start treatment with LHRH analogues

12.7   Skin changes
        A 39-year-old woman joins your practice after relocating to the area.
        She comes to see you for a new patient check and to ask about fertility
        treatment. She is nulliparous and has diabetes mellitus, for which she takes
        metformin. You note that she has acne and is obese, and that she has
        hirsutism with dark skin in her axillae. Which ONE of the following is the
        SINGLE MOST likely cause of her symptoms? Select ONE option only.

        O   A   Addison's disease

        O   B   Cushing's disease

        O   C   Cushing syndrome

        O   D   Hypopituitarism

        O   E   Polycystic ovary syndrome

12.8   Leg pain
        A 27-year-old woman of south Asian origin is brought to see you
        complaining of chronic pain in her legs. This seems to have started
        insidiously and there is no history of trauma. She lives according to strict
        cultural rules and wears full Muslim dress. You arrange for an X-ray and
        blood tests. These both show evidence of osteomalacia. What would be
        the SINGLE MOST appropriate next step in her management?

        O   A   Arrange for DEXA scan

        O   B   Investigate for causes of vitamin D deficiency

        O   C   Prescribe bisphosphonates

        O   D   Prescribe calcium and vitamin D supplements

        O   E   Refer to social services

12.9   Breast symptoms
        A 21-year-old woman presents with a non-tender, firm, mobile, 2-cm lump
        in the upper inner quadrant of the right breast. She has been on oral
        contraception for 5 years. Select the SINGLE MOST likely cause of her
        symptoms from the following options.

        O   A   Breast carcinoma

        O   B   Breast cyst

        O   C   Fibroadenoma

        O   D   Galactocele

        O   E   Gynaecomastia

12.10   **Lump in breast**
A 79-year-old woman in a residential home was found by her carers
to have a painless lump in the lower inner quadrant of the left breast.
Clinically, there is a 4-cm lump adherent to the overlying skin, with nipple
retraction on extending the arm. Select the SINGLE MOST likely diagnosis
from the list below.

- O   A   Breast carcinoma
- O   B   Breast cyst
- O   C   Fat necrosis
- O   D   Fibroadenoma
- O   E   Mastitis

12.11   **Neck lump**
A 34-year-old woman who has recently arrived from India attends for a
new patient check. You note an asymmetrical goitre, shown below.

**Which ONE of the following statements with regard to this situation is
correct?**

- O   A   If she is asymptomatic, no treatment or investigation is needed
- O   B   She is probably suffering from endemic goitre and should receive
iodine supplementation
- O   C   She should be referred for surgical assessment
- O   D   She should be started on carbimazole
- O   E   She should have thyroid function tests carried out and if these are
normal she can be reassured

12.12 Neck lumps

Indicate at which one of the options A–E would be the most likely location for a thyroglossal cyst, on the picture below.

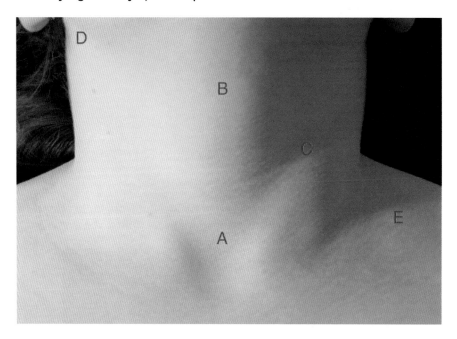

12.13 Stepwise management of type 2 diabetes mellitus

SELECT the rank order of the options (1–4) that best fulfils the requirements given in the question.

The following is a list of treatments used in the management of a patient newly diagnosed with type 2 diabetes mellitus:

1 Exenatide
2 Gliclazide
3 Insulin
4 Metformin

The responses (A–E) rank the treatments in the management of type 2 diabetes mellitus in various orders. Select the response that places the options (1–4) in the order of the **first** treatment to **last**.

Select one rank order only.

○ A: 2, 4, 1, 3

○ B: 4, 2, 1, 3

○ C: 2, 1, 3, 4

○ D: 4, 1, 2, 3

○ E: 1, 4, 2, 3

12.14 Management of diabetes in pregnancy
Which ONE of the following statements is true with regard to recent developments in the management of diabetes in pregnancy? Select ONE option only.

O A Mild gestational diabetes should be monitored initially rather than treated aggressively

O B Pregnancy outcomes are similar in diabetic and non-diabetic women

O C Screening for gestational diabetes based on clinical risk factors is more effective than universal screening

O D The rates of caesarean section in diabetic women are approximately twice the rate in non-diabetic women

O E Two-thirds of pregnant women with diabetes have an HbA1c >7% in the first trimester

Extended matching questions

Breast pain

12.15–12.18

Options

A Benign breast change
B Blunt injury
C Breast abscess
D Breast carcinoma
E Breast engorgement
F Breast hypertrophy
G Gynaecomastia
H Haematoma
I Mondor's disease
J Shingles (herpes zoster)

For each of the scenarios described below, select the SINGLE MOST appropriate diagnosis from the list above. Each option can be used once, more than once or not at all.

12.15 A 19-year-old man complains of a diffuse swelling and discomfort of the right breast over a 9-month period. Clinically and on ultrasound scanning there is no discrete lesion.

12.16 A 22-year-old woman presents in the immediate postpartum period with moderately severe bilateral breast pain and swelling; she is unable to initiate lactation.

12.17 A 53-year-old woman presents with a 4-day history of severe left-sided breast pain and the appearance of a red rash and blisters over the breast.

12.18 A 38-year-old woman who underwent excision of a large fibroadenoma of the left breast 10 days ago complains of pain, swelling and bruising at the operation site.

Blood tests in endocrinology

12.19–12.23

Options

A   Addison's disease
B   Clinical hypothyroidism
C   Cushing's disease
D   Hypercalcaemia
E   Hyperparathyroidism
F   Hyperthyroidism
G   Hypocalcaemia
H   Hypopituitarism
I   Menopause
J   Subclinical hypothyroidism

For each of the blood result profiles below, select the SINGLE MOST likely diagnosis from the list above. Each option may be used once, more than once or not at all.

12.19   Raised TSH, normal T_4.
12.20   Low sodium, raised potassium, raised ACTH with low cortisol.
12.21   Raised follicle-stimulating hormone (FSH), low estrogen.
12.22   Low levels of T_4, T_3, TSH, prolactin, sodium and potassium.
12.23   Low TSH, raised T_4.

Assessing the risk of diabetes

12.24–12.28

Options

A	HbA1c <30 mmol/mol
B	HbA1c <42 mmol/mol
C	HbA1c <48 mmol/mol
D	HbA1c 42–47 mmol/mol
E	HbA1c 48–54 mmol/mol
F	HbA1c > 48 mmol/mol
G	HbA1c > 54 mmol/mol
H	Reassess BMI and HbA1c annually
I	Reassess BMI and HbA1c every 3 years
J	Reassess risk every 3 years
K	Reassess risk every 5 years

The flowchart below is used to classify patients screened for diabetes. From the list of options above, COMPLETE the flowchart.

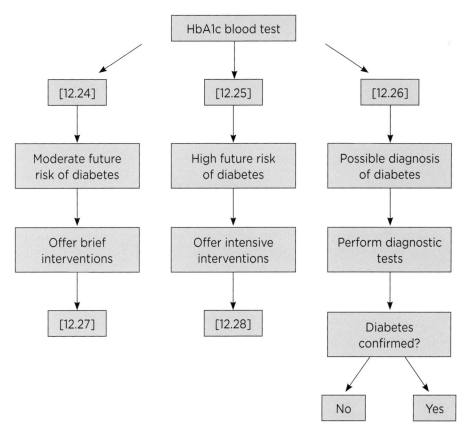

Breast pain

12.29-12.33

Options

A   Combined oral contraceptive
B   Fluoxetine
C   GnRH analogue
D   NSAID
E   Reassure, lifestyle advice and supportive bra
F   Routine referral
G   Urgent referral
H   Vitamin B complex

Complete the algorithm below describing the management of patients presenting with breast pain in primary care, using the list of options above. Each option may be used once, more than once, or not at all.

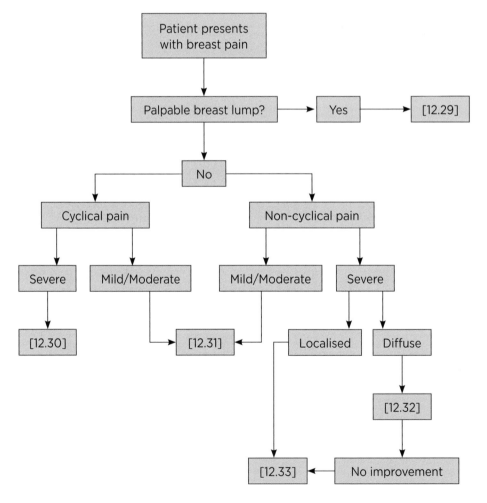

Data interpretation question

12.34   Interpreting blood test results

A 46-year-old woman presents with a 3-month history of weight gain, tiredness and irritability with night sweats. She reports that her periods have been rather irregular for the last 6 months but that she had not had any missed periods. She says that she is not depressed. Blood tests are taken which give the following results:

Haemoglobin	13.2 g/dl
White cell count	$5.2 \times 10^9/l$
Platelet count	$232 \times 10^9/l$
Glucose	4.8 mmol/l
TSH	3.7 mU/l (normal range 0.5–4.5 mU/l)
FT_4	11 pmol/l (normal range 10–24 pmol/l)
FSH	12.8 U/l
bhCG	<1 U/l

FT_4, free thyroxine; FSH, follicle-stimulating hormone; bhCG, β human chorionic gonadotrophin.

Normal range for FSH: follicular phase = 3.5–12.5 U/l; ovulatory phase = 4.7–21.5 U/l; luteal phase = 1.7–7.7 U/l; postmenopausal range = 25.8–134.8 U/l.

What is the SINGLE MOST likely diagnosis? Select ONE option only.

O   A   Clinical hypothyroidism

O   B   Depression

O   C   Hyperthyroidism

O   D   Perimenopause

O   E   Pregnancy

Free-text question

12.35 Insulin dose

You see a patient with type 2 diabetes who has an HbA1c of 93 mmol/mol despite maximum tolerated doses of a biguanide, sulfonylurea and glitazone. You decide to initiate once-daily insulin taken at night, to supplement his oral hypoglycaemics. The patient weighs 100 kg.

Daily insulin requirement = 0.5 U/kg

Basal requirement = 50% of daily insulin requirement

Safe starting dose = 60% of basal requirement

What would be the safe starting basal insulin dose, in units?

Type your answer in the following text box. Use figures NOT words. Percentages and fractions are NOT acceptable.

12.1   D: Ranitidine

Gynaecomastia can be caused by a number of medications, the most common being antacids such as PPIs and H_2-receptor antagonists. Other causes include hormone manipulation for benign and malignant prostatic conditions, recreational drug use such as marijuana or anabolic steroids. Gynaecomastia is common at puberty. Breast cancer tends to cause non-tender enlargement.

12.2   C: Cushing syndrome

This patient has symptoms of Cushing syndrome, which is usually iatrogenic due to long-term steroid use. There is characteristic 'orange on a stick' appearance of central obesity and a buffalo hump with muscle weakness, striae and thinning of skin. Cushing's disease is caused by excessive production of cortisol from the adrenals due in most cases to excessive pituitary ACTH secretion. Addison's disease is due to adrenal insufficiency and cortisol levels are low. Hypothyroidism may cause some of the symptoms of Cushing syndrome but can be differentiated on testing thyroid function, whereas elevated blood glucose in patients on steroids is often secondary to steroid therapy and resolves when doses are reduced.

12.3   C: Primary hypogonadism

This man has symptoms of hypogonadism. In the absence of obvious causes such as mumps orchitis, chemotherapy or other medication, or testicular surgery in his previous medical history, it is likely to be primary rather than secondary. Primary hypogonadism is suggested by raised FSH and LH with low testosterone, whereas secondary hypogonadism would be associated with low FSH/LH with low testosterone. He should have a karyotype to exclude Klinefelter syndrome (prevalence 1:700) and be assessed for osteoporosis. Any signs of pituitary disease should prompt referral for CT scan.

12.4   Insulin

Speed of action	Insulin brand
Biphasic	NovoMix
Long acting	Lantus
Short acting	Actrapid
Very rapidly acting	Humalog

Very rapidly acting insulin has an onset of action within 15 min and lasts 2–5 h. Short-acting insulins start to act within 30–60 min and last 2–6 h. They are often given 20–30 min before a meal. Long-acting insulins such as Lantus (insulin glargine) have prolonged absorption without a peak effect, making them suitable for once-daily dosing. Biphasic insulin combines a long- and a short-acting insulin and can be given twice daily.

12.5   A: Calcium and vitamin D supplements

This patient has osteopenia rather than osteoporosis. Treatment should be aimed at lifestyle measures, calcium supplementation and reassurance. Where there are underlying risk factors such as coeliac disease these should be treated. Bisphosphonates are indicated only in otherwise healthy patients where osteoporosis is confirmed, or for prophylaxis in patients on steroids. Teriparatide is useful only in patients who do not respond to bisphosphonates.

12.6   B: Prescribe sildenafil at 25 mg initially and review in 2 weeks

If there are symptoms or signs of hypogonadism, checking FSH levels will differentiate between primary or secondary causes. A drug history should be taken to exclude reversible causes such as steroids, β-blockers, spironolactone or drugs of abuse such as marijuana. In the absence of contraindications, a trial of sildenafil starting at 25 mg is appropriate.

12.7   E: Polycystic ovary syndrome

This patient has symptoms of PCOS. The diagnosis can be confirmed with blood tests during the first week of her period. PCOS is associated with raised free testosterone, raised LH and normal FSH. Primary Cushing's disease is rare and is caused by pituitary-dependent adrenal hyperplasia. Treatment of Cushing syndrome should be by gradual reduction of steroids and replacement where possible with steroid-sparing agents. Addison's disease is caused by a deficiency of steroids and causes low blood pressure, lassitude and depression.

12.8   B: Investigate for causes of vitamin D deficiency

Osteomalacia is characterised by abnormal mineralisation of bone and is usually caused by vitamin D deficiency in adults. It can be difficult to differentiate from osteopenia and osteoporosis, but there are typically Looser's zones evident on X-ray, and blood tests reveal reduced calcium, phosphate and vitamin D levels with raised alkaline phosphatase. It is often caused by low sunlight or poor diet, but investigation should aim to exclude secondary causes such as coeliac disease or inherited disorders of vitamin D metabolism. Treatment is usually with dietary supplements once other causes have been excluded.

12.9   C: Fibroadenoma

Fibroadenomas are not uncommon in premenopausal women and are usually transient. They are small mobile lumps with a smooth surface. However, once they exceed 3 cm in size they seldom regress; rarely, they may grow into a giant fibroadenoma or a phyllodes tumour.

12.10   A: Breast carcinoma

A solid lump with overlying skin tethering or nipple retraction is clinically diagnostic of an infiltrating ductal carcinoma. In elderly people these tumours are usually slow growing and slow to metastasise. They are usually hormone receptor positive and respond well to tamoxifen, letrozole or anastrozole therapy.

12.11   C: She should be referred for surgical assessment

All patients with goitre should have their thyroid function tested. Where there is asymmetry, referral is indicated to exclude cancer. Hyperthyroidism is treated with carbimazole initially, although levothyroxine supplementation is often required later under a 'block-and-replace' regimen. Diffuse enlargement with normal thyroid function is usually due to endemic goitre.

12.12   B

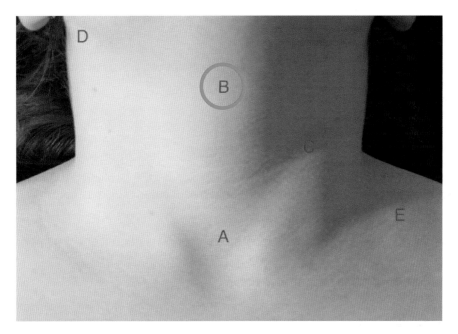

Thyroglossal cysts are usually found along the tract of the thyroglossal duct, from the thyroid to the tongue base. A lump at A is likely to be thyroid, whereas at C it is likely to be a branchial cyst or lymph node. Lumps at D are likely to be either lymph nodes or enlarged parotid gland.

12.13   B: 4, 2, 1, 3

Rank ordering: 4 Metformin; 2 Gliclazide; 1 Exenatide; 3 Insulin

All patients with type 2 diabetes should receive lifestyle advice with regard to exercise, diet and weight loss. Metformin should be used if diet fails to control sugar levels, unless contraindicated. Second-line oral treatment is usually a sulphonylurea. Failure to respond to this should prompt an additional oral treatment such as a glitazone or gliptin. If these are ineffective, injectable treatment with exenatide may be used as an alternative to insulin.

12.14   E: Two-thirds of pregnant women with diabetes have an HbA1c >7% in the first trimester

Pregnancy care for diabetic women should start before conception, with joined-up care involving primary care, obstetricians and endocrinologists. Close control of diabetes is associated with lowered perinatal mortality and lowered risk of congenital malformation. The ACHOIS trial (the Australian Carbohydrate Intolerance Study) demonstrated the benefits of treating mild gestational diabetes, and therefore supports the argument for universal screening, particularly because relying on clinical risk factors alone has been shown to miss up to 50% of cases of gestational diabetes in some groups. The caesarean section rate is 60–70% in diabetic women and current NICE guidelines suggest that women should be offered delivery at 38 weeks to reduce the risk of shoulder dystocia and subsequent emergency section.

Breast pain

12.15   G: Gynaecomastia

Gynaecomastia in adolescence is due to unopposed estrogenic activity; it is usually self-limiting and resolves after puberty. Occasionally the swelling persists and when it is cosmetically unacceptable it is treated by subcutaneous mastectomy.

12.16   E: Breast engorgement

Breast engorgement in the early postpartum period is not uncommon in primips; it is also associated with a poor suckling reflex or inverted nipples.

12.17   J: Shingles (herpes zoster)

Herpes zoster infection presents as a linear subcutaneous rash with overlying blisters along intercostal dermatomes; the breast is not affected. However, the diagnosis can be difficult before the rash appears, as pain may precede the development of vesicles by 24–48 hours.

12.18   H: Haematoma

Postoperative haematoma or a seroma after surgery on the breast usually resolves, provided that the collection is small and uninfected; large collections can require repeated aspiration.

Blood tests in endocrinology

12.19   J: Subclinical hypothyroidism

Subclinical hypothyroidism is associated with raised TSH with normal T_4 and T_3 levels. These patients should be monitored over time because a significant number will become overtly hypothyroid in time.

12.20   A: Addison's disease

Addison's disease is due to adrenal failure, so ACTH is elevated with a normal or low serum cortisol. A short Synacthen test will often confirm hypoadrenalism.

12.21   I: Menopause

Luteinising hormone (LH) and follicle-stimulating hormone (FSH) levels are raised in testicular and ovarian failure, in association with low levels of estrogen or testosterone.

12.22   H: Hypopituitarism

Hypopituitarism should be suspected in patients with signs of hypothyroidism, hypogonadism or growth hormone deficiency; these patients often also have diabetes insipidus. The diagnosis can be confirmed by a combined pituitary test.

12.23   F: Hyperthyroidism

Raised T_4 with suppressed TSH is diagnostic of primary hyperthyroidism. Low TSH with normal T_4 and T_3 is usually caused by excess thyroxine replacement or high-dose steroids.

Assessing risk of diabetes

12.24	B:	HbA1c <42 mmol/mol
12.25	D:	HbA1c 42–47 mmol/mol
12.26	F:	HbA1c > 48 mmol/mol
12.27	J:	Reassess risk every 3 years
12.28	H:	Reassess BMI and HbA1c annually

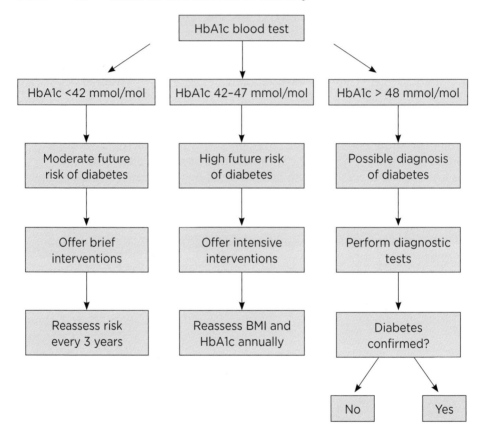

NICE recommend using a diabetes risk assessment tool to stratify risk of diabetes, and the results are then used to screen using HbA1c results. The risk assessment scores are based on age, sex, ethnicity, family history, BMI, waist circumference and history of hypertension. Patients with a low–moderate score should receive brief lifestyle interventions. Those with a high-risk score should be tested for HbA1c.

Breast pain

12.29	G:	Urgent referral
12.30	F:	Routine referral
12.31	E:	Reassure, lifestyle advice and supportive bra
12.32	D:	NSAID
12.33	F:	Routine referral

Breast pain alone is seldom a symptom of breast cancer; however, persistent pain not responding to NSAIDs is an indication for routine referral. Lifestyle changes such as a low-fat diet, evening primrose oil and phytoestrogens may help. Where pain is severe and underlying pathology has been excluded, danazol or tamoxifen may help. Some women also find antidepressants helpful.

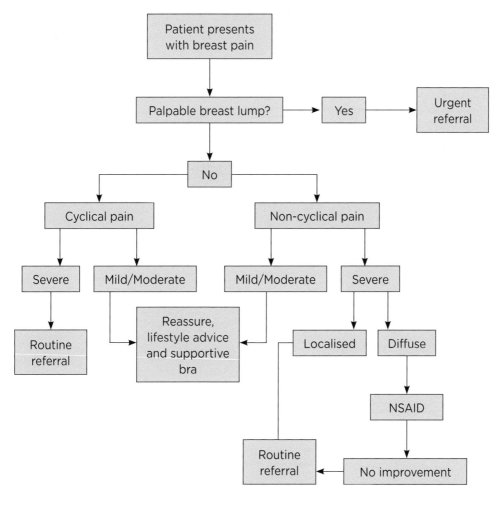

12.34   D: Perimenopause

Blood tests are unreliable in diagnosing the perimenopause and clinicians should rely on a menstrual history and exclusion of other possible causes. Overt hypothyroidism is unlikely with a T_4 in the normal range. Hyperthyroidism would generally cause a raised T_4 and suppressed TSH, whereas pregnancy would cause a raised bhCG. Estradiol levels are unhelpful for diagnosing and monitoring the menopause.

12.35   15 units

Daily insulin requirement = 0.5 × 100 units = 50 units (U)

Basal requirement = 50% of daily insulin requirement = 25 U

Safe starting dose = 60% of basal requirement = 15 U

Chapter 13
Musculoskeletal problems, including trauma

Single best answer questions

13.1 Rheumatoid arthritis

A 67-year-old woman with long-standing rheumatoid arthritis has recently started taking etanercept. She feels that this is working very well but has developed an acutely swollen, red knee. She comes to see you and asks if she can have this aspirated and steroid injected, which has always worked well in the past for exacerbations of her arthritis. Which ONE of the following would be an appropriate action in this situation? Select ONE option only.

O A Aspirate the joint and inject with steroid

O B Increase the dose of etanercept

O C Prescribe oral non-steroidal anti-inflammatories

O D Prescribe oral steroids

O E Stop the etanercept, check blood for inflammatory markers and send aspirate for microscopy

13.2 Back pain

A 34-year-old IT worker comes to you with a 6-month history of back pain, with no recent history of trauma and no red flag symptoms. He has presented in the past with intermittent episodes of back stiffness and occasional neck ache and was treated for plantar fasciitis last year. On examination he has no neurological signs but does have reduced range of movement in his cervical spine, particularly for extension. Which one of the following options is the SINGLE MOST likely diagnosis?

O A Ankylosing spondylitis

O B Mechanical back pain

O C Osteoarthritis

O D Rheumatoid arthritis

O E Wedge fracture

13.3   Hip pain
A 72-year-old man presents with a 1-week history of a pain around his hip, which he tells you he feels most prominently in his right buttock, especially when he is gardening and when he turns on that side in bed. He is normally well and rarely comes to the surgery. He denies trauma, although he has spent the past few weeks digging his new allotment. On examination, leg lengths are equal and straight-leg raising is normal. He is markedly tender over the right hip but he has a normal range of movement in the hip. There is no rash. What is the SINGLE MOST likely diagnosis?

○   A   Myeloma

○   B   Osteoarthritis of hip

○   C   Osteoarthritis of lumbar spine

○   D   Sciatica

○   E   Trochanteric bursitis

13.4   Painful hands
A 53-year-old schoolteacher presents with a history of gradually increasing deformity of the small joints of both her hands, associated with stiffness and swelling. She has found it increasingly difficult to carry textbooks and is often clumsy with coffee cups and pens. She also tells you that she feels tired all the time. There is no relevant medical history and no family history of note. Her metacarpophalangeal joints are red and swollen. What is the SINGLE MOST likely diagnosis?

○   A   Gout

○   B   Osteoarthritis

○   C   Pseudogout

○   D   Rheumatoid arthritis

○   E   Systemic lupus erythematosus

13.5   Ankle injury
Using the Ottawa rules in a patient with ankle pain after an injury, what findings would indicate the need for an X-ray? Select ONE option only.

○   A   Bone tenderness 4 cm above the lateral malleolus

○   B   Bone tenderness at the head of the fifth metatarsal

○   C   Bone tenderness over the cuboid bone

○   D   Patient unable to weight bear at the time of injury but now managing despite some pain

○   E   Tenderness and swelling inferior to the lateral malleolus

13.6   Management of shoulder pain
Which of the following statements about new developments in the
management of shoulder pain is true? Select ONE option only.

○   A   Adhesive capsulitis usually settles after 6 months

○   B   All patients with shoulder pain seen in primary care should have an
X-ray performed

○   C   In the management of rotator cuff disorders, short-term outcomes are
superior for physiotherapy compared with steroid injection

○   D   Red flag symptoms include unexplained wasting and sensory loss

○   E   Steroid injections should not be repeated due to the risk of cartilage
damage

13.7   Hip pain
A 67-year-old man with a history of prostate cancer treated with Zoladex
complains of persistent pain in his right hip for the last few weeks, but
cannot recall any significant injury. On examination, he has a reduced
range of movement in his hip and you arrange an X-ray at the local cottage
hospital. The X-ray is shown below.

Which ONE of the following is the SINGLE MOST likely diagnosis?

○   A   Constipation

○   B   Fractured neck of femur

○   C   Fractured pubic ramus

○   D   Osteoarthritis of the hip

○   E   Perthes' disease

13.8   Hand injuries
        At which site would tenderness be felt in a scaphoid fracture? Select ONE
        option from A to E shown on the image below.

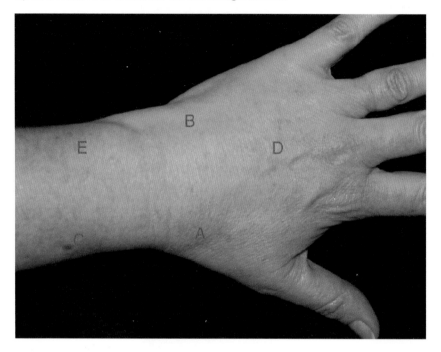

Extended matching questions

Soft-tissue rheumatism

13.9–13.11

Options

A   De Quervain's tenosynovitis
B   Dorsal tenosynovitis
C   Fibromyalgia
D   Flexor tenosynovitis
E   Golfer's elbow
F   Osgood–Schlätter disease
G   Polymyalgia rheumatica
H   Tennis elbow
I   Trigger finger
J   Trochanteric bursitis

For each of the scenarios below, select the most appropriate diagnosis from the list above. Each option may be used once, more than once or not at all.

13.9   A 53-year-old woman complains of pain in her back, neck and abdomen over a period of several months. This seems to be worse in cold weather and she reports being very tender, particularly over her bony prominences. She gets headaches and sleeps badly. Examination is unremarkable apart from generalised tenderness. Blood tests are normal.

13.10   A 34-year-old baker complains of pain in the medial part of his elbow. On examination he is tender over the medial epicondyle, with pain on resisted pronation.

13.11   A 45-year-old housewife complains of pain and reduced movement of her thumb after spending the afternoon pruning roses. On examination there is pain on resisted abduction of the thumb and pain and tenderness on the radial side of the thumb proximal to the thumb base.

Rheumatological problems

13.12-13.15

Options

A Gout
B Polymyalgia rheumatica
C Primary nodal osteoarthritis
D Pseudogout
E Systemic lupus erythematosus
F Rheumatoid arthritis
G None of the above

For each of the signs shown below select the SINGLE condition from the list above most often associated with this sign. Each option may be used once, more than once, or not at all.

[13.12]   [13.13]

[13.14]   [13.15]

Management of osteoarthritis of the knee

13.16–13.21

Options

A   Chondroitin
B   Exercise
C   Glucosamine
D   Intra-articular hyaluronic acid injections
E   NSAID
F   Opioids
G   Paracetamol
H   Refer for surgery
I   Weight loss

In conjunction with the local physiotherapy service, your practice has developed a flow chart to standardise the management of osteoarthritis of the knee. Complete the following flow chart with the SINGLE MOST appropriate item from the list of options given above. Each option can be used once, more than once or not at all.

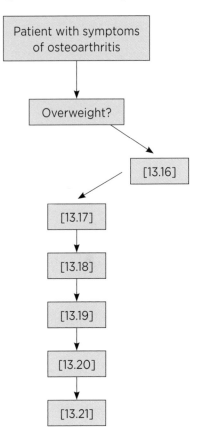

Data interpretation question

13.22 Interpretation of blood results

What is the SINGLE MOST likely metabolic bone disease in a patient with the following results?

Calcium (corrected)	2.34 (2.10–2.55) mmol/l
Phosphate	1.23 (0.8–1.45) mmol/l
Vitamin D	63 (50–140) nmol/l
Parathyroid hormone	34 (10–72) ng/l
Alkaline phosphatase	221 (30–126) U/l

○ A   Osteomalacia

○ B   Osteoporosis

○ C   Paget's disease

○ D   Primary hyperparathyroidism

○ E   Renal disease

Free-text question

13.23 Shoulder pain

A 32-year-old man attends the local minor injury unit complaining of pain in his right shoulder after falling off his mountain bike. On examination he has pain and swelling over the upper outer part of his back and, although he can move his shoulder, it is painful. You arrange an X-ray, which is shown below:

What is the diagnosis? Write the answer in words in the box below.

13.1   E: Stop the etanercept, check blood for inflammatory markers and send aspirate for microscopy

Anti-tumour necrosis factor (anti-TNF) treatments are associated with septic arthritis and can mask the severity of this complication. In any patient on anti-TNF treatment where infection is suspected, the treatment should be stopped and the infection investigated and treated. Before starting treatment with an anti-TNF you should ensure that vaccinations are up to date and patients should be warned of the possibility of infection and advised what to do if they develop symptoms and/or signs of infection. There should be a low threshold for admission in these patients.

13.2   A: Ankylosing spondylitis

Ankylosing spondylitis has a prevalence of approximately 1 in 2200 and affects men twice as frequently as women. It tends to present in young men with morning back pain and stiffness. As progressive spinal fusion occurs there can be reduced spinal movement, with kyphosis and sacroiliac joint pain. It is associated with plantar fasciitis, lung fibrosis, inflammatory bowel disease and amyloidosis. X-ray of the spine might show a 'bamboo spine', with vertebral fusion. The disease is associated with HLA-B27 positivity.

13.3   E: Trochanteric bursitis

Trochanteric bursitis is the most likely diagnosis, given the information provided in the history. One would expect to find tenderness on palpation of the affected side but a full range of movement. The pain is often felt deep in the buttock. Repeated trauma can result in inflammation of the bursa. Treatment options include NSAIDs and physiotherapy; corticosteroid injections can be useful for chronic episodes.

13.4   D: Rheumatoid arthritis

This is a classic presentation of rheumatoid arthritis in a middle-aged woman – symptoms affecting the small joints of her hands symmetrically, with pain, stiffness, swelling and loss of function. This can be associated with tiredness, malaise and other non-articular features, such as fever, weight loss, pleural effusion, mouth ulcers and dry eyes. Gout usually affects only one joint and pseudogout more typically affects the knee. This woman needs to be referred to a rheumatologist because early treatment with disease-modifying drugs can alter the progression of the disease and help to minimise the progression to involvement of larger joints.

13.5   A: Bone tenderness 4 cm above the lateral malleolus

X-ray if there is pain in the malleolar area or midfoot and bone tenderness in one or more of the following:

- Lower 6 cm of the distal fibula above the lateral malleolus

- Distal tibia above the medial malleolus

- The navicular bone

- The fifth metatarsal base.

Also X-ray if the patient is unable to weight bear at the time of the injury and subsequently.

13.6   D: Red flag symptoms include unexplained wasting and sensory loss

Adhesive capsulitis usually resolves after 18–24 months. Red flag symptoms include systemic signs of infection, bony abnormality (eg undisplaced fracture), history of cancer and neurological signs. Systematic reviews suggest equivalent short-term benefit for steroids and physiotherapy. Steroid injections can be repeated up to three times, but should not be used in the presence of a large tear.

13.7   B: Fractured neck of femur

This X-ray shows a right-sided fractured neck of femur. In the context of minor trauma there should be a high degree of suspicion that this is a pathological fracture. In this case it was due to bony metastases and he received radiotherapy to the hip after a surgical repair of the fracture.

13.8   A

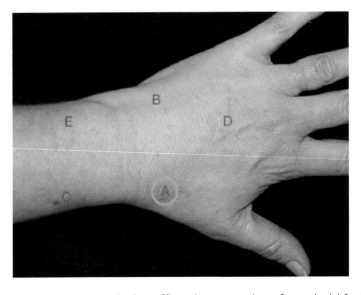

Tenderness in the anatomical snuffbox is suggestive of scaphoid fracture. Tenderness at D would suggest a metacarpal injury whereas tenderness at C or E would suggest the possibility of a radial or ulnar injury.

Soft-tissue rheumatism

13.9   C: Fibromyalgia

Fibromyalgia is usually diagnosed on the basis of the history and lack of any evidence of other causes of symptoms. The American College of Rheumatology diagnostic criteria state that pain should be present in all 4 quarters of the body and should be present in at least 11 of 18 trigger points. Graded exercise and low-dose amitriptyline are helpful.

13.10   E: Golfer's elbow

Golfer's elbow is caused by inflammation over the flexor origin at the medial epicondyle. Treatment involves rest and support. If this doesn't help (together with the avoidance of exacerbating factors), steroid injections might help.

13.11   A: De Quervain's tenosynovitis

De Quervain's tenosynovitis is caused by inflammation of the extensor pollicis brevis and abductor pollicis longus tendons resulting from repetitive activity. It usually settles with rest and sometimes steroid injection, but surgery might be needed if it becomes chronic.

Rheumatological problems

13.12   C: Primary nodal osteoarthritis

Primary nodal osteoarthritis affects the distal interphalangeal joint, causing Heberden's nodes to form. It affects women (10:1) predominantly and there is usually a positive family history.

13.13   F: Rheumatoid arthritis

Rheumatoid arthritis causes swan neck deformity, hyperextension of the PIP joint with flexion of the DIP joint.

13.14   A: Gout

Untreated hyperuricaemia will in time cause gouty tophi to develop.

13.15   E: Systemic lupus erythematosus

SLE is often associated with a vasculitic rash.

Management of osteoarthritis of the knee

13.16   I: Weight loss

13.17   G: Paracetamol

13.18   B: Exercise

13.19   E: NSAID

13.20   F: Opioids

13.21   H: Refer for surgery

13.22   C: Paget's disease

Paget's disease is characterised by excessive and disorganised resorption and formation of bone. This is reflected by high levels of alkaline phosphatase. Osteomalacia often shows low calcium, phosphate and vitamin D levels. Alkaline phosphatase and PTH levels can be raised in osteomalacia but the best marker of disease is the serum vitamin D level. In osteoporosis there are usually normal levels of all these minerals and hormones.

13.23   Fracture of the scapula

Fracture of the scapula is usually due to a high-velocity impact, such as a direct blow or falling backwards on to the shoulder. There may be a typical triangular bruise over the scapula. It is often associated with fractured ribs and dislocation of the sternoclavicular joint. Reduction is not usually necessary and most patients can be managed with a sling and physiotherapy. Where there is an associated glenoid fracture, reduction and fixation may be needed.

Chapter 14
Neurological problems

Single best answer questions

14.1 Swallowing problems
A 57-year-old woman complains that for the last few months she has been getting increasingly frequent attacks of choking when eating and drinking. Her family have also commented that she is losing weight and her voice sounds more nasal than usual. She is otherwise fit and well and takes no regular medications. On examination her tongue looks thin and fasciculates, and she is unable to poke her tongue out for you to examine her throat. Her speech sounds slurred and you notice twitching in her eyelids. Which ONE of the following is the SINGLE MOST likely diagnosis?

- O A Brain tumour
- O B Guillain–Barré syndrome
- O C Motor neurone disease
- O D Multiple sclerosis
- O E Myasthenia gravis

14.2 Headache
A 35-year-old man complains of 2 weeks of daily headaches, starting around the same time of day. The pain starts around his right orbit and rapidly escalates, becoming unbearable, and lasts 45–60 minutes. Which ONE of the following is the MOST APPROPRIATE acute treatment for this patient? Select ONE option only.

- O A Indometacin
- O B Morphine
- O C Oxygen
- O D Paracetamol
- O E Tramadol

14.3   Epilepsy
You are asked to do a tutorial for your final year medical student on the impact on patients and their families of a diagnosis of epilepsy. Which ONE of the following statements is correct with regard to epilepsy? Select ONE option only.

O   A   Epilepsy is a rare condition in the UK

O   B   Epilepsy is usually an isolated diagnosis

O   C   Most cases of epilepsy are inherited as autosomal recessive traits

O   D   Up to 75% of patients become seizure free on treatment

O   E   With good treatment compliance patients with epilepsy have normal morbidity and mortality when compared with patients without epilepsy

14.4   Blurred vision
A 35-year-old woman complains that for the last few weeks she has been aware of blurred vision and slurred speech when she is tired, and has noticed that her eyelids seem to be droopy. She is easily fatigued, but reports that she feels well when she wakes in the morning. She has no history of recent travel and no previous medical history of note. Examination shows normal reflexes and tone, and normal sensation, but bilateral ptosis and no cranial nerve signs. What is the SINGLE MOST likely diagnosis? Select ONE option only.

O   A   Depression

O   B   Lyme disease

O   C   Motor neurone disease

O   D   Multiple sclerosis

O   E   Myasthenia gravis

14.5   Pins and needles
A 34-year-old man complains of 6 months of gradual onset of burning pain in both feet with numbness on both sides. He takes no regular medicine although he has been treated in the past for intravenous drug abuse. Examination shows reduced sensation on both feet but normal reflexes power and tone. Which ONE of the following statements with regard to his management is correct?

O   A   He should be admitted as an emergency

O   B   He should be reassured that his symptoms will settle in time

O   C   He should be referred for an outpatient MRI

O   D   He should be referred initially for nerve conduction studies

O   E   He should be tested for HIV infection

14.6   Gilles de la Tourette syndrome
       Which of the following statements is correct with regard to the
       management of patients with Gilles de la Tourette syndrome? Select ONE
       option only.

   O   A   Aripiprazole is the drug of choice in children

   O   B   Cognitive-behavioural therapy is the only treatment modality proven
           to be effective

   O   C   Eye movement desensitisation and reprocessing are effective in
           patients with tics

   O   D   Haloperidol is effective but may cause unacceptable side effects

   O   E   There is no place for pharmacological therapy in management

14.7   Twitching
       A 23-year-old girl presents with recurrent twitching of her face and
       abdomen, which started after one of her friends gave her a pill for travel
       sickness. On examination, she has repetitive twitching movements of her
       face and both arms and abdomen, every 20–30 seconds. Examination
       is otherwise normal. Which of the following is the SINGLE MOST likely
       diagnosis? Select ONE option only.

   O   A   Jacksonian epilepsy

   O   B   Multiple sclerosis

   O   C   Non-organic symptoms

   O   D   Tardive dyskinesia

   O   E   Temporal lobe epilepsy

14.8   Dementia
       According to NICE guidance, which ONE of the following would be
       appropriate treatment for a patient with uncomplicated moderate
       Alzheimer's disease who is intolerant of acetylcholinesterase inhibitors?
       Select ONE option only.

   O   A   Citalopram

   O   B   Clopixol

   O   C   Memantine

   O   D   Olanzapine

   O   E   Risperidone

14.9 Pins and needles

A 40-year-old man complains of numbness and paraesthesia of the left thumb, index and middle fingers, and half of the ring finger over a period of several weeks. Initially the symptoms were present only at night, but now he is starting to get symptoms in the daytime and is getting pain in his shoulder. On examination he has wasting and weakened abduction of the thumb, but no fasciculation. He has diet-controlled diabetes but no other history of note. What is the SINGLE MOST likely diagnosis?

- A   Carpal tunnel syndrome
- B   Cervical radiculopathy
- C   Diabetic neuropathy
- D   Motor neurone disease
- E   Multiple sclerosis

14.10 Motor neurone disease

One of your patients has just been diagnosed with motor neurone disease and comes to see you to discuss the diagnosis. Which ONE of the following statements about the management of this condition is true? Select ONE option only.

- A   All patients should have a tracheostomy performed to prevent aspiration
- B   Baclofen does not help in the treatment of spasticity
- C   NICE guidance does not support the use of riluzole in motor neurone disease
- D   Riluzole has been shown to bring about remission in 25% of patients
- E   Riluzole increases the period of time to need for ventilation but does not improve prognosis

14.11 Suspected meningitis

Which of the following statements about the initial management of suspected meningitis is correct? Select ONE option only.

- A   A stat dose of ciprofloxacin is effective prophylaxis in close contacts
- B   Cefotaxime can be used safely in patients known to have anaphylaxis with penicillin
- C   Dexamethasone should be given with the first dose of antibiotics
- D   Intravenous amoxicillin is the first-line empirical treatment for suspected meningitis
- E   Treatment should be guided by the results of blood culture

14.12   Trigeminal neuralgia
Which of the following statements about trigeminal neuralgia is true?
Select ONE option only.

O   A   Amitriptyline is the most effective treatment

O   B   It always affects the mandibular branch of the trigeminal nerve

O   C   It can be associated with a facial nerve palsy

O   D   It is typically relapsing and remitting

O   E   Paroxysms of pain usually last at least 30 minutes

14.13   Headache prophylaxis
According to current NICE guidance, the following are recommended prophylactic treatments for headache.

MATCH each prophylactic treatment to the MOST APPROPRIATE column with regard to the headache type. All four must be correctly matched to score ONE mark.

A   Botulinum toxin
B   Drug withdrawal
C   Verapamil
D   Zolmitriptan

Headache type	Prophylactic treatment
Chronic migraine	
Menstrual migraine	
Cluster headache	
Medication-overuse headache	

14.14 Epilepsy
Consider the graph shown below, which illustrates the epidemiology of epilepsy.

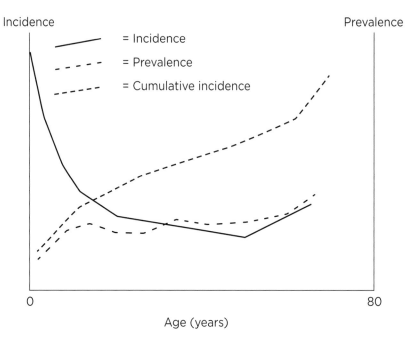

Which ONE of the following statements about these data is true?

O   A   The fact that the cumulative incidence is higher than the prevalence in middle to older age suggests that most people enter remission at some stage

O   B   The fall in incidence in early to middle age is due to the high mortality of childhood epilepsy

O   C   The graph shows that most patients with epilepsy have the condition all their lives

O   D   The increase in incidence in old age is due to an increase in idiopathic epilepsy

O   E   The increase in prevalence in old age is due to physiological changes affecting seizure threshold

Extended matching questions

Headache

14.15–14.18

Options

A   Analgesic overuse headache
B   Brain tumour
C   Chronic paroxysmal hemicrania
D   Chronic sinusitis
E   Cluster headache
F   Giant-cell arteritis
G   Migraine
H   Postcoital cephalgia
I   Subarachnoid haemorrhage
J   Temporal lobe epilepsy
K   Tension-type headache
L   Transient global amnesia
M   Transient ischaemic attack

For each of the descriptions below, select the SINGLE MOST appropriate diagnosis from the list above. Each option can be used once, more than once or not at all.

14.15   A 67-year-old man with a history of several weeks of malaise, now complains of headache and scalp tenderness on the sides of his head, together with pain in his scalp on eating.

14.16   A 44-year-old man complains of daily headaches that are centred around his right eye over the past 2 months. These are severe and are not improving despite taking paracetamol and ibuprofen every day. They are associated with nasal congestion and epiphora.

14.17   A 73-year-old woman presents with 2 months of headaches, worse in the morning, but usually improve by mid-afternoon. They are getting gradually worse, and seem particularly bad when she bends over. She feels nauseous with them and experiences visual disturbances at times.

14.18   A 23-year-old woman who takes the combined oral contraceptive pill complains of severe headache with flashing lights and loss of vision in one eye. She reports that she felt 'out of sorts' immediately before with hypersensitivity to lights and sound started.

New-onset seizure

14.19–14.23

Options

A   Epilepsy likely
B   Epilepsy unlikely
C   Incontinence
D   No
E   Petit mal
F   Syncope likely
G   Syncope unlikely
H   Tongue biting
I   Yes

The differentiation of epilepsy from syncope can be difficult. The following flowchart has been developed to simplify the diagnosis. From the list of options above, select the SINGLE MOST appropriate choice for each question in the flowchart.

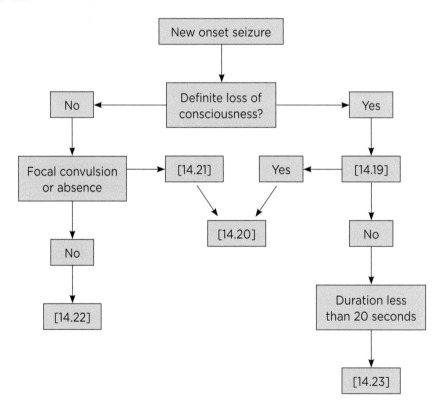

Free-text question

14.24   Tardive dyskinesia
A 24-year-old woman develops symptoms of tardive dyskinesia after taking metoclopramide. What drug would be most appropriate to treat this symptom? Write your answer in the box below, in words.

14.1   C: Motor neurone disease

This patient has symptoms of a bulbar palsy. The progressive nature suggests that this is most likely to be due to motor neurone disease. Guillain–Barré usually causes an ascending paralysis rather than starting with bulbar symptoms. Unlike multiple sclerosis there is no sensory or cognitive loss and the sphincters and ocular muscles are unaffected, distinguishing the condition from myasthenia gravis. A brain tumour would normally cause symptoms of raised intracranial pressure.

14.2   C: Oxygen

This patient has a cluster headache. NICE guidance (CG 150) suggests using subcutaneous or nasal triptans, or high-flow 100% oxygen, 12 L/min, and consideration of referral for imaging in new-onset headaches. Patients with cluster headache should be offered home oxygen and triptans to use at the onset of headache. Opioids, oral triptans, NSAIDs and paracetamol are not recommended.

14.3   D: Up to 75% of patients become seizure free on treatment

Epilepsy affects 400 000 people in the UK. It is often seen in association with other conditions such as cerebral palsy or tuberous sclerosis, or in later life as a result of cerebrovascular disease. About 40% of cases of epilepsy have a generic component. Epilepsy is associated with two to three times higher morbidity and mortality rates due to both epilepsy itself (sudden unexpected death and seizures) and to accidents, eg drowning.

14.4   E: Myasthenia gravis

Myasthenia gravis typically presents with weakness, usually of the ocular, bulbar, facial and girdle muscles. Patients are easily fatigued and usually first notice blurred vision or ptosis. The condition affects 1:20 000 people and can be associated with thymoma. Autoantibodies against acetylcholinesterase receptors are positive in 75% of cases, and diagnosis can be confirmed with a Tensilon test. Treatment is with oral pyridostigmine with treatment of any associated thymoma. Where thymoma is present, the 5-year survival rate is 30%; for non-thymoma cases 80% respond well to oral treatment.

14.5   E: He should be tested for HIV infection

Peripheral neuropathy is common, and investigation should be directed to the most common causes. Patients should have a history and examination to identify potential underlying disease and be tested accordingly. The most common causes are diabetes, alcohol use, vitamin B_{12} deficiency and HIV. All patients should have a biochemical screening and treatment initiated with either a tricyclic antidepressant or anticonvulsant. Nerve conduction studies may be helpful where there is diagnostic doubt. Cauda equina symptoms should prompt emergency admission.

14.6   D: Haloperidol is effective but may cause unacceptable side effects

There is good evidence for the use of neuroleptics alongside CBT in Gilles de la Tourette syndrome, with the strongest evidence for haloperidol and pimozide. Aripiprazole is effective with a favourable side-effect profile but is unsuitable for use in children. Eye movement desensitisation is used in post-traumatic stress disorder. Where haloperidol is not tolerated atypical neuroleptics such as risperidone may be useful.

14.7   D: Tardive dyskinesia

Tardive dyskinesia is characterised by repetitive facial grimaces and choreoathetoid movements of the upper limbs, and is usually seen after neuroleptic use, although it can occur after taking antiemetics or over-the-counter medications. It is more common in females and usually settles with drug withdrawal, although 40% still have symptoms after 3 years. Anticholinergics (eg Kemadrin) or benzodiazepines usually help with symptoms. Jacksonian epilepsy is a condition where seizures are initially localised but spread to become a generalised tonic–clonic seizure; temporal lobe epilepsy is characterised by unusual behaviour or hallucinations.

14.8   C: Memantine

NICE recommend memantine as second-line treatment for patients with mild-to-moderate dementia who are intolerant of acetylcholinesterase inhibitors, or who have severe dementia. The guidance suggests that antipsychotics should be used only in exceptional circumstances in elderly patients with dementia due to increased risk of side effects and death. The risks are particularly high in Lewy body dementia, in which irreversible parkinsonism and neuroleptic malignant syndrome occur.

14.9   A: Carpal tunnel syndrome

Carpal tunnel syndrome is caused by compression of the median nerve at the wrist. Diagnosis can be confirmed by Phalen's or Tinel's tests, or by nerve conduction studies where there is doubt. Treatment is with steroid injection, although surgery is often required when there is muscle wasting.

14.10   E: Riluzole increases the period of time to need for ventilation but does not improve prognosis

Riluzole has been shown to increase the mean time to need for ventilation but does not affect the final outcome. The multidisciplinary approach involving occupational therapy and physiotherapy as well as speech and language therapy can lead to significant benefits, and symptomatic drug treatments such as benztropine for drooling and baclofen or diazepam for spasticity are very helpful. The decision to ventilate is one that must be made with the patient because this will often be seen as simply prolonging the patient's suffering.

14.11   A: A stat dose of ciprofloxacin is effective prophylaxis in close contacts

Rifampicin is traditionally used for prophylaxis but ciprofloxacin has fewer side effects and interactions, although is it is unlicensed for this use. Intravenous or intramuscular benzylpenicillin should be used for suspected meningitis, or cefotaxime if there is a history of drug reaction with penicillin. In cases of anaphylaxis, however, chloramphenicol should be used. Amoxicillin is the treatment of choice for listeria meningitis. Meningitis is a life-threatening condition and treatment should not be delayed for blood cultures. Polymerase chain reaction (PCR) testing will often confirm the diagnosis after initiation of therapy, regardless of antibiotic use.

14.12   D: It is typically relapsing and remitting

Trigeminal neuralgia is a relapsing and remitting neuralgic pain in any of the branches of the trigeminal nerve, nearly always unilateral and characterised by paroxysms lasting <2 minutes. Associated neurological signs suggest the presence of alternative causes such as tumour. Carbamazepine is effective in 70% of patients and gabapentin is often used as an alternative. Refractory cases can be treated with surgery.

14.13   Headache prophylaxis

Headache type	Prophylactic treatment
Chronic migraine	Botulinum toxin (**A**)
Menstrual migraine	Zolmitriptan (**D**)
Cluster headache	Verapamil (**C**)
Medication-overuse headache	Drug withdrawal (**B**)

NICE guidance (CG 150) recommends topiramate and propranolol for prophylaxis of migraine. Where this is ineffective, acupuncture or Botox injections may be tried. Menstrual migraine with aura that does not respond to usual prophylaxis may be treated with zolmitriptan 2.5 mg two to three times daily on days when migraine is expected. Verapamil may be effective as prophylaxis for cluster headache. Medication-overuse headache should be treated by drug withdrawal, followed by adequate treatment of the underlying cause of the headache.

14.14   A: The fact that the cumulative incidence is higher than the prevalence in middle to older age suggests that most people enter remission at some stage

The risk of recurrence after a single seizure is approximately 50–70% but the long-term prognosis is good. Retrospective studies suggest that, after 20 years, 76% of patients had at least one 5-year period of complete freedom from seizures, and 70% remained seizure free. Approximately 50% were in remission of at least 5 years' duration and had been off all antiepileptic drugs for at least 5 years. The cumulative incidence of epilepsy is considerably higher than the prevalence, suggesting that most patients enter long-term remission at some stage.

Headache

14.15　F:　Giant-cell arteritis

Giant-cell arteritis causes a prodromal illness of malaise, anorexia and weight loss, followed by temporal headache and scalp tenderness. Jaw claudication is pathognomonic of this condition. Late features include visual loss and severe temporal tenderness.

14.16　E:　Cluster headache

Cluster headache typically affects men in their 40s and causes daily severe headaches, often with associated watering of the eye and nasal symptoms. The headaches are severe and last 1–2 hours. They are often triggered by alcohol.

14.17　B:　Brain tumour

These symptoms are consistent with raised intracranial pressure (ICP). Common chronic causes include brain tumour but, when presenting acutely, a colloid cyst or intracranial bleed should be excluded.

14.18　G:　Migraine

This is a typical history of focal migraine, with a prodrome, aura and headache, followed by resolution. Treatment is aimed at avoiding provoking factors (including the pill) where appropriate and treating symptoms, often with a triptan.

New-onset seizure

14.19　H:　Tongue biting

14.20　A:　Epilepsy likely

14.21　I:　Yes

14.22　B:　Epilepsy unlikely

14.23　F:　Syncope likely

Syncope can cause stiffening of the body, twitching of the limbs and occasional incontinence. These symptoms are not therefore always useful in differentiating epilepsy from syncope. Attempt to identify a precipitating factor for syncope, such as standing for long periods (particularly if the ambient temperature is high), pain, strong emotion, micturition, diarrhoea or vomiting. It is uncommon for syncope to occur without some warning symptoms, usually including some combination of nausea, blurred vision, light-headedness and a sensation of muffled hearing. Syncope is often accompanied by pallor and sweating, whereas cyanosis is usual in the early stages of generalised tonic–clonic seizures. The actual duration of the loss of consciousness in syncope usually amounts to a few seconds only; it can, however, be longer if the patient is supported in the upright position after fainting. The postictal phase after syncope does not involve prolonged drowsiness and confusion, and recovery is generally rapid, although the patient might feel a sense of malaise for some time. Tongue biting suggests a seizure.

14.24   Procyclidine or benztropine

Either drug may be used for the emergency treatment of acute drug-induced dystonias. Tardive dyskinesia is characterised by oral grimaces and chewing or sucking movements, with choreoathetoid movements of the arms. It is more common in women and the risk is greatest with conventional antipsychotics.

Chapter 15
Palliative and end-of-life care

Single best answer questions

15.1 **Confusion**

A 91-year-old woman with a previous history of hypertension and breast cancer is brought in by her daughter, who is concerned that she is depressed. Further questioning reveals constipation, nausea, lethargy and weakness, and significant worsening of her short-term memory and concentration. Which ONE of the following is the MOST LIKELY cause of her symptoms? Select ONE option only.

- O A Dementia
- O B Depression
- O C Hypercalcaemia
- O D Hypothyroidism
- O E Urinary tract infection

15.2 **Breathlessness**

A 79-year-old man with end-stage heart failure is having palliative care in a local nursing home. He gets very distressed at night due to breathlessness, despite having home oxygen. The staff request medication to use on an as-needed basis for this. Which ONE of the following would be most appropriate in this situation? Select ONE option only.

- O A Amitriptyline
- O B Dexamethasone
- O C MST
- O D Oramorph as needed
- O E Zopiclone at night

15.3   Headache
A 47-year-old man is being treated for a brain tumour. His latest scans show that his tumour has not responded to treatment and he has opted for palliative care. He complains of a worsening headache, especially in the morning, which is aggravated by bending over. Which ONE of the following would be the SINGLE MOST APPROPRIATE treatment? Select ONE option only.

○ A   Amitriptyline

○ B   Dexamethasone

○ C   Gabapentin

○ D   Indometacin

○ E   Morphine

15.4   Bereavement

1   Acceptance
2   Despair and depression
3   Pain of separation
4   Resolution and reorganisation
5   Shock

Which ONE of the following correctly describes the normal stages of bereavement from the list above after the death of a loved one? Select ONE option only.

○ A   2 5 3 1 4

○ B   3 5 2 4 1

○ C   4 5 2 3 1

○ D   5 3 2 1 4

○ E   5 3 2 4 1

15.5   Wound management in palliative care
A 91-year-old woman has a fungating tumour of her breast. She is very conscious of the smell and asks for treatment for this. Which ONE of the following is the SINGLE MOST APPROPRIATE initial treatment in this case? Select ONE option only.

○ A   Activated charcoal

○ B   Occlusive dressings

○ C   Radiotherapy

○ D   Topical metronidazole

○ E   Topical tranexamic acid

Multiple best answer questions

15.6 and 15.7   End-of-life symptomatic care

A 78-year-old man is in the last stages of metastatic colon cancer. He is very drowsy and on a syringe driver, but his family are distressed by rattling noises from upper respiratory secretions. Which TWO of the following are the most appropriate first-line treatment choices at this stage? Select TWO options only.

O   A   Amitriptyline

O   B   Glycopyrronium

O   C   Haloperdol

O   D   Hyoscine butylbromide

O   E   Levomepromazine

O   F   Octreotide

15.8 and 15.9   End-of-life care planning

Which TWO of the following statements are true with regard to do not attempt resuscitation (DNAR) forms? Select TWO OPTIONS ONLY.

O   A   Any member of the medical or nursing team can complete a DNAR form, as long as the patient has capacity

O   B   DNAR forms are valid for 12 months

O   C   DNAR forms should be stored in the patient's hospital records at all times

O   D   Patients aged 16 and 17 with capacity are considered as adults for the purposes of consent

O   E   Where a patient lacks capacity but has a valid advance directive, this cannot be ignored even if the treating clinician feels it is in the best interests of the patient to do so

O   F   When a patient lacks capacity, a DNAR form cannot be completed

Extended matching questions

Palliative care prescribing

15.10–15.15

Options

A   Baclofen
B   Buscopan
C   Dexamethasone
D   Lidocaine patches
E   Non-steroidal anti-inflammatories
F   Regional anaesthesia

For each symptom listed below, select the SINGLE MOST APPROPRIATE treatment from the list above. Each option may be used once, more than once or not at all.

15.10	Pain from bony metastases
15.11	Liver capsule pain in patients with liver metastases
15.12	Smooth muscle spasm
15.13	Muscle pain and spasms
15.14	Upper abdominal pain in patients with pancreatic cancer
15.15	Pathological rib fracture where non-steroidal anti-inflammatories are contraindicated

Transdermal medication in palliative care

15.16–15.19

Options

A   12 hours
B   24 hours
C   36 hours
D   48 hours
E   72 hours
F   10–25%
G   25–50%
H   50–75%
I   Buprenorphine
J   Codeine
K   Fentanyl
L   Oxycodone

From the list of options complete the algorithm for initiating transdermal opioids in palliative care.

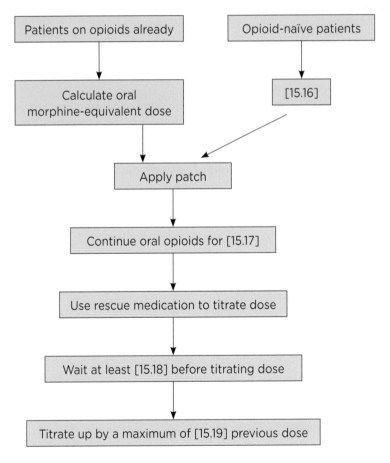

Data interpretation questions

15.20 Transdermal drug doses
Patients with chronic pain who have previously been on weak opioids only may be treated with transdermal buprenorphine. The dose required is dependent on their previous opioid use.

MATCH each drug dose to the appropriate buprenorphine patch strength from the list of options below, to complete the table. Each option will be used once. All SIX options must be correctly to score ONE mark.

A   30–60 mg/day
B   <50 mg/day
C   50–100 mg/day
D   60–120 mg/day
E   100–150 mg/day
F   120–180 mg/day

	Buprenorphine 5 µg/h	Buprenorphine 10 µg/h	Buprenorphine 20 µg/h
Tramadol (mg/day)			
Codeine (mg/day)			

15.21 Analgesic choice in palliative care
A 78-year-old man is dying of metastatic bladder cancer. This has caused hydronephrosis and he has chosen not to have further treatment for his renal impairment. He is taking sustained-release morphine tablets 60 mg twice daily and Oramorph 10 mg/5 ml, 5–10 ml as needed for breakthrough pain. He has been using his Oramorph on average four times a day. His most recent blood tests are shown below:

Na+	137 mmol/l
K+	5.5 mmol/l
Creatinine	167 µmol/l
eGFR	21 = ml/min

Which ONE of the following would be appropriate in this situation?

○ A   Change the morphine to buprenorphine

○ B   Change the morphine to diamorphine

○ C   Change the morphine to oxycodone

○ D   Increase the dose of morphine tablets

○ E   Reduce the dose of morphine tablets

Free-text question

15.22 Backache
A 73-year-old man who has been treated for prostate cancer for 12 years complains of severe unremitting lower spinal pain for the last 10 days. This is aggravated by coughing or sneezing and is keeping him awake at night. On examination he has localised bony tenderness, difficulty in walking and sensory loss below the site of the pain.

What is the most likely diagnosis? White your answer in the box below.

15.1   C: Hypercalcaemia

Mild hypercalcaemia is usually asymptomatic but moderate-to-severe hypercalcaemia causes abdominal symptoms, such as: pain, constipation, nausea and pancreatitis; depression, weakness, anorexia and impaired cognition; bone pain and arthritis; renal stones and polyuria; hypertension and prolonged Q–T interval. 80% of cases are due to primary hyperparathyroidism, whereas 20–30% are due to malignancy. Investigation is aimed at the underlying cause, and treatment is usually with rehydration and bisphosphonates where necessary.

15.2   D: Oramorph as needed

Immediate-release morphine is very effective at reducing the sensation of breathlessness in heart failure, and may also help with cough. MST will not be effective due to its slow onset of action. Dexamethasone, cyclizines and NSAIDs exacerbate heart failure due to fluid retention and these should be stopped where possible. Sedatives help with sleep but do not help the subjective sensation of breathlessness.

15.3   B: Dexamethasone

These are typical symptoms of raised intracranial pressure. This usually responds very quickly to dexamethasone 8–16 mg a day. Amitriptyline is useful for chronic daily headache or tension-type headache. Morphine may be required but usually causes sedation.

15.4   D: 5 3 2 1 4

There are many different descriptions of the grief process. This model uses 'tasks' of grief. It should be understood that grieving may take place before death and often the bereaved will oscillate between loss-oriented states such as grieving, letting go, breaking bonds, and restoration-oriented work such as trying new things, investing in new relationships. Bereavement is very much a dual process of coping with pain and loss, at the same time as building a new life.

15.5   D: Topical metronidazole

Fungating tumours often smell and metronidazole topically is the first-line treatment for this. If widespread, systemic metronidazole may be required. Topical adrenaline, alginates, tranexamic acid, cautery or radiotherapy may be used for persistent bleeding. Where the tumour itself is painful, topical morphine may help.

15.6 and 15.7   End-of-life symptomatic care

B: Glycopyrronium;
D: Hyoscine butylbromide

Amitriptyline is useful for drooling but not in an end-of-life setting because it is usually taken orally. Haloperidol and levomepromazine are treatments for agitation and nausea, whereas octreotide is used for intestinal obstruction. Some centres use hyoscine hydrobromide first line, but this can cause worsening of agitation. Hyoscine butylbromide is also helpful for intestinal colic.

15.8 and 15.9   End-of-life care planning

> D: Patients aged 16 and 17 with capacity are considered as adults for the purposes of consent;
> E: Where a patient lacks capacity but has a valid advance directive, this cannot be ignored even if the treating clinician feels it is in the best interests of the patient to do so

The BMA, Resuscitation Council and Royal College of Nursing have released guidance on DNAR decision-making (see www.resus.org.uk). It should be noted that a valid advance directive is legally binding regardless of whether the treating physician agrees with it, as long as the patient had capacity at the time it was completed. Children aged 16 and 17 with capacity are adults in terms of consent, but parents have parental responsibility so should be consulted as long as the child agrees. DNAR forms do not have a time limit for validity, but it is good practice to review them periodically. Where a patient lacks capacity, a previously appointed attorney (under the power of attorney rules) should be consulted. If not available friends and family should be asked what the patient would probably have decided if he or she could express him- or herself. All discussions should be scrupulously documented and this should be by the most senior clinician available.

Palliative care prescribing

15.10   E: Non-steroidal anti-inflammatories

Bone pain often responds well to NSAIDs. Second-line options are bisphosphonates, denosumab, surgical fixation or single fraction radiotherapy.

15.11   C: Dexamethasone

This is often helpful for liver capsule pain, characterised by right upper quadrant or shoulder-tip pain. Response should be assessed after 5 days.

15.12   B: Buscopan

This is useful for smooth muscle spasm, characterised by colicky cramp-like pains. Medication should be reviewed because prokinetic agents such as domperidone and metoclopramide may be the cause.

15.13   A: Baclofen

Stiff aching muscles with spasms, often worse in the morning are sometimes seen in motor neurone disease and Parkinson's disease. They often respond to baclofen, diazepam, clonazepam or tizanidine.

15.14   F: Regional anaesthesia

Upper abdominal pain is often seen in advanced pancreatic cancer. This responds to coeliac axis neurolysis in 80% of cases. Regional anaesthesia is also helpful for Pancoast's tumour, rib involvement and chest wall pain due to mesothelioma.

15.15   D: Lidocaine patches

These may be helpful with chest wall pain.

Transdermal medication in palliative care

15.16   I: Buprenorphine

15.17   A: 12 hours

15.18   E: 72 hours

15.19   G: 25–50%

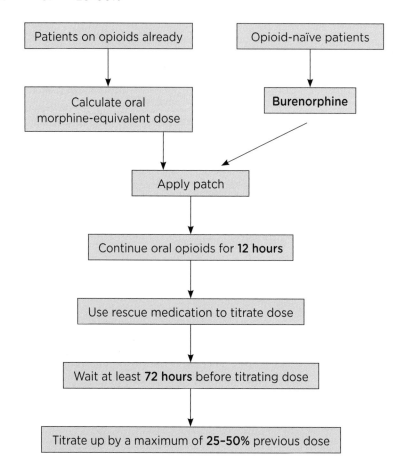

15.20   Transdermal drug doses

	Buprenorphine 5 µg/h	Buprenorphine 10 µg/h	Buprenorphine 20 µg/h
Tramadol (mg/day)	<50 (**B**)	50–100 (**C**)	100–150 (**E**)
Codeine (mg/day)	30–60 (**A**)	60–120 (**D**)	120–180 (**F**)

Transdermal opioids should be used for chronic pain. Their onset of action is too slow to be used for acute pain. Caution should be exercised when initiating them, especially with fentanyl in opioid-naïve patients. Nausea may be seen in the first 7 days and buprenorphine transdermal patches may cause a local rash. Increased temperature, eg hot water bottle, bath or heat pad, may increase the rate of absorption, increasing the risk of toxicity and reducing the duration of action of the patch.

15.21   C: Change the morphine to oxycodone

Morphine, diamorphine and codeine should be avoided in patients with an eGFR <30 ml/min per 1.73 m^2 due to reduced excretion and the tendency for active metabolites to accumulate. The metabolites of oxycodone are less toxic and this, or fentanyl, is the usual treatment of choice in renal impairment. Buprenorphine is relatively safe but would not provide adequate equivalent analgesia to this dose of MST.

15.22   Spinal cord compression

Any patient with a history of cancer who complains of severe back pain with neurological symptoms or signs should be assessed as soon as possible to exclude malignant spinal cord compression. Early detection is crucial to prevent permanent spinal cord damage. There are usually lower motor neurone signs at the level of the lesion and upper motor neurone signs below that. Urinary or faecal incontinence is usually a late sign. Metastatic disease is the most common cause of acute cord compression.

Chapter 16
Pharmacotherapeutics

Single best answer questions

16.1   Antidepressant safety
A 48-year-old man who has been taking citalopram for 18 months comes to see you concerned about media reports regarding the safety of this drug. Which ONE of the following statements is true with regard to the safety of this drug? Select ONE option only.

○   A   Citalopram has been shown to cause hepatic impairment

○   B   Citalopram has been shown to cause renal impairment

○   C   Citalopram is associated with increased risk of suicide compared with other SSRIs

○   D   Citalopram is associated with prolonged QT interval at higher doses

○   E   Citalopram should not be used in patients aged >65

16.2   Constipation in palliative care
A 74-year-old woman currently in the local cottage hospital is taking morphine orally for bone pain from her myeloma. She has been constipated for 1 week despite enemas, Movicol and bisacodyl. She is in a great deal of discomfort. On examination she is constipated but there are no signs of bowel obstruction. Which ONE of the following would be appropriate in this situation? Select ONE option only.

○   A   Change morphine to oxycodone/naloxone

○   B   Fybogel

○   C   Lactulose

○   D   Methylnaltrexone

○   E   Sodium picosulfate

16.3   **Prescribing for children**
       With regard to the prescribing of medications to children, which ONE of
       the following statements is true? Select ONE option only.

O   A   Intramuscular injections are preferable to intravenous injections in
        small children because of the difficulty in achieving venous access

O   B   Quantities of medicine of <5 ml should be given by syringe rather than
        by spoon

O   C   The small quantity of sugar in medicine is unlikely to cause tooth
        decay

O   D   The use of unlicensed medications in children is strictly forbidden

O   E   To ensure compliance with unpalatable medicines, these should be
        mixed in with food (eg mashed potato)

16.4   **Drug treatment of osteoporosis**
       With regard to drug treatments for osteoporosis, which ONE of the
       following statements is true? Select ONE option only.

O   A   Bisphosphonates can only be given either daily or weekly

O   B   Calcitonin is taken orally

O   C   Patients with poor dental hygiene should see their dentist before
        starting bisphosphonate therapy

O   D   Strontium is taken as a once-weekly preparation

O   E   Teriparatide can be used to prevent osteoporosis in those at high risk

16.5 Rash
A 78-year-old woman with dementia is brought to see you by her carer after he noticed a rash on her back. He thinks that she is on some medication for her dementia but is not sure what this is. The rash is shown below.

What is the SINGLE MOST likely cause of her rash? Select ONE option only.

O   A   Contact dermatitis

O   B   Erythema multiforme

O   C   Erythema nodosum

O   D   Non-accidental injury

O   E   Shingles

16.6   Drug treatment of eczema
        Select the rank order of the options (1-4) that best fulfils the requirements
        given in the question.

The following is a list of eczema treatment options:

1   Beclomethasone cream
2   Clobetasol cream
3   Hydrocortisone cream
4   Mometasone cream

The responses (A-E) rank the treatment options in various orders. Select
the response that places the treatment options (1-4) in the order of
potency, with the **weakest** cream first to the **strongest** cream last.

Select one rank order only.

○   A: 2, 3, 1, 4

○   B: 3, 1, 4, 2

○   C: 3, 1, 2, 4

○   D: 1, 3, 4, 2

○   E: 1, 3, 2, 4

16.7   Common drug interactions
        MATCH EACH drug to the MOST LIKELY interaction. Each drug must be
        correctly matched to score ONE Mark.

A   Verapamil
B   Pregabalin
C   Clopidogrel
D   Simvastatin

Interaction	Most likely drug
Effect is inhibited by omeprazole	
Risk of toxicity is increased by amlodipine	
Causes bradycardia when given with β blockers	
Increases the risk of side effects of tramadol	

Extended matching questions

Adverse drug reactions

16.8–16.12

Options

A   Amiloride
B   Amiodarone
C   Azithromycin
D   Bendroflumethiazide
E   Colchicine
F   Diclofenac
G   Indometacin
H   Methotrexate
I   Prednisolone
J   Sulfasalazine

For each of the scenarios described below, select the SINGLE drug most likely to be responsible from the list above. Each option can be used once, more than once or not at all.

16.8   A man who has inflammatory arthritis starts a new medication, but it has to be withdrawn promptly by the specialist when the patient develops a dry cough, fever and breathlessness.

16.9   A woman with rheumatoid arthritis starts taking a new daily medication but has to stop it after developing neutropenia.

16.10   A woman develops dizziness after starting a medication prescribed by her GP for an acutely swollen and painful metatarsophalangeal joint.

16.11   A patient develops severe diarrhoea after starting a medication prescribed for an acutely swollen and painful metatarsophalangeal joint.

16.12   A patient develops hypothyroidism 6 months after starting this new medication.

Suspected adverse reaction

16.13–16.17

Options

A	Black triangle drug
B	Consider reporting
C	No
D	Paediatric drug
E	Report under yellow card scheme
F	Serious reaction
G	Yes

The following flow chart illustrates the hierarchy of actions that should be taken in the event of a suspected adverse drug reaction.

For each of the numbered spaces in the flow chart, select the SINGLE MOST appropriate option from the list above. Each option can be used once, more than once or not at all.

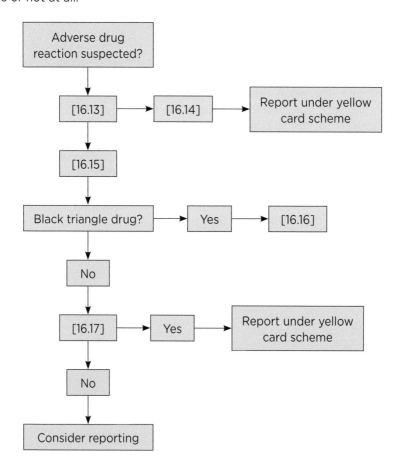

Management of diabetic neuropathy

16.18–16.22

Options

A   Amitriptyline
B   Carbamazepine
C   Duloxetine
D   Fentanyl
E   Gabapentin
F   Morphine
G   Pregabalin
H   Topical lidocaine
I   Tramadol
J   None of the above

Complete the table below describing the stepwise approach to the management of painful diabetic neuropathy, using the list of option above.

Each option may be used once, more than once or not at all.

	First-line treatment	Second-line treatment	Third-line treatment
No contraindications	[16.18]	[16.20]	[16.21]
Alternative if contraindications	[16.19]		[16.22]

Data interpretation question

16.23   Interpretation of lithium levels
A 67-year-old woman who suffers from bipolar disorder has been taking
lithium for 6 months. She attends for routine blood tests and the following
results are obtained:

Lithium	1.6 mmol/l (normal range 0.4–1.0 mmol/l)
Creatinine	112 bmol/l (normal range 60–110 bmol/l)
eGFR	57 ml/min per 1.73m²
TSH	5.3 mU/l (normal range 0.5–4.5 mU/l)
FT4	13 pmol/l (normal range 10–24 pmol/l)

What action should be taken? Select ONE option only.

○   A   Check compliance

○   B   Increase dose of lithium

○   C   Reduce dose of lithium

○   D   Start an ACE inhibitor for chronic renal impairment

○   E   Start levothyroxine 50 mg/day and repeat thyroid function in 3 months

Free-text questions

16.24   Travel advice
A 19-year-old man with no previous history of note comes to see you
for advice about his forthcoming gap year trip. He is planning to trek to
Everest base camp in Nepal and would like to take prophylaxis against
altitude sickness. Which drug would you recommend? Write your answer in
the box below.

16.25 and 16.26   Foot pain

A 73-year-old man with a previous history of congestive heart failure and atrial fibrillation takes bendroflumethiazide and warfarin. He complains of an acutely red, swollen first metatarsophalangeal joint. His temperature is 36.7°C. You arrange for a blood test. The results are shown below:

Hb	13.5 g/dl
WBCs	13.5 × 10⁹/l
Platelets	356 × 10⁹/l
CRP	7 mg/l
Urate	397 µmol/l (<417 µmol/l)

Part A

What is the SINGLE MOST likely diagnosis? Write your answer in the box below.

Part B

He is intolerant of colchicine. Which ONE of the following would be the most appropriate treatment for his acute gout? Select ONE option only.

A   Allopurinol
B   Indometacin
C   Naproxen
D   Paracetamol
E   Prednisolone

16.1 D: Citalopram is associated with prolonged Q–T interval at higher doses

Citalopram has a dose-dependent effect on Q–T interval and should not be used in patients taking other drugs that have the same effect, such as amiodarone. The maximum dose in those >65 or those with pre-existing heart disease is 20 mg (10 mg for escitalopram) and 40 mg for those <65 without heart disease. Patients with a history of heart disease should have an ECG and blood tests before starting treatment.

16.2 D: Methylnaltrexone

For severe opioid-induced constipation not responding to oral or rectal treatment, an injection of methylnaltrexone is often helpful. This is a peripherally acting opioid antagonist that reverses constipation without causing withdrawal or loss of analgesic affect. It is given parenterally and works within 30 minutes. Once the acute constipation has been dealt with, changing to oxycodone/naloxone might be effective in preventing recurrence but this can take 1–2 weeks for the bowels to return to normal. Co-prescription of Fybogel, lactulose and Movicol is often helpful in patients who wish to stay on morphine.

16.3 B: Quantities of medicine <5 ml should be given by syringe rather than by spoon

The BNF for children has a wealth of advice on prescribing for children. Unpalatable medicines can be mixed with small quantities of food but not with a large amount because of the risk of not taking the full dose, and the risk of developing an aversion to the food if there is an unpalatable taste. There is a risk of dental caries if frequent medication needs to be taken and sugar-free preparations should be used wherever possible. Many common medicines are unlicensed in children, but their use is acceptable where there is a body of evidence that it is appropriate to do so and the prescriber accepts the professional responsibility and potential liability.

16.4 C: Patients with poor dental hygiene should see their dentist before starting bisphosphonate therapy

Strontium is taken as an oral suspension, 2 g/day. It is useful in those who cannot tolerate bisphosphonates and promotes new bone growth as well as reducing resorption. Bisphosphonates are associated with osteonecrosis of the mandible and patients should have regular dental follow-up. Ibandronic acid is given monthly as an oral tablet or 3-monthly by intravenous infusion. Teriparatide is initiated by specialists and only in patients who are intolerant of bisphosphonates, or where these have failed to prevent a fracture and the patient has either extremely low bone mineral density or very low bone density, and has had fractures and risk factors such as low BMI. Calcitonin is taken as either an injection or a nasal spray.

16.5   A: Contact dermatitis

This woman is using rivastigmine patches and has had a reaction to the adhesive in the patch. This is a common side effect of patches and can be reduced by rotation of sites but, as shown here, this does not always prove effective. Changing the patient to oral treatment results in resolution. Patients should be warned about this side effect. With some drugs (eg transdermal buprenorphine) co-prescription of antihistamines is recommended initially.

16.6   B: 3, 1, 4, 2

Rank ordering: 3 Hydrocortisone cream; 1 Beclomethasone cream; 4 Mometasone cream; 2 Clobetasol cream

Eczema should be treated with the mildest treatment possible, to avoid steroid-related side effects. Treatment with potent and very potent steroids should be for short periods of 1–2 weeks at a time. Where this fails to control symptoms referral for systemic immunosuppressants should be considered.

16.7   Common drug interactions

Interaction	Most likely drug
Effect is inhibited by omeprazole	Clopidogrel (**C**)
Risk of toxicity is increased by amlodipine	Simvastatin (**D**)
Causes bradycardia when given with β blockers	Verapamil (**A**)
Increases the risk of side effects of tramadol	Pregabalin (**B**)

Omeprazole inhibits the enzymes that convert the prodrug clopidogrel to its active form, and has thus been shown to reduce platelet inhibition by 30%. The co-prescription of omeprazole and clopidogrel should be avoided. Amlodipine increases the risk of myopathy and rhabdomyolysis when taken with doses of simvastatin ≥40 mg. Pregabalin potentiates the side effects of tramadol, and this may cause drowsiness and confusion in elderly people, and makes the combination popular with those who misuse prescription drugs. Verapamil and β blockers taken together can cause marked bradycardia.

Adverse drug reactions

16.8   H: Methotrexate

Methotrexate can cause pneumonitis. This can be fatal and methotrexate needs to be withdrawn and corticosteroids administered under specialist supervision in hospital. Other side effects of methotrexate include pulmonary fibrosis and blood dyscrasias.

16.9   J: Sulfasalazine

Sulfasalazine is known to cause blood dyscrasias, including neutropenia, particularly in patients with rheumatoid arthritis. Methotrexate is also used in rheumatoid arthritis and can cause neutropenia, but is given weekly rather than daily.

16.10   G: Indometacin

This patient has arthritis affecting her metatarsophalangeal joint, the classic joint affected by gout. NSAIDs are used in the treatment of gout. Indometacin can cause dizziness as a side effect and the BNF recommends that patients are warned that this can affect the performance of skilled tasks (eg driving).

16.11   E: Colchicine

Colchicine is used in the treatment and prevention of gout. Nausea and vomiting and profuse diarrhoea are well-recognised side effects.

16.12   B: Amiodarone

Both hypo- and hyperthyroidism are recognised adverse effects of amiodarone treatment. Thyroid function tests should be performed before commencing treatment and after 6 months.

Suspected adverse reaction

16.13   F: Serious reaction

16.14   G: Yes

16.15   C: No

16.16   E: Report under yellow card scheme

16.17   D: Paediatric drug

Management of diabetic neuropathy

16.18	C:	Duloxetine
16.19	A:	Amitriptyline
16.20	G:	Pregabalin
16.21	I:	Tramadol
16.22	H:	Topical lidocaine

	First-line treatment	Second-line treatment	Third-line treatment
No contraindications	Duloxetine	Pregabalin	Tramadol
Alternative if contraindications	Amitriptyline		Topical lidocaine

NICE guidance (CG96) on managing painful diabetic neuropathy suggests duloxetine as first line, unless contraindicated, in which case amitriptyline should be used. Second-line treatment should involve addition of pregabalin on its own or in combination with the first-line treatment. Failure to improve on maximally tolerated doses is usually an indication for specialist referral, but tramadol or topical lidocaine may be useful while specialist review is awaited. The guidelines suggest that strong opioids should not be used.

16.23 C: Reduce dose of lithium

These blood tests show stage 3 chronic kidney disease and subclinical hypothyroidism with elevated lithium levels. Lithium is toxic to the thyroid and kidneys, and at higher doses causes increasing confusion, disorientation and hyperreflexia, and eventually convulsions and death. Regular monitoring of renal and thyroid function, together with lithium levels, is necessary in all patients.

16.24 Acetazolamide

Acetazolamide 250 mg/day in divided doses is recommended for prophylaxis of acute mountain sickness, whereas a dose of 250 mg twice daily is used for treatment. An alternative where rapid ascent is needed and acetazolamide is not appropriate (eg sulphonamide allergy) would be dexamethasone, but the side-effect profile of dexamethasone makes it unsuitable for routine use.

16.25 and 16.26   Foot pain

Part A   Gout

Acute gout affects the first MTP in 75% of cases and is acutely tender, often to the point at which patients cannot even bear to have a sheet on their toes. Uric acids may fall in acute gout, but a raised CRP and leukocytes are suggestive. If there is diagnostic doubt, aspiration and microscopy of synovial fluids are diagnostic. Radiology can show suggestive signs but is not diagnostic.

Part B   E: Prednisolone

NSAIDs are first-line treatment, but caution should be used where there is a risk of GI bleeding or exacerbation of pre-existing renal or heart disease. Colchicine is effective but may cause diarrhoea. Prednisolone orally or intra-articular steroids are rapidly effective in acute gout, but should not be used if there is any possibility of a septic arthritis. Allopurinol should not be used in acute gout because it may prolong the attack or precipitate a further acute attack.

Chapter 17
Renal problems

Single best answer questions

17.1   Renal colic
A 37-year-old man with a history of renal calculi asks for a home visit for a severe attack of colic. He has tried some paracetamol and codeine but vomited. On examination he is flushed and tachycardic, and has tenderness in his right loin area. Urinalysis is strongly positive for blood. His blood pressure is 100/70 mmHg and his temperature is 37.6°C. Which one of the following would be the SINGLE MOST appropriate option in his management at this point?

O   A   Hospital admission

O   B   Intramuscular diclofenac 75 mg stat and review in 2 hours

O   C   Intramuscular morphine 2.5 mg stat and review in 2 hours

O   D   Oral morphine sulphate 10–20 mg 3 hourly and review if no better

O   E   Rectal diclofenac 100 mg stat and review if no better

17.2   Renal side effects
Which ONE of the following statements is correct regarding the effect of analgesics on renal function? Select ONE option only.

O   A   NSAIDs are safe if used on an as required basis only

O   B   Co-prescription of ACE inhibitors or ARBs is associated with reduced risk of NSAID-associated acute kidney injury

O   C   Dual therapy with ACE Inhibitors or ARBs and diuretics significantly increases susceptibility to NSAID-associated renal damage

O   D   Risk of NSAID-associated renal damage increases with duration of use beyond 30 days

O   E   Sustained-release NSAID preparations are associated with lower risk of renal damage than standard preparations.

17.3   **Polycystic kidneys**

One of your patients is in her second pregnancy and has just had a growth scan at 30 weeks which has shown that her baby has polycystic kidneys. She has researched this on the internet and is worried that her 6-year-old son will have inherited the condition. She comes to see you to discuss this situation. Which ONE of the following statements is true with regard to this situation?

- O   A   Childhood polycystic kidney disease is inherited as an autosomal recessive trait

- O   B   Many patients with polycystic kidneys are asymptomatic

- O   C   She can be reassured that infantile polycystic kidney disease is always present on prenatal ultrasound and so her other child will not be affected

- O   D   She should be advised that her other child has a 50% chance of being affected

- O   E   With medical treatment from an early age most children have a normal life expectancy

17.4   **Chronic renal impairment**

You see a 69-year-old man with diabetes for his annual review. He was noted to have stage 3 chronic renal impairment 2 years ago and, although his estimated glomerular filtration rate (eGFR) has been stable, his haemoglobin has dropped over that period to 10.1 g/dl. He has had a colonoscopy and gastroscopy, and been told that his anaemia is due to his chronic renal impairment. According to NICE guidelines, which ONE of the following statements about his management is correct?

- O   A   Anaemia in chronic renal disease is usually macrocytic, so folic acid should be prescribed

- O   B   He should be referred for erythropoietin injections

- O   C   He should have regular blood transfusions

- O   D   No treatment is necessary as long as his haemoglobin is >10 g/dl

- O   E   Oral iron supplements should be prescribed

17.5   Urinary tract infection

A 67-year-old man comes to see you with his third proteus urinary tract infection in 3 months. These infections seem to settle down with antibiotics but he does report that he gets a persistent ache in his back between attacks, and often notices blood in his urine. Clinical examination is unremarkable apart from microscopic haematuria. Urine cytology is positive for blood but shows no atypical cells. You arrange an ultrasound scan, which shows unilateral hydronephrosis. What is the SINGLE MOST likely diagnosis? Select ONE option only.

  ○ A   Chronic renal failure

  ○ B   Prostatic enlargement

  ○ C   Renal calculus

  ○ D   Schistosomiasis

  ○ E   Urethral valves

17.6   Dysuria

A 19-year-old man has had perineal pain for the past 3 days and has developed a fever. He also describes dysuria. On rectal examination he is found to have a tender, boggy prostate gland. Which ONE of the following actions is the SINGLE MOST appropriate next step?

  ○ A   An HIV test should be organised as soon as possible

  ○ B   A urine sample should be obtained for culture

  ○ C   Antibiotics should be started only after any culture results have been received

  ○ D   Rectal tissue should be swabbed and sent to the laboratory

  ○ E   The prostate should be massaged to obtain prostatic fluid for culture

17.7   Renal calculi

Which ONE of the following microorganisms is most likely to be associated with struvite (mixed infective) renal calculi?

  ○ A   *Candida albicans*

  ○ B   Enterococci

  ○ C   *Escherichia coli*

  ○ D   *Proteus* sp.

  ○ E   Streptococci

17.8   Monitoring renal function
A 78-year-old man comes to see you for his annual check-up. He has
been treated for hypertension for some years and it has always been well
controlled. On checking his BP you find the systolic persistently raised
>170 mmHg. You arrange for some blood tests, which show a reduced
eGFR. An ECG is normal and urine dipstick testing is negative for protein.
Reviewing his records there seems to have been something of a decrease
in his eGFR over the last 2 years. He is otherwise well, apart from some
nocturia, dribbling and poor flow, which he feels is normal at his age. A
graph showing his recent eGFR results is shown on the following page.

Which ONE of the following is the SINGLE MOST appropriate action at this
point?

○   A   Introduce a calcium antagonist to improve BP control

○   B   Refer for renal ultrasound

○   C   Refer to cardiology for advice on further antihypertensive treatment

○   D   Start finasteride

○   E   Start ramipril and repeat renal function test in 1 week

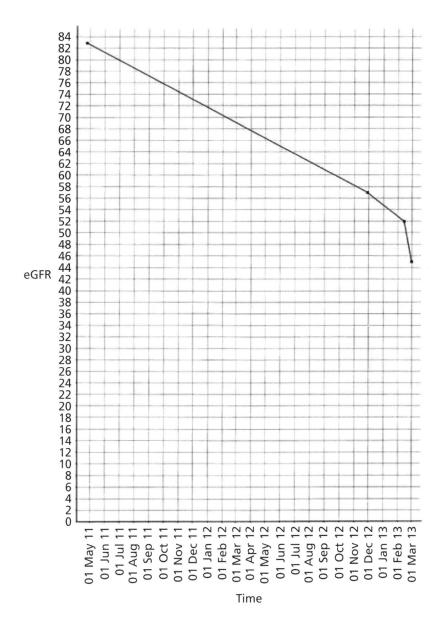

Extended matching questions

Loin pain

17.9–17.12

Options

A   Adrenal cortical necrosis
B   Aortic aneurysm
C   Polycystic kidneys
D   Pelviureteric junction obstruction
E   Pyelonephritis
F   Renal adenocarcinoma
G   Renal haemangioma
H   Renal vein thrombosis
I   Retroperitoneal haemorrhage
J   Ureteric calculus

For each of the scenarios below, select the SINGLE MOST appropriate diagnosis from the list above. Each option can be used once, more than once or not at all.

17.9   A 56-year-old man on long-term warfarin therapy after prosthetic heart valve replacement complains of right-sided back pain, hip weakness and malaise for the past week. He has a pulse of 110 beats/min, and a BP of 110/80 mmHg.

17.10   A 48-year-old man presents with a 3-month history of intermittent haematuria and discomfort in the left loin. A mass is palpable in the left upper quadrant.

17.11   A 30-year-old woman presents with acute right-sided loin pain, which comes in waves and radiates to her groin, with vomiting. Abdominal examination is negative and urinalysis shows microscopic haematuria.

17.12   A 67-year-old man presents with sudden-onset, severe left loin pain that is radiating to the left groin, with nausea and dizziness. He has a pulse of 136 beats/min and a BP of 90/60 mmHg.

The management of chronic renal impairment in primary care

17.13–17.17

Options

A   Aim for BP <125/75 mmHg
B   Aim for BP <130/80 mmHg
C   Aim for BP <140/80 mmHg
D   Aim for BP <150/90 mmHg
E   Check phosphate levels
F   Check urine for protein
G   eGFR <15 ml/min
H   eGFR <30 ml/min
I   eGFR 30–60 ml/min
J   eGFR >60 ml/min
K   eGFR >90 ml/min
L   Refer to renal physician

Complete the following algorithm, which describes the management of chronic renal impairment in primary care, from the list of options above (CKD is chronic kidney disease). Each option can be used once, more than once or not at all.

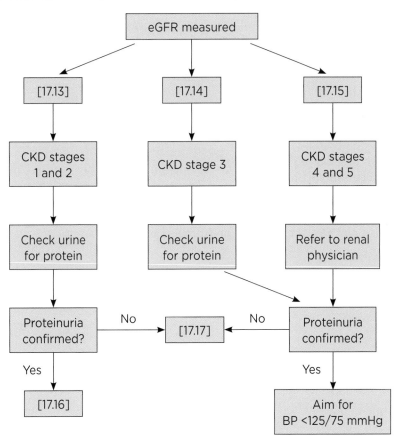

Data interpretation questions

17.18 and 17.19   Renal disease

A 56-year-old man who takes atenolol for hypertension sees the nurse for his annual check-up. She takes blood and finds his blood pressure to be elevated at 164/80 mmHg. His blood tests show the following results:

Sodium	139 mmol/l
Potassium	4.0 mmol/l
Creatinine	73 µmol/l

You prescribe ramipril and ask him to return in 1 week. After 36 hours he complains of nausea and anorexia. You arrange repeat blood tests with the following results:

Sodium	141 mmol/l
Potassium	5.6 mmol/l
Creatinine	120 µmol/l

Part A

Which is the SINGLE MOST likely diagnosis? Select ONE option from A–E only.

A   Acute kidney injury
B   Chronic kidney disease
C   Hepatorenal syndrome
D   Hypertensive nephropathy
E   Obstructive uropathy

Part B

Which is the SINGLE MOST appropriate first line investigation to carry out at this point? Select ONE option from F–J only.

F   Chest X-ray
G   CT of the kidney, ureters and bladder (KUB)
H   Renal biopsy
I   Ultrasound scan of kidneys, ureters and bladder
J   Urinalysis

17.20   **Prostate problems**
According to NICE guidance on the management of lower urinary tract symptoms (LUTSs) in men, the following is a list of medications used for this condition.

MATCH each drug to the MOST APPROPRIATE column with regard to indication. All six must be correctly matched to score ONE mark.

A   5α-Reductase inhibitor
B   α Blocker
C   Anticholinergic and α blocker
D   Combination of 5α-reductase inhibitor and α blocker
E   Desmopressin
F   Loop diuretic

Indication	Drug choice
First-line, moderate LUTSs, normal prostate	
Moderate LUTSs, enlarged prostate	
Moderate-to-severe LUTSs, enlarged prostate	
Storage symptoms despite α blocker	
Nocturnal polyuria	
Resistant nocturnal polyuria	

17.1   A: Hospital admission

Although most patients with renal colic can be managed at home with oral or rectal analgesics and NSAIDs, patients with symptoms or signs or urinary sepsis should be admitted as an emergency due to a high risk of overwhelming sepsis developing. Patients in whom the diagnosis of renal colic is uncertain should also be considered for admission, eg to exclude aortic aneurysm. Patients managed at home should have urgent outpatient imaging.

17.2   C: Dual therapy with ACE inhibitors or ARBs and diuretics significantly increases susceptibility to NSAID-associated renal damage.

Data from the UK general practice database has shown that dual therapy with diuretics and ACE inhibitors/ARBs increases the risk of acute kidney injury by 31%, and the effect is most marked (twofold) in the first 30 days. Monotherapy with ACE inhibitors/ARBs does not increase risk compared with NSAIDs alone.

17.3   A: Childhood polycystic kidney disease is inherited as an autosomal recessive trait

Childhood polycystic kidney disease is inherited as an autosomal recessive trait, with an incidence of 1 in 40 000. Most children with the condition are diagnosed antenatally with ultrasound but, less commonly, they can present later in childhood with an abdominal mass. Prognosis is poor, with renal transplantation the only realistic option for most patients. There are often associated hepatic cysts and subsequent portal hypertension and splenomegaly. Adult polycystic kidney disease is inherited as an autosomal dominant trait. It is less severe but 45% of patients will develop renal failure by the age of 60. It is always bilateral and can be associated with liver cysts; berry aneurysms are found in 40% of patients with the adult form of the condition.

17.4   B: He should be referred for erythropoietin injections

NICE guidelines say that a target haemoglobin of between 10.5 g/dl and 12.5 g/dl is ideal, and patients should be referred to the renal anaemia team if their haemoglobin is <11 g/dl. If patients have low iron stores, supplementary iron might be needed and this is usually in the form of parenteral supplements. Folate supplements are not necessary unless there is coexistent folate deficiency (eg due to poor diet or alcoholism).

17.5   C: Renal calculus

Renal tract calculi cause different symptoms depending on their anatomical location. Lower ureteric stones can impact at the vesicoureteric junction and cause hydronephrosis. Other significant causes to consider in this case are tumour of the bladder or ureter. Prostatic hypertrophy (either benign or malignant) and urethral strictures can cause bilateral hydronephrosis. *Proteus* infections are associated with renal tract calculi. Schistosomiasis is a common cause of haematuria in north Africa but is not common in the UK.

17.6   B: A urine sample should be obtained for culture

This patient has symptoms consistent with acute prostatitis. Fever, arthralgia, low abdominal or perineal pain, and a urethral discharge are all common symptoms. Diagnosis is made by urine culture. Prostatic massage should be avoided because it can allow the infection to disseminate, and will be painful for the patient. Treatment with quinolone antibiotics is usually effective.

17.7   D: *Proteus* sp.

Renal calculi are common, affecting approximately 2% of the UK population, although most are asymptomatic. Symptomatic patients often present with severe, colicky abdominal pain that causes difficulty lying still. The pain often radiates to the testes or labia; haematuria is also a common feature. Most calculi are composed of calcium oxalate or calcium phosphate. Around 15–20% of renal calculi are known as 'mixed infective' or 'struvite' calculi. They are associated with chronic urinary tract infection. These calculi are composed of magnesium ammonium phosphate. Urease-producing bacteria break down urea to form this compound. *Proteus* and *Klebsiella* spp. produce urease enzyme and are common causes of struvite calculi.

17.8   B: Refer for renal ultrasound

Unexplained deterioration in eGFR or an unexpected change in the BP should prompt a search for causes of secondary hypertension. This patient had an enlarged prostate causing bladder outflow obstruction and progressive hydronephrosis. Management of the hydronephrosis followed by treatment of the prostatism restored renal function to normal.

Loin pain

17.9   I: Retroperitoneal haemorrhage

Poorly controlled anticoagulant therapy results in bleeding into the renal and gastrointestinal tracts. Retroperitoneal bleeding is uncommon and can present as hip weakness due to femoral nerve paresis. A retroperitoneal haematoma might be palpable over the psoas.

17.10   F: Renal adenocarcinoma

Renal cell carcinoma is usually of insidious onset. Loin pain occurs when the renal capsule is stretched or invaded, and haematuria occurs when the tumour erodes into the pelvicalyceal system.

17.11   J: Ureteric calculus

Ureteric colic from calculus obstruction can present as an acute abdomen with normal serum inflammatory markers and amylase. There is usually microscopic haematuria.

17.12   B: Aortic aneurysm

A leaking abdominal aortic aneurysm can present as left loin pain radiating to the groin and can be mistaken for ureteric calculus obstruction. There might be guarding/rigidity and a pulsatile mass is sometimes present. An absent or diminished femoral pulse on that side with early signs of hypovolaemia should point to an impending catastrophe.

The management of chronic renal impairment in primary care

17.13	J:	eGFR ≥60 ml/min
17.14	I:	eGFR 30–60 ml/min
17.15	H:	eGFR <30 ml/min
17.16	A:	Aim for BP <125/75 mmHg
17.17	B:	Aim for BP <130/80 mmHg

17.18 and 17.19   Renal disease

Part A   A: Acute kidney injury

Part B   J: Urinalysis

Acute kidney injury is defined as an increase in serum creatinine >26 µmol/l or >1.5 times baseline within 48 hours, oliguria (<0.5 ml/kg per h for 6 ≥h) or a 25% or greater fall in eGFR in the last 7 days. Causes may be prerenal (eg hypovolaemia), renal (eg acute tubular necrosis, drugs such as NSAIDs, aminoglycosides or ACE inhibitors) or postrenal (eg renal calculi, prostatic obstruction). Initial assessment should include urine dipstick for proteinuria, blood and microscopy for casts, and culture for infection. Further tests such as X-rays should be directed at probable causes.

17.20   Prostate problems

The principal treatments for BPH are α blockers, which relax the urethra, and 5α-reductase inhibitors, which cause the prostate to shrink in time. NICE recommend assessing prostatic size or carrying out a prostate-specific antigen (PSA) measurement to guide treatment: with a PSA >1.4 ng/ml and a high risk of progression, eg older men – an indication for the use of 5α-reductase inhibitors.

Indication	Drug choice
First-line, moderate LUTSs, normal prostate	α Blocker
Moderate LUTSs, enlarged prostate	5α-Reductase inhibitor
Moderate-to-severe LUTSs, enlarged prostate	Combination of 5α-reductase inhibitor and α blocker
Storage symptoms despite α blocker	Anticholinergic and α blocker
Nocturnal polyuria	Loop diuretic
Resistant nocturnal polyuria	Desmopressin

Chapter 18
Respiratory problems

Single best answer questions

18.1   Fibrosing alveolitis
A 57-year-old man is newly diagnosed with cryptogenic fibrosing alveolitis.
He comes to see you to discuss his condition and asks about his prognosis.
Which ONE of the following statements is correct with regard to this issue?

O   A   He has a significantly increased risk of developing lung cancer

O   B   Most patients do not experience any functional limitation

O   C   The majority of patients respond to treatment

O   D   The mean life expectancy from diagnosis is 6 months

O   E   Treatment should be aimed at the underlying cause

18.2   Chest tightness
A 24-year-old woman complains of intermittent chest tightness and
wheeze over the past 3 months. Her symptoms have been getting worse
and are troublesome at night. She smokes cigarettes socially. She has a
past history of hay fever. Her respiratory examination is normal. What is
the next best action? Select ONE option only.

O   A   Ask her to keep a diary of her symptoms and review her in 2 weeks

O   B   Issue her a prescription for a salbutamol metered-dose inhaler and
arrange a review in 2 weeks

O   C   Refer her to the hospital as an outpatient for a chest X-ray

O   D   Show her how to use a peak flowmeter and request that she keeps
a record of morning and evening readings for 1 week, then come for
review

O   E   Show her how to use a peak flowmeter and request that she keeps a
record of morning and evening readings for 2 weeks, then come for
review

18.3   Sleep apnoea
A 40-year-old man has recently been diagnosed with mild obstructive sleep apnoea. He works as a handyman for a local school and part-time as a taxi driver. He attends for review. Which one of the following is the SINGLE MOST appropriate course of action?

  ○ A   Advise that he need not inform his car insurance company of his diagnosis as his obstructive sleep apnoea is mild

  ○ B   Ensure that he has been told verbally and in writing that he must inform the Driver and Vehicle Licensing Agency (DVLA) of the diagnosis

  ○ C   Inform him that for now he should not work as a taxi driver. He might be able do so in the future provided that he has no daytime sleepiness over the following month

  ○ D   Inform him that he has a legal obligation to inform the school that he has obstructive sleep apnoea and will not be able to operate machinery until further notice

  ○ E   Inform him that he is likely to require nasal CPAP treatment overnight

18.4   Hoarseness
A 42-year-old man who is an ex-smoker complains of right shoulder pain and hoarseness for 4 weeks. Examination of his shoulder reveals a normal range of movement. His chest is clear, he is not breathless and he has no lymphadenopathy. His voice is hoarse. He does not have finger clubbing. The SINGLE MOST appropriate course of action is:

  ○ A   Organise a chest physician to review him urgently as an outpatient

  ○ B   Organise an urgent cervical spine X-ray

  ○ C   Organise an urgent chest X-ray

  ○ D   Organise a routine chest X-ray

  ○ E   Organise a routine X-ray of his shoulder and review with results

18.5   **Acute breathlessness**
You see a teenager with a history of asthma. On examination, his respiratory rate is 30/min with prolonged expiration; he cannot complete sentences on talking to you, is tachycardic and has wheeze heard throughout his chest. What is the SINGLE MOST appropriate course of action, given the following options? Select ONE option only.

O   A   Give 5 mg salbutamol via oxygen-driven nebuliser and send home if he feels completely back to normal

O   B   Give oxygen via facemask at 10 l/min and call an ambulance

O   C   Give six puffs of salbutamol via a spacer and if the patient starts to improve send him home with a 5-day course of prednisolone

O   D   Give salbutamol nebuliser and prednisolone 40 mg orally; arrange hospital assessment

O   E   Give 10 puffs of salbutamol and 10 puffs of ipratropium; arrange a review the next day with the asthma nurse

18.6   **Respiratory emergencies**
A 14-year-old boy is rushed into the surgery by his mother with sudden-onset abdominal pain and vomiting, and an urticarial skin rash. On examination, you note that he is very breathless with both stridor and wheeze. His lips and tongue are swollen. From the following options, what is the SINGLE MOST appropriate initial drug management? Select ONE option only.

O   A   Administer nebulised 1 in 1000 adrenaline, 2 ml via oxygen-driven nebuliser

O   B   Administer oxygen and give 1 in 1000 adrenaline, 0.1 ml intravenously

O   C   Administer oxygen and give 1 in 1000 adrenaline, 0.5 ml intramuscularly

O   D   Administer oxygen and give 10 puffs of salbutamol via a spacer

O   E   Give nebulised salbutamol 5 mg via oxygen-driven nebuliser

18.7   Drug treatment of COPD
        Your practice holds a clinic for the treatment of patients with known
        COPD. Some patients who are reviewed find that they are still symptomatic
        despite taking single short-acting bronchodilators. According to NICE
        guidelines, what would the SINGLE MOST appropriate next treatment
        option be? Select ONE option only.

O   A   A 4-week trial of combination long-acting β agonist and inhaled
        corticosteroid

O   B   Combined therapy of current short-acting β agonist and theophylline

O   C   Long-acting bronchodilator (β agonist or anticholinergic)

O   D   Mucolytic therapy to reduce the incidence of dry cough

O   E   Oxygen therapy via nasal cannulae at 2 l/min for 15 hours each day

18.8   Cough
        This 64-year-old man has had a productive cough, shortness of breath
        and intermittent fever for the past week. He is a non-smoker. He has had a
        chest X-ray and this is the AP film:

What is the SINGLE MOST likely diagnosis? Select ONE option only.

○ A   Foreign body aspiration

○ B   Pneumonia

○ C   Pneumothorax

○ D   Pulmonary oedema

○ E   Upper respiratory tract infection

18.9   Spirometry
A 45-year-old woman presents with increasing exertional breathlessness over the past 6 months. She has scleroderma. Spirometry shows:

	Measured	Predicted
FVC (litres)	1.98	3.51
FEV_1 (litres)	1.64	2.82
FEV_1/FVC (%)	83	80

FEV_1 = forced expiratory volume in 1 second; FVC = forced vital capacity.

Which of the following is the SINGLE MOST likely diagnosis? Select ONE option only.

○ A   Asthma

○ B   Bronchiectasis

○ C   Extrinsic allergic alveolitis

○ D   Pulmonary fibrosis

○ E   Tracheal stenosis

18.10 **Management of chronic asthma**
Select the rank order of the options (1–4) that best fulfils the requirements given in the question.

The following is a list of management steps in chronic asthma (1–4) for adults and children over 5 years of age:

1   Addition of inhaled corticosteroid
2   Addition of long-acting β agonist
3   Addition of regular oral steroids
4   Bronchodilator as needed

The responses (A–E) rank the management steps in chronic asthma in various orders. Select the response that places the options (1–4) in the order of early management first to **advanced** management last.

Select one rank order only.

○   A: 1, 2, 3, 4
○   B: 2, 1, 3, 4
○   C: 4, 3, 1, 2
○   D: 4, 1, 2, 3
○   E: 3, 1, 2, 4

Extended matching questions

Shortness of breath

18.11–18.15

Options

A   Bronchial carcinoma
B   Bronchiolitis
C   COPD
D   Croup
E   Metastatic lung disease
F   Pneumonia
G   Pneumothorax
H   Pleural effusion
I   Pleurisy
J   Upper respiratory tract infection

Choose the SINGLE MOST likely diagnosis for each patient described below from the list of options above. Each option can be used once, more than once, or not at all.

18.11   A 78-year-old man presents with cough, dyspnoea and weight loss over the past month. He has recent-onset haemoptysis and his nail beds appear spongy. He smokes regularly. On examination, his respiratory rate is 18/min at rest and he has crackles affecting his right lung.

18.12   A 55-year-old man has had a productive cough for the past 3 days. He has right-sided chest pain and feels short of breath. He is a non-smoker. On examination, his respiratory rate is 20/min at rest. Right low chest percussion is dull and he has inspiratory right lower zone crackles. His temperature is 38.5°C.

18.13   A 60-year-old woman complains of a dry cough and sore throat for the past 3 days. She says that she feels breathless for a short while after coughing. She smokes 10 cigarettes a day. On examination, her oropharynx looks injected, her respiratory rate is 14/min, her BP 150/90 mmHg and her pulse 70 beats/min. Her chest is clear to auscultation and she is apyrexial. She has had no previous chest problems.

18.14   A man asks to see one of the nurses at your practice to get a 'cough bottle'. On further questioning, he tells the nurse that he has had a productive cough intermittently for the past 4 years. He is in his late 40s. At present, he smokes cigars regularly and experiences shortness of breath when dressing or walking more than 100 yards on the flat. His weight is steady. He sometimes wheezes on exertion.

18.15   A 6-month-old baby is seen at a general practice with a 3-day history of shortness of breath, reduced feeding and cough. On examination, the child has a respiratory rate of 30/min and his chest examination reveals bilateral coarse inspiratory crepitations. He is afebrile.

Assessment of airflow obstruction in COPD

18.16–18.20

Options

A   Cough and sputum production common
B   Evening cough and sputum production problematic
C   50–80% predicted
D   50–70% predicted
E   33–49% predicted
F   30–49% predicted
G   <33% predicted
H   <30% predicted
I   Severe dyspnoea on minimal exertion
J   Severe dyspnoea prevents even minimal exertion

The following flow chart has been adapted from NICE guidance on classifying COPD.

For each stage of the flow chart, select the SINGLE MOST appropriate option from the list above for measured FEV_1 and likely symptomatology. Each option can be used once, more than once or not at all.

Free-text question

18.21   Steroid doses

A child weighing 21 kg has an acute exacerbation of asthma. He does not need hospital admission but you decide to give him 5 days of oral prednisolone. What daily dose would be appropriate at this age? Write your answer in milligrams, in figures, in the box below.

18.1   A: He has a significantly increased risk of developing lung cancer

Patients with cryptogenic fibrosing alveolitis have a 10-fold increased risk of developing lung cancer. Overall, the prognosis is poor, with only a small proportion responding to treatment and a 5-year survival rate of 40–50%. In most cases a cause cannot be identified and, where steroids and immunosuppression do not work, lung transplantation might be an option. For most patients, however, treatment is symptomatic, with oxygen when necessary.

18.2   E: Show her how to use a peak flowmeter and request that she keeps a record of morning and evening readings for 2 weeks, then come for review

The history is suggestive of asthma and her past history of hay fever suggests atopy, supporting the diagnosis. A 20% or greater diurnal variation in peak flow on 3 days a week for 2 weeks is highly suggestive of asthma. She is unlikely to be able to use an inhaler effectively without training by a healthcare professional. The British Thoracic Society (BTS) guidelines recommend objective tests to confirm the diagnosis of asthma before starting long-term therapy.

18.3   B: Ensure that he has been told verbally and in writing that he must inform the DVLA of the diagnosis

The Scottish Intercollegiate Guidelines Network (SIGN) have produced guidelines for the investigation and management of obstructive sleep apnoea (OSA). OSA can lead to an increased risk of the sufferer having an accident due to sleepiness. It is an offence to fall asleep at the wheel of a car and custodial sentences can be imposed. Patients with OSA can present reporting daytime sleepiness, but can also present with non-specific symptoms such as irritability and poor concentration. The Epworth questionnaire has been used in patients with suspected OSA to measure pre-treatment sleepiness. Moderate-to-severe OSA is treated with nasal CPAP; weight loss should be encouraged in all patients. Patients should not drive if they report daytime sleepiness. Once diagnosed, patients should be told verbally and in writing that they must inform the DVLA. Those working with machinery or driving should be referred to a sleep centre for assessment.

18.4   C: Organise an urgent chest X-ray

The NICE guidelines for the diagnosis and management of suspected lung cancer suggest urgent referral for a chest X-ray in smokers and ex-smokers over the age of 40 with:

- Haemoptysis
- Persistent or unexplained (>3 weeks):
  - cough
  - chest/shoulder pain
  - weight loss
  - dyspnoea
  - chest signs
  - clubbing
  - hoarseness
  - cervical/supraclavicular lymphadenopathy
  - signs of metastatic disease.

18.5   D: Give salbutamol nebuliser and prednisolone 40 mg orally; arrange hospital assessment

The patient has features of acute severe asthma and warrants referral. Features of acute severe asthma include:

- Respiratory rate >25/min
- Inability to complete a sentence in one breath
- Pulse >110 beats/min
- Peak flow 33–50% of best or predicted.

High-flow oxygen should be administered if available. Salbutamol or terbutaline can be administered by spacer or nebuliser as available, with oxygen-driven nebuliser the preferred method. D was the best option out of those given.

18.6   C: Administer oxygen and give 1 in 1000 adrenaline, 0.5 ml intramuscularly

Gastrointestinal manifestations of anaphylaxis include abdominal pain and vomiting, and are more common in cases of food allergy. This child has signs of respiratory compromise and should be given intramuscular adrenaline and oxygen while an ambulance is called. An inhaled β_2 agonist might help if the bronchospasm does not respond to your initial treatment.

18.7 C: Long-acting bronchodilator (β agonist or anticholinergic)

NICE guidelines suggest that patients who are not controlled with a single short-acting bronchodilator can be started on a combination of two short-acting bronchodilators or a single long-acting bronchodilator. Mucolytic therapy is used in patients with chronic cough productive of sputum. Oxygen therapy, inhaled steroids and theophylline are all considered, but as later more invasive treatments.

18.8 B: Pneumonia

The X-ray shows consolidation within the right middle lobe and some patchy airspace consolidation adjacent to the horizontal fissure. The patient needs to be assessed using the CR B-65 scoring system and then treated at home or in hospital as appropriate.

18.9 D: Pulmonary fibrosis

Lung involvement in scleroderma is common and ultimately up to 80% of patients with the condition will develop abnormal pulmonary function tests. The spirometry measurements show a restrictive pattern (FVC and FEV_1 spirometry measurements are reduced and the FEV_1:FVC ratio is normal).

18.10 D: 4, 1, 2, 3

> Rank ordering: 4 Bronchodilator as needed; 1 Addition of inhaled corticosteroid; 2 Addition of long-acting β agonist; 3 Addition of regular oral steroids.

The stepwise approach for chronic asthma involves starting with bronchodilators as required, and then adding to that sequentially until control is established, with regular reviews and stepping down according to symptoms.

Shortness of breath

18.11 A: Bronchial carcinoma

The patient has shortness of breath, haemoptysis and early finger clubbing. Non-small-cell carcinoma presents with finger clubbing more often than small-cell carcinoma. He needs to be referred under the 2 week rule.

18.12 F: Pneumonia

This 55-year-old has signs and symptoms consistent with right-sided pneumonia. His examination findings show that he should be managed in the community. He does not need further investigations such as a chest X-ray at present. A course of amoxicillin should be provided as long as he is not allergic to penicillins. The patient should be advised to rest and drink plenty of fluids.

18.13 J: Upper respiratory tract infection

The patient's chest is clear and her respiratory examination shows only injection of her oropharynx, which is often present during upper respiratory infections. Her upper respiratory tract infection requires only symptomatic relief but she should have her BP rechecked and should be encouraged to attend smoking cessation services.

18.14   C: COPD

This patient needs full investigation and management as he probably has COPD. If COPD is confirmed on further testing, he should stop smoking and is likely to need regular treatment to control his current symptoms.

18.15   B: Bronchiolitis

Bronchiolitis affects babies aged <12 months. Infection with RSV is the most common cause. It classically presents with coryzal symptoms, increased work of breathing, cough and reduced feeding. Infants aged <2 months can present with a history of apnoeic episodes. Treatment is supportive; referral is required if fluid intake is reduced to less than two-thirds of normal or if the child is showing signs of respiratory distress.

Assessment of airflow obstruction in COPD

18.16   C: 50–80% predicted

18.17   E: 33-49% predicted

18.18   G: <33% predicted

18.19   A: Cough and sputum production common

18.20   I: Severe dyspnoea on minimal exertion

Patients with COPD should undergo spirometry testing as part of their diagnosis and also on at least an annual basis. Mild COPD usually causes minimal symptoms, but progression to moderate and severe COPD markedly affects symptomatology. Continuing to smoke is the major cause of disease progression; patients should stop smoking to limit disease progression as soon as possible.

18.21   20 mg

The usual dose is 1 mg/kg for this group. Where patients have a severe exacerbation or are already on steroids by mouth, 2 mg/kg may be appropriate.

Chapter 19
Sexual and reproductive health

Single best answer questions

19.1   **Management of menorrhagia**
        What is the SINGLE MOST effective non-surgical management strategy for menorrhagia?

○   A   Combined oral contraceptive pill

○   B   Mirena (levonorgestrel intrauterine system)

○   C   Depo-Provera

○   D   Progesterone-only pill

○   E   Tranexamic acid

19.2   **Contraception**
        A 26-year-old woman who recently had an ectopic pregnancy treated with laparoscopic salpingectomy visits her GP to discuss contraception. She is keen to try for a baby again but feels that she should leave this for 6 months to get over the operation. Which ONE of the following is the SINGLE MOST appropriate contraceptive method for her?

○   A   Barrier method

○   B   Combined oral contraceptive (COC) pills

○   C   Copper intrauterine contraceptive device (IUCD)

○   D   Depo-Provera

○   E   Mirena coil

19.3 Subfertility

Which ONE of the following statements about the causes of subfertility is true? Select ONE option only.

○ A   A cause is found after standard investigations in only 30% of cases

○ B   Endometriosis is found in about 25% of cases

○ C   Ovulatory failure accounts for about 20% of cases

○ D   Sperm defects are found in about 5% of couples

○ E   Tubal damage is the most common cause in women

19.4 Cervical screening

A 25-year-old woman recently diagnosed with HIV after donating blood attends for her first smear. She is a non-smoker and is otherwise fit. With regard to cervical screening, which of the following is the correct screening regime in this situation? Select ONE option only.

○ A   Cervical smear 3-yearly

○ B   Cervical smear yearly

○ C   Colposcopy and smear every 3 years

○ D   HPV vaccination and 3-yearly cervical smears

○ E   Initial colposcopy and yearly cervical smears

19.5 Pyuria

A 40-year-old woman has recently emigrated to the UK from Asia. At her new patient check she reports that she has recently lost weight and feels tired. She is found to have leukocytes in her urine which persist despite antibiotic treatment. There is no significant bacterial growth on two consecutive urine cultures. What diagnosis do you suspect? Select ONE option only.

○ A   Bladder carcinoma

○ B   Bladder stones

○ C   Contamination from vaginal discharge

○ D   Interstitial cystitis

○ E   Tuberculosis

19.6   Urethritis

Non-gonococcal urethritis may result from infection with which ONE of the following organisms?

O   A   Bifidobacteria

O   B   *Chlamydia psittaci*

O   C   *Mycobacterium bovis*

O   D   *Mycoplasma hominis*

O   E   *Ureaplasma urealyticum*

19.7   Dysuria

A 45-year-old businessman complains of dysuria and discharge after returning from a business trip to Berlin. A swab confirms chlamydial infection but tests for other sexually transmitted infections are negative. What is the SINGLE MOST appropriate treatment for this condition?

O   A   Azithromycin

O   B   Benzylpenicillin

O   C   Ciprofloxacin

O   D   Fluconazole

O   E   Trimethoprim

19.8   Interpretation of antenatal blood results

A 28-year-old primip who is 32 weeks pregnant complains of epigastric pain, nausea and pedal oedema. Her BP is 140/90 mmHg and dipstick analysis of her urine reveals protein++. She feels unwell. Blood tests are taken, the results of which are shown below:

Haemoglobin	10.0 g/dl
Haematocrit	0.35
WCC	$12 \times 10^9/l$
Platelets	$95 \times 10^9/l$
Bilirubin	20 mmol/l
ALP	250 U/l
ALT	76 U/l
Protein	6.6 g/l
LDH	550 U/l
Amylase	35 U/l
Creatinine	60 mmol/l
Urea	4.0 mmol/l
Uric acid	442 mmol/l
Na^+	141 mmol/l
K^+	3.5 mmol/l
Glucose	5 mmol/l

Which ONE of the following is the SINGLE MOST likely diagnosis?

O A   Acute liver failure

O B   Cholecystitis

O C   Fatty liver

O D   HELLP syndrome

O E   Renal failure

Extended matching questions

Female genital mutilation

19.9–19.11

Options

A   Type 1
B   Type 2
C   Type 3
D   Type 4
E   De-infibulation
F   Re-infibulation
G   None of the above

For each description below describing forms of female genital mutilation, select the SINGLE MOST appropriate classification from the list above.

19.9   Excision of the clitoris and labia minora
19.10   Traditionally takes place on the first night of marriage
19.11   Involves suturing of the vaginal edges after childbirth

Emergency contraception

19.12–19.16

Options

A   Barrier contraception
B   Barrier contraception for 7 days + emergency contraception
C   Continue combined oral contraceptive and barrier contraception for 7 days
D   Depo-Provera
E   Offer IUCD
F   Pregnancy test followed by emergency contraception (levonorgestrel) and screen for sexually transmitted infections (STIs)
G   Reassurance
H   Screen for STIs, emergency contraception (levonorgestrel) and barrier contraception for next 7 days
I   Sterilisation

Please choose the SINGLE best management option for the each of the women described in the scenarios below with regard to emergency contraception. Each option can be used once, more than once or not at all.

19.12   A 20-year-old student requests emergency contraception. She had unprotected sexual intercourse after a night out with friends 2 days ago. She does not remember when her last period was but thinks that it was about 3 months ago. She assures you that she has had no other unprotected sexual intercourse since her last period.

19.13   A weight-conscious, married mother of three, whose last child was born only 3 months ago, does not wish to have any further children. She reports a burst condom 24 hours ago, and requests emergency contraception and long-term family planning advice.

19.14   A 17-year-old girl had unplanned sex last night with a stranger. Her last period was 7 days ago. She is on the progesterone-only pill and she took her last pill 36 hours ago.

19.15   A 27-year-old married woman whose last period was 15 days ago is on a combined contraceptive pill. She forgot to take her last pill (which was due 12 hours ago) and had sex 3 hours ago.

19.16   A 30-year-old married woman on the COC pill has had an episode of diarrhoea and vomiting for the last 3 days. Her last period was 9 days ago. She has not had sex since being ill but wonders if it is safe to do so.

Gynaecological emergencies

19.17–19.21

Options

A   Appendicitis
B   Complete miscarriage
C   Constipation
D   Ectopic pregnancy
E   Endometriosis
F   Ovarian hyperstimulation
G   Ovarian torsion
H   Pelvic inflammatory disease
I   Retroverted uterus
J   Syncopal attack
K   Threatened miscarriage
L   Urinary tract infection

For each of the following scenarios, select the SINGLE MOST appropriate diagnosis from the list of options above. Each option can be used once, more than once or not at all.

19.17   A woman who is 8 weeks into her first pregnancy and who had a small fresh vaginal bleed 2 days ago now presents with brownish loss. Her ultrasound scan performed in the early pregnancy assessment clinic 2 days ago showed an intrauterine gestational sac with a normal fetal heartbeat.

19.18   A 20-year-old woman attends the out-of-hours treatment centre with abdominal pain and having fainted. Her last period was 5 weeks ago. Her urine pregnancy test is positive, her blood pressure is 70/40 mmHg and her pulse is 120 beats/min.

19.19   An 18-year-old presents with right iliac fossa pain, diarrhoea and a temperature of 38°C. Vaginal examination reveals slight tenderness on the right side with no palpable masses. She is tender in the right iliac fossa with guarding.

19.20   A 35-year-old being treated for infertility had embryo transfer 5 days ago. She now complains of feeling unwell and breathless. Abdominal examination shows distension and dullness to percussion in the flanks.

19.21   A 20-year-old primip presents with urinary retention. She also complains of tenderness in her loins. Urine dipstick testing is positive for protein. A booking scan 2 weeks ago showed a normal 12-week fetus.

Menopausal symptoms

19.22–19.27

Options

A   12 months postmenopause
B   Continue
C   Continuous combined estrogen/progestogen
D   Lifestyle advice
E   Estrogen only
F   Previous hysterectomy
G   Sequential estrogen/progestogen

Complete the flowchart below for the management of menopausal symptoms, using the list if options above. Each option may be used once, more than once or not at all.

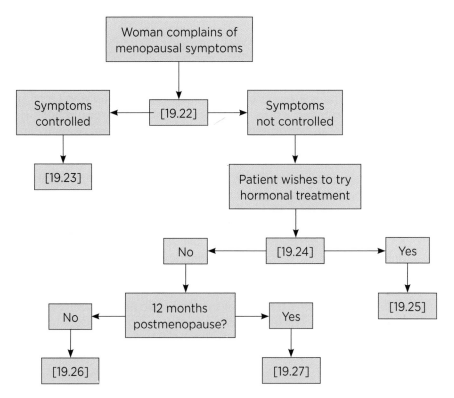

Free-text question

19.28   Period problems
A 27-year-old woman who has one child, now aged 6 years, complains of amenorrhoea for the last 6 months and has recently noticed bilateral white nipple discharge. Clinical examination is unremarkable and bloods tests show normal levels of FSH, LH, oestrogen and TSH. She takes no regular medications and a pregnancy test is negative. What would be the single most appropriate blood test to carry out at this stage in primary care? Write your answer in the box below.

19.1   B: Mirena (levonorgestrel intrauterine system)

This has been shown in a 2-year RCT to be superior to pharmacological treatment with a drop-out rate half of that seen in conventional drug treatment, in patients with menorrhagia (ECLIPSE Study, *New England Journal of Medicine* 2013).

19.2   B: Combined oral contraceptive (COC) pills

IUCDs are not advisable for short-term contraception, and there is a theoretical increased risk of ectopic pregnancy. Depo-Provera is associated with secondary amenorrhoea and can cause delayed return to fertility. Barrier methods are less effective than the combined pill but can be useful if the contraceptive pill is contraindicated.

19.3   C: Ovulatory failure accounts for about 20% of cases

The main causes of infertility are shown below (remember that some couples can have more than one cause):

- Unexplained – 30%
- Sperm defects – 25%
- Ovulatory failure – 20%
- Tubal damage – 15%
- Other – 10%
- Endometriosis – 5%
- Mucus defects – 5%
- Other male problems – 2%
- Coital failure – 2%

19.4   E: Initial colposcopy and yearly cervical smears

HIV-positive patients are at increased risk of developing cervical intraepithelial neoplasia (CIN) and they can progress rapidly from CIN to cervical cancer. It is important to counsel these women adequately regarding the need for initial colposcopy and yearly cervical smears thereafter.

19.5   E: Tuberculosis

Persistent pyuria with negative cultures in a woman from a high-prevalence area should raise the suspicion of tuberculosis. Carcinoma and stones would present with haematuria and can increase the risk of a UTI but cultures would be positive.

19.6   E: *Ureaplasma urealyticum*

Chlamydia trachomatis accounts for up to half of cases of non-specific urethritis. In the remainder, *Ureaplasma urealyticum* and *Mycoplasma genitalium* are pathogens, whereas *Mycoplasma hominis* is not. Bifidobacteria are commensal faecal organisms. *Mycobacterium bovis* causes infection in cattle and *Chlamydia psittaci* causes psittacosis.

19.7   A: Azithromycin

Often patients are infected with more than one pathogen at a time and consideration should be given to treating accordingly. *Chlamydia* sp. is sensitive to doxycycline and azithromycin. Any partners should be treated at the same time, as untreated chlamydia infection can cause infertility in females by damaging the fallopian tubes. Aciclovir is a treatment for herpes; benzylpenicillin can be used to treat syphilis or gonorrhoea. A high index of suspicion for other sexually transmitted infections should prompt screening for co-infection, including HIV. Ciprofloxacin is useful for the management of gonorrhoea but resistance is becoming a problem in some areas of the UK.

19.8   D: HELLP syndrome

HELLP syndrome (haemolysis, elevated liver enzymes, low platelets) is the diagnosis in this patient. The raised LDH and ALT, low platelets and raised bilirubin indicate the need for urgent action. Patients with pre-eclampsia can have this syndrome with even mild elevation of blood pressure. This patient should be delivered after being started on magnesium sulphate because, if it is left untreated, it is associated with high mortality rates.

Female genital mutilation

19.9   B: Type 2

19.10   E: De-infibulation

Women who have undergone infibulation (type 3 female genital mutilation, narrowing of the vaginal opening through creation of an artificial seal) are unable to have sexual intercourse unless they are cut on their first night.

19.11   F: Re-infibulation

In some communities, the vaginal edges of women who have previously had infibulation are sutured again after childbirth, to recreate a small vaginal opening.

Female genital mutilation is practised in a band from east to west across sub-Saharan Africa. Worldwide it is estimated that 100–140 million women have undergone the procedure and, in the UK, 137 000 girls and women are living with the consequences. Type 1 involves removal of the clitoris, type 2 removal of the clitoris and labia minora, type 3 infibulation, narrowing the introitus and creating a seal, and type 4 is any other non-medical procedure on the genital area.

Emergency contraception

19.12   F: Pregnancy test followed by emergency contraception
              (levonorgestrel) and screen for STIs

19.13   E: Offer IUCD

This is the most suitable long-term option in this case.

19.14   H: Screen for STIs, emergency contraception (levonorgestrel) and
              barrier contraception for next 7 days

Patients missing one or more progesterone pills will need emergency contraception
and 7 days of additional cover with barrier contraception, and should also be
advised on future barrier contraception use along with pills.

19.15   G: Reassurance

Patients on the combined pill who forget their pill can take it up to 12 hours late
without problems. If pills are more than 24 hours late or where antibiotics are being
taken, the 7-day rule needs to be applied, with barrier precautions for 7 days.

19.16   C: Continue COC and use barrier contraception for 7 days

Gynaecological emergencies

19.17   K: Threatened miscarriage

19.18   D: Ectopic pregnancy

Any female with vaginal bleeding or symptoms of internal bleeding and a positive
pregnancy test should be considered to have an ectopic pregnancy until proven
otherwise.

19.19   A: Appendicitis

19.20   F: Ovarian hyperstimulation

Ovarian hyperstimulation can present with pleural effusions and ascites.

19.21   I: Retroverted uterus

Menopausal symptoms

19.22	D:	Lifestyle advice
19.23	B:	Continue
19.24	F:	Previous hysterectomy
19.25	E:	Estrogen only
19.26	G:	Sequential estrogen/progestogen
19.27	C:	Continuous combined estrogen/progestogen

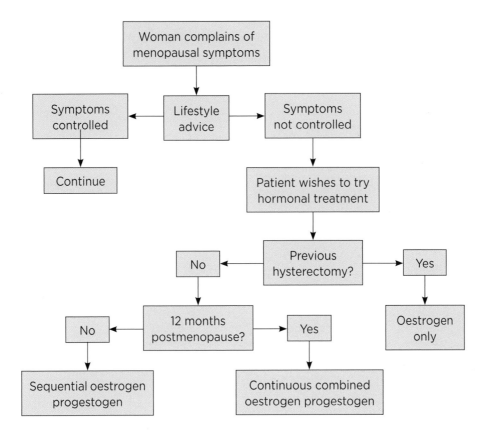

19.28   Prolactin

This patient has symptoms of a prolactinoma. This is the most common form of pituitary tumour and accounts for 50% of pituitary adenomas. Typically presenting with secondary amenorrhoea or galactorrhoea, it may also be caused by pregnancy, hypothyroidism and medications, such as antipsychotics and antiemetics. Initial treatment of uncomplicated prolactinomas is with bromocriptine or cabergoline, and 25% of cases resolve on this treatment within 2 years. Failure to improve on medical treatment is an indication for surgery.

Chapter 20
Skin problems

Single best answer questions

20.1 Urticaria
A 17-year-old boy comes to see you about his recurrent attacks of urticaria. Over the years he has tried excluding possible triggers but is now getting regular attacks. These involve itch and rash but he has no signs of angioedema. He has not tried any prescription medications yet. Which ONE of the following would be appropriate as the next step in his treatment?

 O A Issue an EpiPen with advice on how to use it

 O B Loratadine tablets

 O C Montelukast tablets

 O D Prednisolone to use orally when he develops attacks

 O E Topical steroids to use for short periods

20.2 Psoriasis
Which ONE of the following is the SINGLE MOST appropriate initial treatment for a patient presenting with palmar psoriasis?

 O A Betamethasone valerate ointment

 O B Hydrocortisone 1% ointment

 O C Oral prednisolone

 O D Regular emollients

 O E Tacrolimus cream

20.3 **Prurigo**

A medical student has seen a 40-year-old man with prurigo nodularis. The medical student asks you to explain more about this condition. Which ONE of the following pieces of information is correct?

○ A Hydrocortisone cream often worsens the condition

○ B Patients with the condition often suffer with intense itch that lasts for about 1 day

○ C The majority of patients have a personal or family history of atopy

○ D The trunk is often the most affected area of the patient's body

○ E Young children are more likely to be affected by prurigo nodularis than adults

20.4 **Finger lump**

A 56-year-old man attends having knocked his finger while working in the garage. He reports having had a small lump on his finger for some months and, since knocking his finger, this has been leaking, as shown below.

What is the SINGLE MOST likely diagnosis?

○ A Keratoacanthoma

○ B Myxoid cyst

○ C Pyogenic granuloma

○ D Sebaceous cyst

○ E Wart

20.5 Arm lesion
A 78-year-old retired farmer shows you the lesion below, which he has noticed on his arm.

What would be the SINGLE MOST appropriate management of this lesion?

○ A Cryotherapy

○ B Curettage

○ C Excision biopsy

○ D Shave biopsy

○ E Watchful waiting

20.6   Skin lesion
A 93-year-old man complains that for the last few weeks he has had a
bleeding lesion on his chest that seems to be growing rapidly. The lesion is
shown below.

What is the SINGLE MOST likely diagnosis? Select ONE option only.

○   A   Basal cell carcinoma

○   B   Malignant melanoma

○   C   Seborrheic keratosis

○   D   Squamous cell carcinoma

○   E   Wart

20.7   Skin disease
A 59-year-old woman complains that the skin lesion shown below catches on her clothing. It has been present for several years and is not associated with any other symptoms.

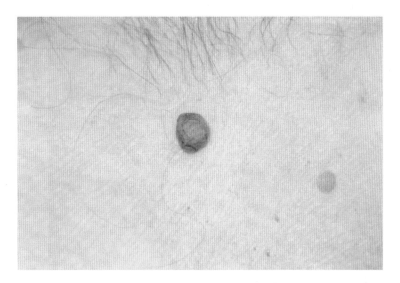

What is the SINGLE MOST likely diagnosis? Select ONE option only.

○   A   Dermatofibroma

○   B   Fibroepithelial polyp

○   C   Keratoacanthoma

○   D   Nodular basal cell carcinoma

○   E   Seborrhoeic keratosis

20.8   Rash affecting the hand
A 23-year-old man complains of an intensely itchy rash on the palms of his hands. This came on without any obvious cause about 2 weeks ago and was initially painful. It is now very itchy and keeping him awake at night. His hand is shown below.

What is the SINGLE MOST likely diagnosis?

O   A   Contact dermatitis

O   B   Eczema

O   C   Hand, foot and mouth disease

O   D   Pompholyx

O   E   Scabies

20.9 Skin lesions

A senior citizen asks you whether you can arrange to have this lesion on his back treated (shown below). He is not sure how long it has been there but he complains that it is now catching on his clothes.

What is the SINGLE MOST appropriate course of action?

○ A Refer to a local minor surgery service for complete excision with 2-mm borders

○ B Refer to dermatology for a routine opinion

○ C Refer to dermatology for an urgent outpatient opinion

○ D Treat with 5-fluorouracil cream

○ E None of the above

20.10 Rashes

A 54-year-old man took paracetamol after a minor injury 3 months ago. He developed a pruritic, oval skin lesion on his right shoulder. The lesion gradually resolved after he stopped the paracetamol. He recently restarted paracetamol for a headache. He quickly developed a recurrent skin lesion affecting his right shoulder (shown below).

Which ONE of the following options is the SINGLE MOST likely skin diagnosis? Select ONE option only.

○ A   Drug hypersensitivity syndrome

○ B   Drug-induced photosensitivity

○ C   Fixed drug eruption

○ D   Gout

○ E   Mycetoma

Extended matching questions

Psoriatic skin diseases

20.11–20.14

Options

A   Acute pustular psoriasis
B   Erythrodermic psoriasis
C   Flexural psoriasis
D   Guttate psoriasis
E   Pustular palmoplantar psoriasis
F   Psoriatic arthritis
G   Psoriasis vulgaris

For each patient described, select the SINGLE MOST likely diagnosis from the list of options above. Each option may be used once, more than once or not at all.

20.11   A 5-year-old boy has been treated for tonsillitis for the last 3 days, and now complains of numerous small, round psoriatic lesions on his trunk and arms

20.12   A 57-year-old man with lifelong psoriasis covering a large portion of his body develops shortness of breath on exertion

20.13   A 43-year-old woman who has been treated for arthritis complains of crumbling fingernails. On examination there is pitting and leukonychia

20.14   A 48-year-old chef complains of blisters on her palms and the soles of her feet. On examination there are numerous small pustules on a background of erythema

Fungal infections

20.15–20.19

Options

A   Oral fluconazole
B   Oral nystatin
C   Oral terbinafine
D   Refer for specialist opinion
E   Topical amorolfine
F   Topical clotrimazole
G   Topical hydrocortisone
H   Topical terbinafine
I   None of the above

For each of the statements below about the management of common fungal infections, select the SINGLE MOST appropriate management from the list above. Each option may be used once, more than once or not at all.

20.15   A 23-year-old woman who has recently had a course of co-amoxiclav now complains of vaginal soreness and discharge. She has not improved with a course of over-the-counter clotrimazole.

20.16   A 34-year-old man with no previous history of note has had a red itchy rash in both sides of his groin for 4 weeks.

20.17   A 3-year-old girl who has been treated for a small patch of suspected ringworm on her scalp has developed a tender, inflamed, cystic lesion on her scalp

20.18   A 39-year-old woman has a discoloured thickened fingernail on her right index finger; her other finger and toenails are normal.

20.19   A 24-year-old amateur footballer has been self-treating his athlete's foot for 2 weeks with topical miconazole. His feet are still intensely itchy and erythematous.

Moles

20.20–20.23

Options

A	Basal cell carcinoma
B	Dermatofibroma
C	Dysplastic naevi
D	Keratoacanthoma
E	Lentigo maligna
F	Malignant melanoma
G	Pyogenic granuloma
H	Squamous cell carcinoma

Complete the table below describing characteristics of skin lesions, from the list of options above. Each option may be used once, more than once or not at all.

Appearance	Usually multiple, irregular outline and pigment	Raised, red, round and bleeds easily; grows rapidly after trauma	Smooth, flesh-coloured, raised lesions on arms and legs	Rapidly growing, raised with a central plug surrounded by a collar
Size (cm)	>1	1	1	>1
Age at onset (years)	<40	Any	<40	40s
Diagnosis	20.20	20.21	20.22	20.23

Acne

20.24-20.28

Options

A   Benzoyl peroxide
B   Benzoyl peroxide plus topical clindamycin
C   Combined oral contraceptive pill
D   Isotretinoin
E   Lymecycline
F   Minocyline
G   Oxytetracycline
H   Secondary care referral
I   Topical clindamycin
J   Topical erythromycin
K   None of the above

Complete the table below detailing the stepwise approach to managing acne, using the list of options above. Each option may be used once, more than once, or not at all.

	Mild	Moderate	Severe
Description	Comedones	Comedones with inflammatory papules and pustules	Comedone, papules, pustules, nodules and cysts with scarring
First line	20.24	Benzoyl peroxide	20.26
		Consider 20.25 in females	Consider COCP in females
Second line	20.27	Benzoyl peroxide plus 20.28	

Free-text question

20.29   Skin conditions
A 45-year-old man complains of an intensely itchy rash on both wrists. On examination he has flat-topped violaceous papules on each wrist and forearms. What is the most likely diagnosis? Write your answer in the box below.

20.1   B: Loratadine tablets

Urticaria has multiple causes and avoidance can be difficult if an obvious precipitant cannot be identified. Symptomatic treatment with oral antihistamines is usually sufficient to control symptoms of simple urticaria but where there is associated angioedema parenteral adrenaline might be needed. Montelukast in association with antihistamines can be useful in refractory cases but is ineffective as monotherapy. In severe cases not responding to oral antihistamines, short courses of steroids orally might be needed but topical steroids are not effective.

20.2   A: Betamethasone valerate ointment

The British Association of Dermatology recommends using potent topical steroids as part of the initial treatment of palmar psoriasis. Keratolytic agents, such as salicylic acid in Lassar's paste, might be required to remove scale from hyperkeratotic skin. Tars and vitamin D analogues can also help. Palms and soles can be difficult areas to treat, and the patient should be referred to a dermatologist if initial treatments fail after 2–3 months or if there is diagnostic uncertainty. Specialists may recommend treatments including clobetasol propionate under occlusion or PUVA.

20.3   C: The majority of patients have a personal or family history of atopy

Prurigo nodularis is an intensely itchy skin condition of unknown aetiology. Adults are affected more frequently than children and the condition is equally distributed between males and females. Affected individuals are likely to have a personal or family history of atopy; up to 80% have a positive history compared with 25% of the normal population. Nodular, itchy lesions, 1–2 cm in diameter, are symmetrically distributed, particularly on the extensor limb surfaces. Itching is often difficult to treat and is commonly a long-standing problem. High-potency corticosteroids can be tried to treat itchy lesions, under occlusive dressings to increase absorption. Many topical and systemic treatments have been tried in the past with limited success.

20.4   B: Myxoid cyst

Myxoid cysts are ganglions of the distal interphalangeal joint. They grow slowly and often cause grooving of the nail as they grow. They are benign, but can become painful. Treatment is by aspiration of the thick jelly inside or injection with steroid, or surgical excision if they recur. A keratoacanthoma has a plug of keratin in the centre whereas a pyogenic granuloma usually grows rapidly at the site of trauma. Sebaceous cysts are not typically seen on digits.

20.5   C: Excision biopsy

Keratin horns should be excised fully including the base to allow histological exclusion of an underlying squamous cell carcinoma. Cryotherapy will not provide tissue for histology and curettage or shave biopsy may yield insufficient depth for diagnosis.

20.6   D: Squamous cell carcinoma

This is a squamous cell carcinoma. The bleeding, rapid growth and irregular surface differentiate from a seborrhoeic keratosis or wart. A basal cell carcinoma usually has a rolled edge.

20.7   B: Fibroepithelial polyp

Fibroepithelial polyps are frequently seen at sites of chafing such as the groin, axilla or neck. They are benign and typically have a narrow stalk. They are occasionally associated with insulin resistance but in most cases are idiopathic. Dermatofibromas are usually seen on the legs or arms and are within the skin. Keratoacanthomas have a central plug of keratin.

20.8   D: Pompholyx

This is a typical appearance of pompholyx, with painful, itchy vesicles on the palms (and sometimes soles). It is difficult to treat without potent topical steroids but usually subsides over 2–3 weeks. Potassium permanganate can be used for treatment if vesicles break down and, in refractory cases, topical calcineurin inhibitors, Botox or PUVA (psoralen plus UVA) can be effective.

20.9   E: None of the above

This is seborrhoeic keratosis, a benign epidermal tumour common in elderly people. Note the characteristic stuck-on appearance and rough, warty surface. Treatment is not necessary unless there is diagnostic uncertainty. Troublesome lesions can be removed by shave excision or curettage; smaller lesions can by treated with cryotherapy. Most commissioners will not authorise removal.

20.10   C: Fixed drug eruption

Fixed drug eruptions manifest as painful oval or round lesions. They characteristically occur at the same site 30 minutes to 8 hours after taking the medication responsible. The lesions sometimes blister and occur most commonly on the hands, feet, glans penis and lips. Many drugs have been implicated.

Psoriatic skin diseases

20.11   D: Guttate psoriasis

Guttate psoriasis is usually self-limiting and occurs in patients with a genetic predisposition, usually triggered by acute group B streptococcal infection. The skin plaques are small, usually centripetal, and may itch. Treatment is with topical steroids and calcipotriol. Recurrent episodes may require tonsillectomy.

20.12   B: Erythrodermic psoriasis

Erythrodermic psoriasis slowly develops over a number of years and plaques may cover 90% of the body. Increased cutaneous blood flow causes high-output heart failure and there is an elevated risk of septicaemia from skin infections. DMARDs such as methotrexate are usually necessary but prognosis is usually poor.

20.13   F: Psoriatic arthritis

Of patients with psoriatic arthritis 70–80% have nail changes, which may be complicated by secondary nail infections. Treatment should be aimed at the underlying arthritis, and patients should be advised to keep their nails short.

20.14   E: Pustular palmoplantar psoriasis

Pustular palmoplantar psoriasis is more common in women between the ages of 40 and 60 who smoke. The pustules in time become scaly and peel off, and nail involvement is common. Combination calcipotriol/steroid cream or coal tar helps.

Fungal infections

20.15   A: Oral fluconazole

Failure to respond to topical antifungals should prompt a review of the diagnosis and if no alternative is suspected a stat dose of fluconazole 150 mg is usually effective.

20.16   H: Topical terbinafine

Topical terbinafine for 2–4 weeks will usually treat tinea cruris. If it fails to respond alternative diagnoses such as erythrasma should be considered.

20.17   D: Refer for specialist opinion

Cases of suspected kerion should be referred for urgent specialist opinion. They are usually caused by zoonotic fungal infections, eg from family pets.

20.18   E: Topical amorolfine

Topical amorolfine can be used for tinea unguium where it is confined to one nail. More widespread disease should be treated with oral antifungals.

20.19   G: Topical hydrocortisone

Addition of topical hydrocortisone to antifungals may help where there is significant inflammation

Moles

20.20   C: Dysplastic naevus

20.21   G: Pyogenic granuloma

20.22   B: Dermatofibroma

20.23   D: Keratoacanthoma

Appearance	Usually multiple, irregular outline and pigment	Raised, red, round and bleeds easily; grows rapidly after trauma	Smooth, flesh-coloured, raised lesions on arms and legs	Rapidly growing, raised with a central plug surrounded by a collar
Size (cm)	>1	1	1	>1
Age at onset (years)	<40	Any	<40	40s
Diagnosis	C Dysplastic naevus	G Pyogenic granuloma	B Dermatofibroma	D Keratoacanthoma

Acne

20.24   A: Benzyl peroxide

20.25   C: Combined oral contraceptive pill

20.26   H: Secondary care referral

20.27   B: Benzoyl peroxide plus topical clindamycin

20.28   E: Lymecyline

	Mild	Moderate	Severe
Description	Comedones	Comedones with inflammatory papules and pustules	Comedone, papules, pustules, nodules and cysts with scarring
First line	Benzoyl peroxide	Benzoyl peroxide Consider COCP in females	Secondary care referral Consider COCP in females
Second line	Benzoyl peroxide plus topical clindamycin	Benzoyl peroxide plusoral lymecycline	

20.29   Lichen planus

Cutaneous lichen planus affects men three times more frequently than women, with a mean age of onset of 40–45. It is intensely itchy and may be widespread. It may also be a sign at sites of previous scarring. It may be associated with hepatitis C infection. Management is with topical steroids. Cases affecting the genital area should be referred for specialist review.

Chapter 21
Children and young people

Single best answer questions

21.1 **Nosebleeds**
A 3-month-old baby boy is brought to see you by his mother. She came home from work after leaving him in the care of her older daughter and found that he had suffered a nosebleed. Her daughter does not recall this happening and says that he has been fine all morning. He was born at term after a normal delivery and is formula fed. On examination the child appears well but there is some dried blood in each nostril. There are no other signs of bleeding. Which ONE of the following would be the SINGLE MOST appropriate action in this situation?

- O   A   Admit under the on-call paediatrician

- O   B   Give vitamin K

- O   C   Prescribe topical antibiotics to use while the nose heals

- O   D   Reassure his mother that the bleeding is likely to be due to a cold and should settle

- O   E   Report the family to social services

21.2 **Six-week check**
While carrying out a routine baby check on a 6-week-old baby you note that there seems to be an absent red reflex in both eyes. The eyes look otherwise normal and the rest of the examination is unremarkable. The mother says that her pregnancy was unremarkable other than a flu-like illness in the second trimester. Which ONE of the following would be an appropriate action in this instance? Select ONE option only.

- O   A   Admit under the on-call paediatrician

- O   B.   Inform the health visitor

- O   C   Reassure mother that this is unlikely to be significant

- O   D   Refer to ophthalmology outpatients

- O   E   Refer to orthoptic clinic

21.3 Kawasaki's disease
You receive a telephone call from one of your patients whose son has been admitted to hospital with suspected Kawasaki's disease. She has been doing some research on the internet and has heard that it has fatal complications. She asks if this is true. Which ONE of the following statements is true in this situation? Select ONE option only.

- O A Of patients 70% develop cardiac complications
- O B Aspirin should not be used due to the risk of Reye syndrome
- O C Kawasaki's disease can cause myocardial infarction
- O D The mortality rate is approximately 20%
- O E Nephrotic syndrome is frequently seen in these patients

21.4 Self-harm
A 12-year-old girl is brought in to see you by her parents after an episode of deliberate self-harm the previous weekend. Her parents are obviously distraught and are terrified that she will do this again and be more successful next time. Which ONE of the following is a risk factor for successful suicide attempt after deliberate self-harm? Select ONE option only.

- O A Drug or alcohol abuse
- O B Early presentation after an episode of deliberate self-harm
- O C High performance at school
- O D Isolated episode of deliberate self-harm
- O E Spontaneous act of deliberate self-harm

21.5 Breathing problems in children
In which ONE of the following situations should a child with bronchiolitis be admitted to hospital? Select ONE option only.

- O A A 7-month-old boy has been monitored at home for several days with coryzal symptoms. His respiratory rate is 36 breaths/min and his saturation rate is 97%

- O B A 6-week-old boy has a temperature of 37.8°C and a cough. His mother reports that she observed him breathholding when sleeping. Examination is normal

- O C A 6-month-old girl has a cough and a respiratory rate of 24 breaths/min. On examination she has fine inspiratory crackles in both lungfields

- O D A 19-month-old girl who has had a cough and cold symptoms for several days has a temperature of 40.8°C. Examination reveals a respiratory rate of 34 breaths/min and bilateral crepitations

- O E A 9-month-old girl who has had a cough and fever for the last few days and has only had one wet nappy in the last 8 hours

21.6   Febrile seizure
An 18-month-old baby has been discharged after a febrile seizure. Which of the following statements about this condition is true? Select ONE option only.

○   A   Sixty per cent of children have recurrent febrile seizures during subsequent illnesses

○   B   A prolonged seizure is a risk factor for further prolonged attacks

○   C   In most cases the seizure lasts 10–15 minutes

○   D   Rigorous attempts should be made to reduce the temperature with ibuprofen and/or paracetamol

○   E   Seizures do not occur until the fever is apparent

21.7   Hip pain
A 4-year-old boy with no history of note comes to see you with a 24-hour history of pain in his right hip and refusal to weight bear. His temperature is 38°C. When you examine him he will not move his hip but there are no signs of bruising and no rash. The SINGLE MOST likely diagnosis is:

○   A   Henoch–Schönlein purpura

○   B   Juvenile rheumatoid arthritis

○   C   Perthes' disease

○   D   Septic arthritis

○   E   Slipped upper femoral epiphysis

21.8   Henoch–Schönlein purpura
A 9-year-old boy has been given a diagnosis of Henoch–Schönlein purpura and has now had the rash for 2 weeks. With regard to his outpatient follow-up, which ONE of the following statements is most appropriate? Select ONE option only.

○   A   He needs no further paediatric follow-up

○   B   He needs to be followed up by the paediatric team until his rash has resolved

○   C   He needs to be seen by an ophthalmologist and a paediatrician within 2 weeks

○   D   He should be followed up by the paediatric team for at least 6 months after the rash has resolved

○   E   He needs no follow-up now that he has had the rash for 2 weeks

21.9 **Croup**

A 14-month-old child is brought to see you out of hours with croup. It is 2am. The child started with symptoms 2 hours ago. He has a barking cough and stridor at rest. He has no other signs of respiratory distress. The SINGLE MOST appropriate course of action would be:

O A Explain the diagnosis to parents and send him home with advice to return if he gets worse

O B Give oral dexamethasone and send him home with advice to return if he gets worse

O C Give oral dexamethasone and send him home with a further dose to be given in a further 12 hours

O D Give oxygen and send to hospital in an ambulance

O E Refer for actue paediatric assessment

21.10 **Unwell child**

This 10-year-old boy attends the surgery. He has been unwell for 4 days, with a high fever, conjunctivitis, sore throat and harsh cough. He is lethargic. The rash started yesterday behind his ears and has now spread to his body. The child is normally well but it is noted that he has never received any immunisations.

Credit: CNRI/SCIENCE PHOTO LIBRARY

What is the SINGLE MOST likely diagnosis?

- ○ A   Measles
- ○ B   Mumps
- ○ C   Parvovirus
- ○ D   Pertussis
- ○ E   Rubella

21.11   **Growth monitoring**

A 9-week-old baby is brought to see you by his mother. She is concerned about the baby's feeding and feels that he has been unsettled and irritable for the last 5 days. He has started to vomit forcefully over the past 24 hours. You cannot find any abnormality on examination. The baby is thriving and height and weight are both on the 25th centile today. The boy's head circumference chart is shown below; the latest measurement is from today.

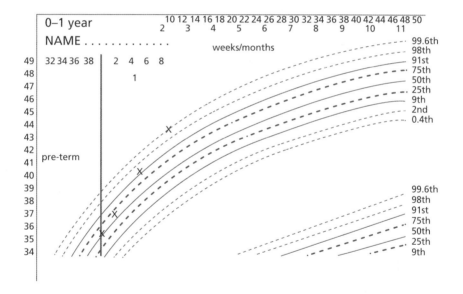

The SINGLE MOST appropriate action would be:

- ○ A   Ask the health visitor to review the child's head circumference in 1 week
- ○ B   Paediatric admission
- ○ C   Reassure mum that all is well
- ○ D   Review the child yourself in 1 week
- ○ E   Routine paediatric outpatient referral

Extended matching questions

Vomiting

21.12–21.15

Options

A   Cows' milk protein intolerance
B   Gastroenteritis
C   Gastro-oesophageal reflux
D   Hiatus hernia
E   Hirschsprung's disease
F   Lactose intolerance
G   Overfeeding
H   Posseting
I   Pyloric stenosis
J   Reduced gastric motility

For each of the following clinical situations, choose the SINGLE MOST likely diagnosis from the list of options given above. Each option can be used once, more than once or not at all.

21.12   A 1-week-old baby is brought in by his mother. He was born at home. Mum is concerned that he is vomiting and not feeding well. On questioning, his mother tells you that she cannot remember her child opening his bowels. On examination, the child appears grey, and his abdomen is distended and firm. He vomits forcefully when you palpate his abdomen.

21.13   A 6-week-old baby is brought to see you with increasing vomiting. His mother reports that he feeds very well and is always hungry. Initially he vomited small amounts after some feeds. Over the last week, he has had large vomits after every feed. On examination, the baby is alert and hungry but appears to have lost weight.

21.14   A 6-week-old baby has a history of vomiting. His mother reports that from the age of 1 week her child has vomited after almost every feed. He is distressed when he vomits and if he is laid flat after a feed. He is thriving and examination is unremarkable.

21.15   A 6-week-old baby has a history of vomiting. His mother reports that he vomits after feeds, two or three times a day. He is described as a hungry baby. He takes 300 ml every 3 hours during the day, having seven feeds in 24 hours. His weight is above the 99th centile. Examination is otherwise unremarkable.

Wheeze

21.16–21.19

Options

A   Anaphylaxis
B   Asthma
C   Bronchiolitis
D   Chronic lung disease
E   Croup
F   Cystic fibrosis
G   Foreign body inhalation
H   Primary ciliary dyskinesia
I   Recurrent aspiration
J   Viral wheeze

For each of the following clinical situations, choose the SINGLE MOST likely diagnosis from the options given above. Each option can be used once, more than once or not at all.

21.16   A 2-year-old child is brought to see you with sudden onset of wheeze and shortness of breath. The symptoms started when the child was at nursery this morning. She has been otherwise well. There is no significant past medical or family history. On examination, she is distressed, with mild subcostal recession; there is an audible wheeze. On auscultation, you can hear wheeze on the right side of the chest, with good air entry throughout.

21.17   A 20-month-old boy is brought to see you with respiratory distress. He has been unwell for 2 days with a runny nose, cough and reduced feeding. He is normally fit and well. On examination, the child is coryzal and has a temperature of 38.1°C. His respiratory rate is 32/min, with mild subcostal recession. Wheeze can be heard throughout the chest with good air entry. He has a blanching maculopapular rash on his trunk.

21.18   A 22-month-old boy is brought to see you by his mother. They have recently moved to the area. His mother tells you that he often needs antibiotics for his chest and that this is why she has brought him in now. On examination, the child is small and thin (weight and height are on the 0.4th centile) with visible Harrison's sulci. He has mild subcostal recession. Wheeze can be heard throughout the chest.

21.19   A 6-week-old baby is brought to see you with breathing difficulties. She was born at 33 weeks' gestation and was discharged home 2 weeks ago. She has a 24-hour history of fast, noisy breathing and reduced feeding and the mother thinks that she might have stopped breathing just now in the waiting room. On examination, there is subcostal recession and wheeze is heard bilaterally.

Telephone triage

21.20–21.26

Your practice is planning to use a telephone triage process for assessment of unwell children. You decide to base this on the NICE guidance CG47 *Feverish Illness in Children*, based on red, amber and green features of the child's illness.

Complete the flowchart below from the list of options. Each option may be used once, more than once or not at all.

Options

A   999 ambulance
B   All features green
C   Amber features present
D   Any red features
E   Face-to-face assessment
F   Manage at home
G   No
H   Urgent face-to-face assessment
I   Yes

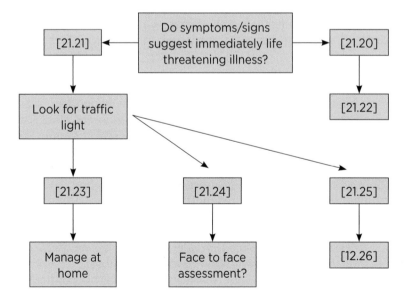

Vesicular rash in children

21.27–21.34

Options

A   Central dimple
B   Contact with disease
C   Crops of lesions
D   Face and hands
E   Limbs
F   May be seriously ill
G   No
H   Trunk
I   Yellow crusting
J   Yes

Complete the table below from the list of options listed above. Each option may be used once, more than once, or not at all.

	Fever	Malaise	Distribution	Pruritus?	Features
Chickenpox	Mild to moderate	Mild	Mainly truncal	Yes	[21.27] [21.28]
Dermatitis herpetiformis	No	No	[21.29]	[21.30]	Sporadic cases
Eczema herpeticum	Moderate to high	Moderate	In areas of eczema	[21.31]	[21.32]
Hand, foot and mouth disease	Mild	Mild	Palms, soles and inside mouth	No	Minor epidemics
Impetigo	No	No	Face and hands	Yes	Vesicles replaced by [21.33]
Molluscum contagiosum	Nil	Nil	Variable	No	Pearly vesicles with [21.34]

Free-text question

21.35   Drug dosage in children
A 5-month-old girl has a viral illness. You recommend ibuprofen at the dose advised in the *British National Formulary* of 30 mg/kg daily in three to four divided doses. She weighs 5 kg.

What is the maximum number of millilitres of ibuprofen suspension 100 mg/5 ml that she could take in a 24-hour period? Type your answer in the following text box. Use figures NOT words.

21.1   A: Admit under the on-call paediatrician

Spontaneous nosebleeds in infants are very rare and this presentation raises concerns over clotting disorders or non-accidental injury. Assessment by a paediatrician will rule out organic causes and allow assessment of possible abuse. Vitamin K-deficient bleeding would be unusual in a bottle-fed baby.

21.2   D: Refer to ophthalmology outpatients

Loss of red reflex can be a sign of congenital cataract or retinoblastoma. Congenital cataract is more likely than retinoblastoma in bilateral cases, although this can be bilateral. Causes of congenital cataract include maternal infection (eg rubella, varicella), hypercalcaemia, Down syndrome, myotonic dystrophy and Alport syndrome. Correction at an early age is necessary to avoid amblyopia.

21.3   C: Kawasaki's disease can cause myocardial infarction

Kawasaki's disease is a vasculitis of unknown origin. It causes a febrile illness in children aged under 5 years that is characterised by fever, polymorphous rash, cervical lymphadenopathy, conjunctival injection, and erythematous desquamation of the hands and feet. Up to a third of untreated patients will develop coronary artery stenosis and aneurysms, and these can lead to myocardial infarction. Treatment is with intravenous immunoglobulin and aspirin and, if aneurysms are found, this treatment should be lifelong. The mortality rate in the UK is <5%.

21.4   A: Drug or alcohol abuse

Risk factors for successful suicide after an episode of deliberate self-harm can be classified as relating to either the current episode or the background of the patient. Factors relating to the current episode that indicate high risk include efforts to avoid being found, planning, use of a dangerous method and refusal of help. Patients who have drug and/or alcohol problems, underlying mental illness or personality disorders, patients who are socially isolated or who have had previous episodes of deliberate self-harm, and older males are higher risk. Between 1% and 2% of patients who deliberately self-harm will be dead within 12 months, and 50% of those who die from suicide have taken a non-fatal overdose previously.

21.5   B: A 6-week-old boy has a temperature of 37.8°C and a cough. His mother reports that she observed him breathholding when sleeping. Examination is normal

Indications for admission to hospital for children with bronchiolitis include apnoea, saturation of <92%, respiratory distress, poor feeding, dehydration with no wet nappies in 12 hours or fluid intake <50–75% normal. At-risk patients should have a lower threshold for admission, eg chronic lung disease, prematurity or immunodeficiency.

21.6   B: A prolonged seizure is a risk factor for further prolonged attacks

A clinical review of febrile seizures in children was published in the *British Medical Journal* in 2007. Seizures can occur before the fever is apparent and can occur early or late in the course of the febrile illness. The fever is usually at least 38°C. In 87% of cases the seizure lasts less than 10 minutes and only 30% of children have recurrent febrile seizures during subsequent illnesses. Rigorous attempts to reduce the temperature with paracetamol or ibuprofen are not recommended because there is no evidence that this decreases recurrence of seizures. Parents should be reassured. Febrile status epilepticus occurs in 5% of affected children and a prolonged seizure is a risk factor for further prolonged attacks.

21.7   D: Septic arthritis

The features of refusal to weight bear and fever warrant immediate referral to rule out septic arthritis. Transient synovitis ('irritable hip') can also present in this way but is a diagnosis of exclusion. Slipped upper femoral epiphysis and Perthes' disease both affect older children. Acute myeloid leukaemia and Henoch–Schönlein purpura can both present with bone and joint pain, but it would be unusual for there to be no other features.

21.8   D: The boy should be followed up by the paediatric team for at least 6 months after the rash has resolved

Henoch–Schönlein purpura is a vasculitic disorder of unknown aetiology. The diagnosis is made clinically on the basis of a characteristic purpuric rash on the lower limbs and buttocks. The disease can affect many systems, most typically causing abdominal pain (which can be due to intussusception) and joint pain and swelling. Rare complications include seizures and strokes. The most common serious complication is renal disease. This occurs in 60% of cases and can progress to end-stage renal failure (1–2% of cases). Renal involvement can occur up to 6 months after the rash has disappeared. All children with Henoch–Schönlein purpura therefore require paediatric follow-up involving urine dipstick and BP monitoring for at least 6 months.

21.9   E: Refer for acute paediatric assessment

This child has acute laryngotracheobronchitis (croup). The presence of stridor at rest indicates that this child requires acute paediatric assessment and at least a period of observation in hospital. Treatment is with oral dexamethasone or nebulised budesonide. Clinical features that suggest at least moderate croup (requiring assessment and treatment in hospital) include: stridor at rest, subcostal recession, tachypnoea or altered conscious level/irritability. Cyanosis is a very late sign and is usually preceded by a period of significant respiratory distress.

21.10   A: Measles

This child has measles, which is a notifiable disease. It is highly infectious from 14 days before the rash appears to 5 days after the onset of the rash. Children are usually unwell, with a high fever. The rash usually starts on the face on day 3 or 4 of the illness, and spreads downwards. Koplik's spots are present before the onset of the rash and are consequently seen only rarely. There is no specific treatment for measles, although complications might require treatment. The illness usually lasts for 7–10 days and most children recover well. Serious complications include pneumonia, seizures, encephalitis, deafness, long-term neurological impairment and, in some cases, death.

21.11   B: Paediatric admission

This child has a rapidly increasing head circumference and symptoms of raised intracranial pressure. He needs to be seen urgently by a paediatrician. Physical signs associated with raised intracranial pressure in a baby can include dilated scalp veins, 'sun-setting' eyes and a bulging fontanelle, although these are usually late signs. A child should have a paediatric assessment if the head circumference crosses two centile lines, or is greater than the 98th centile and not in proportion with height and weight measurements. Children should be seen urgently if there is a rapid change in head circumference or associated physical symptoms or signs.

Vomiting

21.12   E: Hirschsprung's disease

Classically this presents in the neonatal period with failure to pass meconium within 24 hours and features of obstruction. It is caused by aganglionosis of the distal bowel. If only a small segment of large bowel is affected children can present several years later with chronic constipation. Diagnosis is made by rectal biopsy.

21.13   I: Pyloric stenosis

Caused by hypertrophy of the pyloric sphincter. Classically presents at 6 weeks with a preceding history of worsening vomiting as the pylorus becomes increasingly hypertrophied with use. Babies usually feed very well and are very hungry. Weight loss can be dramatic. Management includes stopping feeds, correction of electrolyte imbalance and surgical correction. The prognosis is very good.

21.14   C: Gastro-oesophageal reflux

Common in infancy, due to relatively poor muscle tone. Symptoms improve with age. This is due to stronger muscle tone, introduction of dietary solids and a more upright posture for the baby. In severe cases there can be failure to thrive and feeding aversion because of the distress associated with feeds. There are several management options:

- Keeping the child upright (no proven benefit)
- Propping up the head of the bed (no proven benefit)
- Thickening agents (proven benefit)
- Antacids, eg Gaviscon (no proven benefit)
- Ranitidine (proven benefit)
- Omeprazole and domperidone, often used but not licensed.

21.15   G: Overfeeding

Full-term babies normally require 150 ml/kg per day of milk. Particularly hungry babies might need more than this to settle them but volumes >200 ml/kg per day are not recommended. Overfeeding is common and often results in vomiting.

Wheeze

21.16   G: Foreign body inhalation

A sudden onset of respiratory distress in a child of 18 months to 3 years should raise the suspicion of an inhaled foreign body. If there is a suggestive history and/or unilateral clinical signs it is an important diagnosis to rule out. Urgent paediatric assessment is required.

21.17   J: Viral wheeze

Many children aged <3 years wheeze with viral infections. No treatment is usually necessary. A trial of salbutamol via inhaler and spacer can be given to children aged >1 year if respiratory distress is severe or if there is a strong family history of atopy.

21.18   F: Cystic fibrosis

Recurrent lower respiratory tract infections and poor weight gain warrant further investigation. The most likely diagnosis in the white population is cystic fibrosis. Other pathologies such as immunodeficiencies, congenital lung abnormalities and rarer causes of bronchiectasis such as primary ciliary dyskinesia should be considered if cystic fibrosis testing is negative.

21.19   C: Bronchiolitis

Bronchiolitis is a viral illness affecting infants aged <1 year. It is predominantly caused by respiratory syncytial virus (RSV). Clinical features include respiratory distress, wheeze, coryzal symptoms, low-grade temperature and reduced feeding. Treatment is supportive. Those under the age of 2 months, ex-premature babies and those with existing pathology (eg cardiac disease) are at particular risk and can develop apnoeas. Paluvizumab, a monoclonal antibody against RSV, is now available, although it is very expensive. It is currently offered to premature babies with significant lung disease and to some children with cardiac problems.

Telephone triage

21.20   I: Yes

21.21   G: No

21.22   A: 999 ambulance

21.23   B: All features green

21.24   C: Amber features present

21.25   D: Any red features

21.26   H: Urgent face-to-face assessment

Vesicular rash in children

21.27	B:	Contact with disease
21.28	C:	Crops of lesions
21.29	D:	Face and hands
21.30	J:	Yes
21.31	J:	Yes
21.32	F:	May be seriously ill
21.33	I:	Yellow crusting
21.34	A:	Central dimple

	Fever	Malaise	Distribution	Pruritus?	Features
Chickenpox	Mild to moderate	Mild	Mainly truncal	Yes	Contact with disease Crops of lesions
Dermatitis herpetiformis	No	No	Face and hands	Yes	Sporadic cases
Eczema herpeticum	Moderate to high	Moderate	In areas of eczema	Yes	May be seriously ill
Hand, foot and mouth disease	Mild	Mild	Palms, soles and inside mouth	No	Minor epidemics
Impetigo	No	No	Face and hands	Yes	Vesicles replaced by yellow crusting
Molluscum contagiosum	Nil	Nil	Variable	No	Pearly vesicles with central dimple

21.35   7.5 ml

The total 24-hour dose is 150 mg. This equates to 7.5 ml of 100 mg/5 ml suspension.

Section 2

Chapter 22
Research, statistics and epidemiology

Single best answer questions

22.1   **Statistical definitions**
Which ONE of the following best describes the term 'external validity'?
Select One option only.

○   A   The agreement between two raters using the same test at the same time

○   B   The consistency of a measure used on two separate occasions

○   C   The extent to which one can appropriately apply the results to other populations

○   D   The level of agreement between two or more raters using the same test on two or more separate occasions

○   E   The level of consistency between two separate halves of the same test

22.2   **Cohort study**
Which ONE of the following study designs most accurately describes a cohort study? Select ONE option only.

○   A   A study that aims to establish the normal height of 4-year-old children by measuring heights at school entry

○   B   A study that compares a group of children whose heights are below the 10th centile with a group of matched controls of normal height, aiming to identify possible causative factors

○   C   A study that compares two groups of 4-year-olds with similar characteristics: one group is given a drug and the other a placebo, and the growth of each group is measured after this intervention

○   D   A study that compares the height of a group of 4-year-olds living near a nuclear plant with the height of a group of 4-year-olds who live elsewhere

○   E   A study that looks at all children born at one hospital in 1 year and measures their height at intervals up to 4 years of age

22.3   Morbidity and mortality

You attend a presentation by the local public health team at which the data are presented on the top three causes of child deaths in your locality over the last 30 years. The data are presented below, with the most common cause of death first.

	1989	1999	2009
First	Trauma	Trauma	Neoplasm
Second	Infection	Neoplasm	Trauma
Third	Neoplasm	Infection	Infection

Which ONE of the following statements is correct with regard to these data? Select ONE option only.

○   A   No conclusions can be drawn on changes in incidence

○   B   The data confirm that child mortality is falling

○   C   The data suggest that the incidence of childhood cancer is increasing

○   D   The data suggest that the incidence of serious accidents is falling

○   E   The decrease in mortality from infection reflects increased immunisation coverage

22.4   Alcohol and mortality

Consider the graph below, which shows alcohol consumption and all-cause mortality.

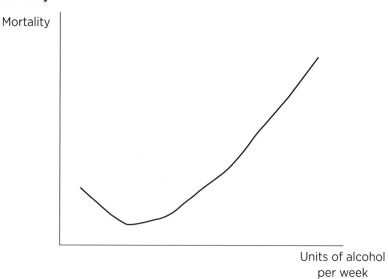

Which ONE of the following is a correct interpretation of this graph? Select ONE option only.

○ A   Alcohol in moderate doses is beneficial to health

○ B   Avoidance of alcohol is more dangerous than moderate consumption

○ C   Heavy drinkers who reduce their alcohol consumption can reduce their risk of dying

○ D   There is no question that high levels of alcohol consumption increase mortality

○ E   These data demonstrate an association rather than a causal relationship

22.5 **Epidemiology**
The graph below shows the standardised (for age, sex and ethnic group) incidence ratios of three different cancers in patients followed up for 10 years after exposure to a potential carcinogen.

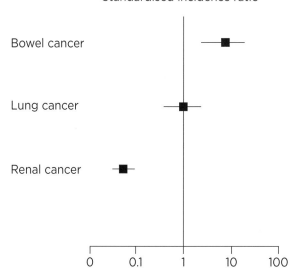

Standardised incidence ratio

Which ONE of the following statements is correct with regard to interpretation of these data? Select ONE option only.

○ A   The confidence intervals for all three cancers are wide so there might not be a true increase in incidence

○ B   The incidence of all three cancers is increased

○ C   The incidence of bowel cancer is increased, whereas the incidence of renal cancer is reduced

○ D   The incidence of renal cancer is increased, whereas the incidence of bowel cancer is reduced in this cohort of patients

○ E   These data confirm that the chemical causes cancer

22.6 Interpretation of symptom scores

After a 6-month pilot project to assess the impact of a nurse practitioner on the management of prostatic symptoms in primary care, the following results for cost and impact on mean symptom score are presented:

	Cost per patient (£)			Symptom score		
	Nurse practitioner care	Standard care	Difference	Intervention	Standard care	Difference
Baseline	0	0	0	5	5	0
6 months	200	100	100	1	3	-2

Which ONE of the following is correct with regard to the cost-effectiveness of this service compared with standard care? Select ONE option only.

○ A   The additional cost per unit change in symptom score is £200

○ B   The additional cost per unit change in symptom score is £100

○ C   The additional cost per unit change in symptom score is £50

○ D   The data suggest that the intervention is cost-effective

○ E   There is a net reduction in costs

22.7 Drug safety data

A study is carried out into drug use in the 3 months before an admission with acute upper gastrointestinal bleeding. The results of this are shown below.

	Drug A	Drug B	Ulcer-healing drugs
Incidence of gastrointestinal bleeding (odds ratio)	2.1	1.9	3.4

Based on these data, which ONE of the following are valid conclusions? Select ONE option only.

○ A   Drug A is more likely to cause gastrointestinal bleeding than drug B

○ B   Drug B is more likely to cause gastrointestinal bleeding than drug A

○ C   These results are not statistically significant

○ D   The use of ulcer-healing drugs is likely to be a confounding variable

○ E   Ulcer-healing drugs are a proven cause of gastrointestinal bleeding

22.8 **Fracture prevention**
Your practice is reviewing the prescribing of calcium and vitamin D in patients at risk of fracture. You decide to look into the data on fracture prevention with different preparations and come across the following data from the DIPART group (*British Medical Journal* 2010;340:b5463).

All trials	0.95 (0.09 to 1.01)
Calcium/D trials	0.92 (0.86 to 0.99)
Vitamin D trials	1.01 (0.92 to 1.12)

0.5   1.0   1.5

Risk of fracture (hazard ratio)

Which ONE of the following is a correct interpretation of these results? Select ONE option only.

○ A   Calcium alone will lead to a statistically significant reduction in fractures

○ B   Co-administration of calcium and vitamin D is necessary to prevent fractures

○ C   Meta-analysis of all trials of calcium and vitamin D confirm efficacy in preventing fractures

○ D   Vitamin D alone will prevent fractures

○ E   Vitamin D use is associated with a statistically significant increase in the risk of fracture

22.9   Mortality in diabetes

Consider the following data from a study of mortality and mean HbA1c levels:

Hazard ratio

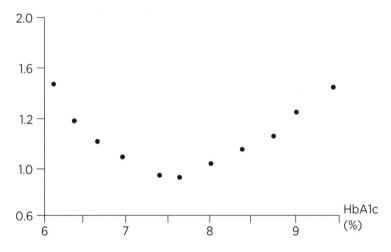

Which ONE of the following is a correct interpretation of these data? Select ONE option only.

○   A   An HbA1c of 7.5% is associated with the highest mortality

○   B   An HbA1c of 7.5% is associated with the lowest mortality

○   C   Intensive glycaemic control is associated with lower mortality

○   D   Intensive glycaemic control is associated with lower morbidity

○   E   There is a direct relationship between glycaemic control and mortality

22.10 **Diet treatment in sleep apnoea**
A trial carried out to assess the impact of a very-low-energy diet on moderate and severe sleep apnoea in obese men (*British Medical Journal* 2009;339:b4609) gives the results below after a 9-week period:

	Intervention	Control	Mean difference	P
Apnoea:hypopnoea index (AHI)	–25	–2	–23 (–30 to –15)	<0.001
Weight (kg)	–18.7	1.1	–19.8 (–21.4 to –18.2)	<0.001

Which ONE of the following statements about these data is correct? Select ONE option only.

O A The intervention improved daytime symptoms

O B The intervention improved night-time symptoms

O C The results suggest that weight loss is an effective treatment for snoring

O D Weight loss provides lasting relief of symptoms

O E Weight loss reduces long-term complications of sleep apnoea

22.11 **Qualitative research**
Your commissioning group decides to audit its nurse-led, walk-in centre. It carries this out by doing semi-structured interviews with a nurse practitioner who works in the clinic. She selects 50 patients over a 4-week period and assesses their satisfaction with various aspects of their care. The results are shown below:

Number of patients completing the interview = 50
Number of patients expressing overall satisfaction = 49
Number of patients who found that the visit satisfied their needs = 49
Number of patients who, when asked, felt that their visit was superior to normal GP care = 44

The group announce that on the basis of these results they will introduce more walk-in centres. Which ONE of the following statements is true with regard to the validity of this study? Select ONE option only.

O A Extremely high satisfaction rates suggest inclusion bias

O B This methodology is a bias-free method of collecting data

O C The data confirm that nurse-led care is superior to GP care

O D The methodology is designed to ensure a representative range of participants

O E This study is a quantitative study

22.12 Drug treatment in arthritis

The results of a trial of treatment for arthritis with drug X compared with ibuprofen are shown below (CI confidence interval; WOMAC Western Ontario and McMaster Universities Index of Osteoarthritis):

Mean reduction in WOMAC score after 4 weeks:
Patients taking drug X = 2.4 (95% CI 1.7–2.6, $P = 0.66$)
Patients taking ibuprofen = 1.8 (95% CI 1.6–2.2, $P = 0.57$)

Cumulative incidence of gastrointestinal side effects after 4 weeks:
Patients taking drug X = 6% (95% CI 3.0–8.4%, $P = 0.04$)
Patients taking ibuprofen = 4% (95% CI 2.2–5.4%, $P = 0.05$)

Which ONE of the following statements about these data is true?

○ A   Drug X has a significantly greater anti-inflammatory effect than ibuprofen

○ B   Drug X has a superior long- and short-term safety profile

○ C   Drug X improves quality of life to a much greater extent than ibuprofen

○ D   Drug X is significantly safer than ibuprofen

○ E   The reductions in WOMAC scores are not statistically significant

22.13 Screening tests

A new test to screen for cystic fibrosis carriers is being considered. Preliminary results for the test in 100 children, in comparison with the gold standard of chromosome analysis, are shown below.

	Gold standard	
	Positive chromosome analysis	Negative chromosome analysis
New test positive	4	8
New test negative	1	87

Based on this information, which ONE of the following claims about the new test is correct? Select ONE option only.

○ A   The accuracy of the test is 91%

○ B   The new test is better than the gold standard test

○ C   The positive predictive value is 80%

○ D   The sensitivity is 96%

○ E   The specificity is 87%

22.14 **Population studies**
Consider the graph below, which summarises the relative risk of
macrosomia for pregnant diabetic mothers according to the 20-week
fasting glucose levels:

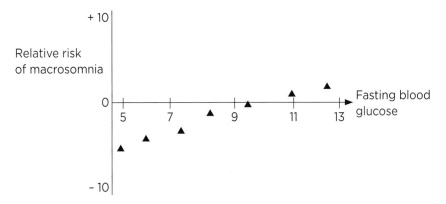

Which ONE of the following statements is true with regard to the
interpretation of these data? Select ONE option only.

○ A   Caesarean section is significantly more likely in diabetic women

○ B   Gestational diabetes is becoming more common with time

○ C   Glucose levels <10 mmol/l are never associated with macrosomia

○ D   Low blood sugar levels are associated with small babies, ie intrauterine
        growth retardation

○ E   Tight control of blood sugar reduces the risk of macrosomia

22.15 Treatment efficacy
A new statin has just been launched with the following advertisement:

'Lowers death rate from myocardial infarction by 33%'

Closer inspection of the original paper reveals the following data:

Number of patients in treatment arm = 200

Number of patients in control arm = 200

Number of patients experiencing MI in treatment arm = 6

Number of patient experiencing MI in the control arm = 7

Number of patients who die as a result of MI in the treatment arm = 4

Number of patients who die as a result of MI in the control arm = 6

Which ONE of the following statements about these data is true? Select ONE option only.

- ○ A The absolute risk reduction for death by MI is 33%
- ○ B The number needed to harm with the new drug is 100
- ○ C The number needed to treat (NNT) with the new drug to prevent one death from MI is 3
- ○ D The NNT with the new drug to prevent one MI is 200
- ○ E The relative risk reduction for MI is 33%

22.16   Diagnostic tests

A trial is conducted to determine which symptoms and signs have the most impact on the diagnosis of pneumonia in patients with respiratory symptoms presenting in primary care. The results are presented below:

Symptom/sign	Likelihood ratio for diagnosis
Fever	0.94
Cough	1.00
Abnormal chest examination	1.25
Tachypnoea	1.34
Otalgia	0.07

Which ONE of the following statements with regard to these results is true? Select ONE option only.

○ A   An abnormal chest examination increases the probability that a patient has pneumonia by 25%

○ B   Tachypnoea has a negative association with the diagnosis of pneumonia

○ C   The presence of cough increases the likelihood that a patient has pneumonia by 100%

○ D   The presence of fever makes the diagnosis of pneumonia more likely in patients with respiratory disease

○ E   These results allow the diagnosis of pneumonia to be made without examining the patient

22.17   Homeopathic studies

A trial is conducted of blood pressure treatment with homeopathic remedies. One group of patients is treated with homeopathic treatment whereas the other group has no treatment. Both groups are monitored by a nurse for BP and side effects at monthly intervals. The data are shown below:

	Number of patients with raised BP in the homeopathy group	Number of patients with raised BP in the control group
Baseline	100	100
1 month	75	85
3 months	74	83
6 months	72	84
12 months	75	87

Which ONE of the following statements is a correct interpretation of these results? Select ONE option only.

○   A   Homeopathy has a statistically significant effect on BP

○   B   Homeopathy is well tolerated

○   C   The results in the control group are due to the Hawthorne effect

○   D   These data suggest that the effect of homeopathy on BP is purely a placebo effect

○   E   This trial is a randomised, double-blind, controlled trial and the results are therefore 'gold standard'

22.18 Kaplan–Meier plots

Consider the Kaplan–Meier survival plot below, taken from a paper comparing the use of a novel treatment for osteoarthritis with conventional treatment. The end-point in the trial was the need for joint replacement.

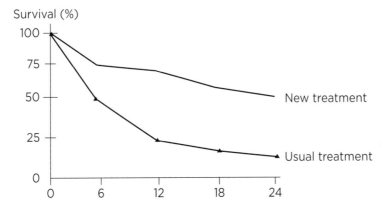

Which ONE of the following statements about these data is true? Select ONE option only.

○ A   At 12 months 75% of the usual treatment group have died

○ B   At 6 months 50% of the new treatment group have had joint surgery

○ C   At 12 months a patient receiving the usual treatment is three times as likely to have had surgery as a patient on the new treatment

○ D   The flattening off of the curves in later months shows that the effects of the treatments wear off with time

○ E   The new treatment is better tolerated than the usual treatment

22.19 Meta-analysis

The results of a meta-analysis comparing drug A with drug B are shown below:

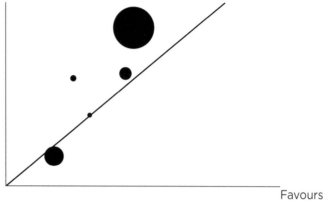

Which ONE of the following statements about these data is true? Select ONE option only.

O   A   As some of trial data cross the line of no effect, larger trials are needed to determine the true effect

O   B   The majority of the trials suggest that drug B is favourable

O   C   There is no difference between drug A and drug B

O   D   The results unequivocally support drug A

O   E   The size of the circles represents the size of individual trials

22.20 Relative risk
A study compares the suicide risk in adolescents and adults who are taking two different classes of antidepressants. The standardised incidence of suicide is shown in the table below:

	Number of suicides in patients on drug A	Number of suicides in patients on drug B
Adolescents	150	100
Adults	50	100

Which ONE of the following statements with regard to these data is correct? Select ONE option only.

○ A The relative risk (RR) of suicide for drug A in adolescents compared with drug B is 1.5

○ B The RR of suicide for drug A in adolescents compared with drug B is 3

○ C The RR of suicide for drug A compared with drug B in adults is 2

○ D The RR of suicide for drug A compared with drug B is higher for adults than for adolescents

○ E The results show a clear association with suicide for both drugs

22.21 Screening
A study looks at the association between certain symptoms and a disease to see if any of these are useful as a screening tool. The following results are obtained:

	Number with symptom	Number without symptom
Patients with disease	60	40
Patients without disease	40	60

What is the likelihood ratio that a patient with the symptom will have the disease? Select ONE option only.

○ A 0.66

○ B 1.5

○ C 40%

○ D 60%

○ E 100%

22.22 Mortality in the UK

Select the rank order of the options (1–4) that best fulfils the requirements given in the question. The following is a list of causes of death in the UK (options 1–4):

1   Cancer
2   Circulatory disease
3   Mental and behavioural illness
4   Respiratory disease

The responses (A–E) rank the causes of death options in various orders. Select the response that places the options (1–4) in the order of least common cause of death first to the most common cause of death last. Select one rank order only.

○ A: 2, 4, 3, 1

○ B: 2, 3, 1, 4

○ C: 3, 4, 2, 1

○ D: 3, 2, 4, 1

○ E: 3, 1, 2, 4

22.23 Epidemiology

Over a 6-month period, your practice diagnoses scarlet fever in 60 children under the age of 10. The number of patients registered at the practice aged <10 years is 1000 out of a total list size of 10 000. Which ONE of the following is CORRECT with regard to these data? Select ONE option only.

○ A   The incidence of scarlet fever in the under-10 age group is 6/1000 per year

○ B   The incidence of scarlet fever in the under-10 age group is 60/1000 per year

○ C   The incidence of scarlet fever in the under-10 age group is 60/10 000 per year

○ D   The incidence of scarlet fever in the under-10 age group is 120/1000 per year

○ E   The incidence of scarlet fever in the under-10 age group is 120/10 000 per year

22.24 Cancer survival

The graph below shows trends in 10-year survival for five common cancers in the UK, between 1971 and 2007.

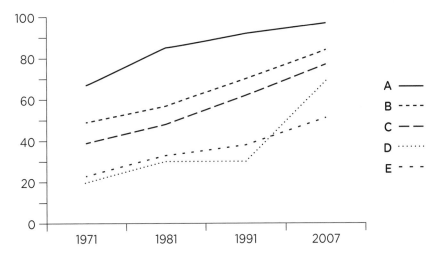

A   Breast
B   Colon
C   Melanoma
D   Prostate
E   Testis

Place each of the cancers listed above in the table below, to indicate which line on the graph represents that cancer. All FIVE must be correctly matched to score ONE mark.

Data	Cancer
A	
B	
C	
D	
E	

22.25 Interpreting test results

A new test is proposed to diagnose coeliac disease, compared to the gold standard of intestinal biopsy. The likelihood ratio is calculated for the test. Which ONE of the following statements is CORRECT with regard to likelihood ratios? Select ONE option only.

○ A   If the likelihood ratio = 1, a positive test result is associated with the presence of the disease

○ B   If the likelihood ratio <1, a positive test result is associated with the presence of the disease

○ C   A likelihood ratio of 0.1 suggests a positive test is strongly associated with the presence of the disease

○ D   A likelihood ratio of 10 suggests a positive test is strongly associated with the presence of the disease

○ E   None of the above

22.26 Testing for disease

The prevalence of a disease in the general population is 3%. A blood test can confirm the diagnosis with a 99% sensitivity and specificity. An audit of patients presenting with symptoms, who are then tested with the blood test, finds that 25% of patients with that symptom are confirmed as having the disease. Which ONE of the following statements is CORRECT with regard to the blood test for this disease? Select ONE option only.

○ A   The pre-test probability in asymptomatic patients is 3%

○ B   The pre-test probability in asymptomatic patients is 25%

○ C   The pre-test probability in symptomatic patients is 99%

○ D   The post-test probability in asymptomatic patients is 3%

○ E   None of the above

Multiple best answer questions

22.27 and 22.28   Population screening

Which TWO of the following are Wilson and Jungner criteria for population screening? Select TWO options only.

○ A   Case finding should be a one-off process

○ B   Costs involved in screening and treating positives should be equal or less than the cost of treating the disease

○ C   Population screening should be used only for fatal disease

○ D   The screening test should be non-invasive

○ E   There should be a recognised latent phase

Free-text questions

22.29 **Meta-analysis**

The graph below shows the results of a meta-analysis of studies of a putative risk factor for stroke.

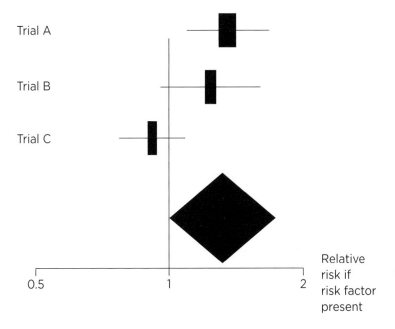

In the box below, write a best estimate for the relative risk of stroke for patients with the risk factor.

22.30 and 22.31 Statistical calculations

A trial is conducted to look at the benefits of a new treatment to reduce stroke. Data from the trial are shown below.

	Treatment arm	Control arm	Total
Number of strokes	20	40	60
Number not suffering strokes	80	60	140
Number of patients suffering side effects	2	1	3
Total in group	100	100	

Part A

What is the number needed to treat (NNN) to prevent one stroke?

Write your answer in the box below, in figures.

Part B

What is the number needed to harm (NNH)?

Write your answer in the box below, in figures.

22.32 and 22.33   Predictive values

An audit is carried out to determine how accurate dipstick testing is at diagnosing urine infection. All urine specimens were tested by dipstick and then sent for culture. The results are shown below:

	Dipstick positive	Dipstick negative
Urine culture positive	60	30
Urine culture negative	40	70

Part A

What is the positive predictive value of dipstick testing for the diagnosis of urine infection? Write the answer in the box below, in figures, as a percentage.

Part B

What is the negative predictive value of dipstick testing for the exclusion of urine infection? Write the answer in the box below, in figures, as a percentage.

22.34 and 22.35   Case–control studies

A study looks at whether a new vaccine has resulted in an increase in neurological side effects. The results are shown below.

	Side effects	No side effects	Total
Vaccinated	20	500	520
Not vaccinated	2	1000	1002
Totals	22	1500	

Part A

Calculate the odds ratio for people who have been vaccinated developing neurological side effects. Write your answer in the box below, in figures.

Part B

Which ONE of the following statements is CORRECT with regard to this result? Select ONE option only.

○ A   It is not possible to determine whether there is an increase or a decrease in the risk of side effects from these data

○ B   There is a significant increase in side effects in the control group

○ C   There is a significant increase in side effects in the treatment group

○ D   There is no significant difference between treatment and control groups

○ E   None of the above

22.36–22.39   Analysing trial data

A trial is conducted of a new treatment for the secondary prevention of myocardial infarction. A trial has been carried out, for 5 years, of 1000 patients who had had a myocardial infarction; 500 patients were randomly allocated to standard care and 500 were allocated the new treatment. Analysis was on an intention-to-treat basis.

After 5 years the following results were obtained:

Usual treatment arm
Number of patients at enrolment = 500
Number of heart attacks during 5-year period = 75
Number of deaths during 5-year period = 50
Number of patients remaining in study at 5 years = 427

New treatment arm
Number of patients at enrolment = 500
Number of heart attacks during 5-year period = 50
Number of deaths during 5-year period = 73
Number of patients remaining in study at 5 years = 387

Part A

What is the absolute risk reduction (ARR) for myocardial infarction with the new treatment, compared with standard treatment? Write your answer in the box below, in figures, as a percentage.

Part B

What is the relative risk reduction (RRR) for myocardial infarction with the new treatment, compared with the standard treatment? Write your answer in the box below, in figures, as a percentage.

Part C

Which ONE of the following is a valid conclusion, drawn from the data above? Select ONE option ONLY.

- O A These data confirm that the new treatment is a safe and effective treatment for the secondary prevention of myocardial infarction
- O B These data suggest that the new treatment is better tolerated than the usual treatment
- O C These data suggest that the new treatment may be associated with significant adverse outcomes
- O D These data suggest that the new treatment significantly reduces cardiac deaths compared with the usual treatment
- O E None of the above

Part D

What is the NNT for the new treatment compared with the standard treatment? Write your answer, in figures, in the box below.

22.40 and 22.41   Screening tests

A new blood test is designed to screen for deep vein thrombosis. Patients who screen positive with the blood test have confirmation with a Doppler ultrasound scan. The results of a trial are shown below:

- 100 patients test positive on the blood test; of these 75 had a DVT on the ultrasound scan, whereas 25 did not

- 100 patients test negative on the blood test; of these 10 had a DVT on the ultrasound scan, whereas 90 did not

Part A

What is the percentage sensitivity of this test in diagnosing DVT? Write the answer in the box below, in figures, as a percentage.

Part B

What is the percentage specificity of this test in diagnosing DVT? Write the answer in the box below, in figures, as a percentage.

22.1   C: The extent to which one can appropriately apply the results to other populations

Answer B describes test–retest reliability, answer E is split-half reliability, answer A is inter-rater reliability and answer D describes intra-rater reliability.

22.2   C: A study that compares two groups of 4-year-olds with similar characteristics: one group is given a drug and the other a placebo, and the growth of each group is measured after this intervention

Study A is a cross-sectional study, study B is a case–control study, study C is a cohort study, study D is a controlled trial and study E is a longitudinal study.

22.3   A: No conclusions can be drawn on changes in incidence

The table shows relative incidence only, rather than absolute incidence. The decrease of trauma from first place in 1999 to second place in 2009 could be due to a fall in absolute incidence of trauma, but could also represent an increase in the incidence of neoplasms.

22.4   E: These data demonstrate an association rather than a causal relationship

These data appear to suggest that there is an association between mortality and alcohol consumption. It is not possible to say, however, that this is a causal relationship because of the need to remove confounding variables. Alcohol consumption could be a cause of increased mortality but it could equally be a surrogate marker for an unhealthy lifestyle. Drinkers are more likely to be obese and smokers, and take little exercise. There is also a possible confounding effect of class because alcohol consumption varies with social class. The graph is a population survey and does not give information on longitudinal outcomes, so conclusions cannot be made on the effects of changing consumption for individuals.

22.5   C: The incidence of bowel cancer is increased, whereas the incidence of renal cancer is reduced

Standardised incidence ratios (SIRs) compare the incidence of a condition in a patient under study with that of 'equivalent' patients. An SIR of 1.0 suggests that the incidence is the same as in an unexposed population. An SIR >1.0 suggests an increased risk, whereas an SIR <1.0 suggests a reduced risk. The results of studies like this suggest association rather than confirm causation.

22.6   C: The additional cost per unit change in symptom score is £50

The intervention produces a reduction in average symptom score of 4 points, whereas standard care reduces the symptom score by 2 points, a difference of 2. The intervention cost, however, is £100 more per patient, making the cost per additional point reduction £50. These data cannot be used alone to judge the cost-effectiveness of an intervention because this requires agreement of an acceptable cost per improvement in symptom control, which commissioners and patients would need to agree. There is a net increase in costs.

22.7   D: The use of ulcer-healing drugs is likely to be a confounding variable

Patients at high risk of upper gastrointestinal bleeding will often use ulcer-healing drugs because of previous bleeding or the development of new symptoms. The finding that the use of these drugs is three times more common in those admitted with an acute gastrointestinal bleed is therefore not unexpected, and use of ulcer-healing drugs is likely to be a confounding variable. There is unlikely to be a significant difference between drug A and drug B, although no comment can be made without information on confidence intervals and P values.

22.8   B: Co-administration of calcium and vitamin D is necessary to prevent fractures

The data suggest that trials of vitamin D alone show a non-significant increase in the risk of fracture, whereas calcium and vitamin D in combination will reduce fractures and this finding is statistically significant. There are no trials of calcium alone in the data so conclusions cannot be drawn about this. Meta-analysis of all trials shows a non-significant reduction in fracture rate.

22.9   B: An HbA1c of 7.5% is associated with the lowest mortality

These data show a U-shaped association between HbA1c levels and mortality, with the lowest mortality associated with an HbA1c around 7.5%, whereas higher mortality is associated with very low and very high HbA1c levels. Hazard ratios are higher in patients at higher risk of an outcome, in this case mortality, so the lowest mortality is associated with the lowest point on the graph. These data apply only to mortality, so conclusions on morbidity cannot be made. Again, conclusions on causation of this effect cannot be made because these data reflect all-cause mortality and this could include death from hypoglycaemic attack as well as from diabetic ketoacidosis.

22.10   B: The intervention improved night-time symptoms

Obstructive sleep apnoea causes night-time symptoms of apnoea and wakening, which can be quantified with the apnoea:hypopnoea index (AHI), and daytime fatigue, which is assessed with the Epworth score. This study measured effect of a very-low-energy diet on the AHI rather than on the Epworth score. It is assumed that daytime symptoms correlate with night-time symptom severity, and it could therefore be assumed that daytime symptoms are improved, but that has not been measured as an outcome in this trial. The data are measured only after 9 weeks and no long-term conclusions can be drawn. Snoring is a clinical entity that is distinct from sleep apnoea and it is not possible to draw conclusions on the effects of this intervention on snoring on the basis of these data. There are no outcome measures relating to complications in this study.

22.11 A: Extremely high satisfaction rates suggest inclusion bias

Qualitative studies are fraught with methodological difficulties and should be used only in appropriate studies, eg when canvassing opinions that cannot be quantified as hard data. Semi-structured interviews are frequently used but the study needs to be well designed to avoid reporting bias or leading questions. Patients should, however, still be selected on a structured basis to ensure that participants are representative of the wider population and not selected on a whim, resulting in inclusion bias. A suitable model might be to enrol every third patient. Ideally, the people working in the clinic should not be aware that they are being audited to avoid 'playing up' to the study. The opinions of patients with regard to their experience of care cannot be extrapolated to determine whether one form of care is superior to another because this was not studied.

22.12 E: The reductions in WOMAC scores are not statistically significant

The reductions in WOMAC scores (a quantitative assessment of symptoms and handicap) show a benefit for drug X but the 95% confidence interval is wide and the limits overlap those of ibuprofen, with P values >0.05, meaning that the results do not achieve statistical significance. The results for gastrointestinal side effects also overlap but P for drug X is 0.04 (ie the true result is likely to lie in the range 3.0–8.4); again, these 95% CIs overlap those of ibuprofen and it cannot be said that there is a true difference between the two groups. A larger study would have greater power to detect these small differences. No long-term safety data are presented here, so no conclusions can be drawn in this area.

22.13 A: The accuracy of the test is 91%

	Gold standard	
	Positive	Negative
New test positive	a	b
New test negative	c	d

Accuracy is the proportion of tests that have given the correct result, ie
$(a + d)/(a + b + c + d)$, so 91/100 = 91%.

Sensitivity is the true-positive rate, ie
$a/(a + c)$, so 4/5 = 80%.

Specificity is the true-negative rate, ie
$d/(b + d)$, so 87/95 = 92%.

Positive predictive value is the probability of having the condition, once the test is positive, ie
$a/(a + b)$, so 4/12 = 33%.

Negative predictive value is the probability of not having the condition, once the test is negative, ie
$d/(c + d)$, so 87/88 = 99%.

22.14   E: Tight control of blood sugar reduces the risk of macrosomia

These data support a link between the risk of large babies and fasting blood glucose levels. Large babies are associated with difficult labour and probably with increased caesarean section rates, but that observation cannot be confirmed from these data. Similarly, a low risk of macrosomia is not the same as a high risk of intrauterine growth retardation, because this would be based on an assumption that the same disease mechanisms apply to both clinical situations. These data do suggest an association between fasting glucose at 20 weeks and macrosomia, so it is reasonable to conclude that tight control of sugar will reduce macrosomia. These data do not provide any time frame, however, so no conclusions on incidence can be made.

22.15   D: The NNT with the new drug to prevent one MI is 200

The number needed to harm cannot be calculated from these data as no adverse outcome data are presented. The results are therefore:

ARR for death by MI = 3% – 2% = 1%
ARR for all MI = 3.5% – 3% = 0.5%
NNT for prevention of death by MI = 1/0.01 = 100
NNT for all MI = 1/0.005 = 200
RRR for death by MI = 1/3 = 33%

22.16   A: An abnormal chest examination increases the probability that a patient has pneumonia by 25%

Likelihood ratios are used to determine the impact of a finding on the outcome. The results are expressed as a ratio: a score of 1 makes both outcomes (presence or absence of disease) equally likely, whereas a likelihood ratio >1 makes the diagnosis more likely and a likelihood ratio <1 makes the diagnosis less likely. In these results the presence of otalgia and fever have likelihood ratios of <1, making them unhelpful in differentiating pneumonia from other infections, but the presence of tachypnoea and abnormal chest examination have likelihood ratios of >1, making a diagnosis of pneumonia more likely. Cough alone has a likelihood ratio of 1.00, making a diagnosis neither more nor less likely, meaning that it is unhelpful in excluding or confirming a diagnosis.

22.17   C: The results in the control group are due to the Hawthorne effect

The control group have no treatment but are monitored. The phenomenon whereby observed outcomes improve merely as a result of being observed is called the 'Hawthorne effect' and is a form of placebo effect. The data presented do not provide any indication of statistical significance or tolerability. This trial is not blinded in any way.

22.18   C: At 12 months a patient receiving the usual treatment is three times as likely to have had surgery as a patient on the new treatment

The Kaplan–Meier curves demonstrate the proportion of patients who have not met the endpoint, meaning survival without treatment rather than true survival. The rate of decline in the new treatment group is slower than in the usual treatment group, implying that this treatment protects patients from reaching the end-point of joint replacement. The flattening of the curves later on in the trial suggests that those patients who need surgery will have it early on. The study does not measure side effects, so no comment can be made on tolerability. At 12 months, 25% of the new treatment group have had surgery, compared with 75% of the usual treatment group.

22.19   E: The size of the circles represents the size of individual trials

This is a L'Abbé plot. Each circle represents a trial and the size of each circle represents the size of the trial. The line bisecting the plot is the 'line of no effect'. Data to the right favour drug B and to the left favour drug A. The further away from the line the more significant the effect, so circles crossing the line do not show a net effect.

22.20   A: The relative risk (RR) of suicide for drug A in adolescents compared with drug B is 1.5

The relative risk is the number of events in the treatment group divided by the number of events in the control group. In this example drug A has a higher RR of suicide in adolescents than drug B but in adults the RR is lower (1.5 in adolescents versus 0.5 in adults). No inference can be made as to causation because there is no true control group in this study, ie the rate in a control group might be higher than both groups if both drugs reduce suicide but by differing degrees.

22.21   B: 1.5

The likelihood ratio is the ratio of the probability that an individual with the target condition has a specified symptom (or test result) to the probability that an individual without the target condition has the same specified symptom. It is used to determine the validity of association between symptoms or tests and disease, eg headache and brain tumour. In this example the probability that the individual with the symptom has the condition is 60%, whereas the probability that a patient with the symptom does not have the condition is 40%. The likelihood ratio is therefore 60/40 or 1.5.

22.22   C: 3, 4, 2, 1

Rank ordering: 3 Mental and behavioural illness; 4 Respiratory disease; 2 Circulatory disease; 1 Cancer

The Office for National Statistics records data on causes of death in the UK. Cancer is the leading cause, with circulatory disease a close second.

22.23   D: The incidence of scarlet fever in the <10 age group is 120 per 1000 per year

Incidence is the number of new cases diagnosed in a given period of time for a given proportion. It is usually expressed as an annual rate for a specified number of patients.

Number of cases in 6 months = 60

Annualised number of cases = 60 × 2 = 120

Target population (<10 years old) = 1000

Incidence = 120/1000 per year

Incidence can also be expressed as a percentage, ie

Incidence (%) = 100% × 120/100

Incidence = 12%

The key issue is to ensure that the time period and target population are specified correctly.

22.24

Data	Cancer
A	Testis
B	Melanoma
C	Breast
D	Prostate
E	Colon

22.25   D: A likelihood ratio of 10 suggests that a positive test is strongly associated with the presence of the disease

Likelihood ratio = probability of a positive result being found in patients with disease/probability of a positive result being found in patients without disease. It can be calculated from the sensitivity and specificity of a test, according to whether the test is being used to rule in or rule out a disease.

Likelihood ratio for a positive test result = sensitivity/(1 − specificity)

Likelihood ratio for a negative test result = (1 − sensitivity)/specificity

A likelihood ratio of 1 suggests no association, either positive or negative. A likelihood ratio <1 suggests a negative association and >1 a positive association. A likelihood ratio of 0.1 or 10 suggests a strong positive or negative association.

22.26   A: The pre-test probability in asymptomatic patients is 3%

Pre-test probability is the likelihood that a test will be positive in a population. If asymptomatic, ie they are being screened rather than diagnosed, the pre-test probability will be approximately the same as the prevalence in the general population. Symptomatic patients have a higher risk than the general population, 25% in this example, so the pre-test probability in this group will be nearer 25%. The post-test probability depends on the likelihood ratio for that test and cannot be calculated without a normogram, and knowledge of both the pre-test probability and the likelihood ratio for that test and that condition.

22.27 and 22.28   Population screening
B: Costs involved in screening and treating positives should be equal or less than the cost of treating the disease;
E: There should be a recognised latent phase

The original Wilson and Jungner criteria for population screening state that: the condition sought should be an important health problem; there should be an accepted treatment for the disease; facilities for diagnosis and treatment should be available; there should be a recognisable latent phase; there should be a suitable screening test acceptable to the population; the natural history should be understood; there should be consensus on who to treat as patients; costs of case finding and treating cases should compare well with costs of treating the disease; and case finding should be a continuing process. The criteria have since been expanded to include a need for a defined population with equity of access, ongoing education, and quality assurance with informed choice and respect for autonomy. Above all, the benefits of screening should outweigh the harms.

22.29   1.4

The pooled studies shown in the lozenge give a peak risk at around 1.4, ie patients with the risk factor are 1.4 times as likely to have a stroke as patients without the risk factor. The individual studies give inconclusive results but the pooled studies give a positive result with the lower 95% CI >1, suggesting a true-positive result.

22.30 and 22.31   Statistical calculations

Part A   5

The NNT or NNH is given by the formula:

NNT = 1/(control event rate − experimental event rate)

The control event rate (CER) = number of strokes in control group/number of participants in that group:

CER = 40/100 = 0.4

The experimental event rate (EER) = number of strokes in treatment group/number of participants in that group:

EER = 20/100 = 0.2

Therefore NNT = 1/(0.4 − 0.2)

= 1/0.2

This gives the answer: NNT = 5

Part B 100

To calculate the NNH the same formula is used, with the rate of side effects rather than the rate of strokes. This time, however, the sum is reversed because the increase in side effects is calculated rather than the reduction in events:

NNH = 1/(experimental side effect rate – control side effect rate)

The control side effect rate or CER = number of side effects in control group/ number of

CER = 1/100
CER = 0.01

The experimental side effect rate or EER = number of side effects in treatment group/number of participants in that group:

EER = 2/100
EER = 0.02

The NNH = 1/(0.02 – 0.01)

NNH = 1/0.0.1

This gives the answer NNH = 100

22.32 and 22.33 Predictive values

The positive predictive value of a test is how likely someone who tests positive is to actually have the condition being tested for. The negative predictive value of a test is how likely someone who tests negative is to actually not have the condition.

	Dipstick positive	Dipstick negative
Urine culture positive	60	30
Urine culture negative	40	70

Part A 60%

PPV = true positives/(true positives plus false positives)
PPV = 60/(60 + 40)
PPV = 60/100
PPV = 60%

Part B 70%

NPV = true negatives/(true negatives plus false negatives)
NPV = 70/(70 + 30)
NPV = 70/100
NPV = 70%

22.34 and 22.35   Case-control studies

Part A   20

The odds ratio can be calculated accordingly:

	Disease present	Disease absent
Suspected cause present	*a*	*b*
Suspected cause absent	*c*	*d*

Odds ratio (OR) = (*a*/*c*)/(*b*/*d*) or can be rewritten as *ad*/*bc*

In this situation

OR = (20 × 1000)/(500 × 2)
OR = 20 000/1000
OR = 20

Part B   C: There is a significant increase in side effects in the treatment group

Where the OR = 1 (or the confidence interval includes 1), there is no difference in risk between the intervention and control group. Where the OR >1 (and the confidence interval given does not include 1) events are significantly more likely in the treatment group than in the control group. Where the OR <1 (and the confidence interval does not include 1) events are significantly less likely in the treatment group than the control group, ie the intervention is protective.

22.36-22.39   Analysing trial data

Part A   5%

ARC = number of events in control group/number of people in that group:

ARC = 75/500 = 0.15 = 15%

ART = number of events in treatment group/number of people in that group:

ART = 50/500 = 0.1 = 10%

Absolute risk reduction (ARR) = absolute risk in control group (ARC) – absolute risk in treatment group (ART)

Therefore: ARR = 15 – 10% = 5%

Part B   33%

Relative risk (RR) = ART/ARC

RR = 0.1/0.15 = 0.67 = 67%

Relative risk reduction (RRR) = 1 – RR

Therefore: RRR = 1 – 0.67 = 0.33 = 33%

Part C   C: These data suggest that the new treatment may be associated with significant adverse outcomes

There are fewer myocardial infarctions in the new treatment arm but there is also a higher drop-out rate and more deaths in that group. Cardiac deaths are not listed in the data. These data might indicate that the drug causes significant adverse outcomes resulting in death, and may also signify that there are unpleasant side effects which cause patients to stop taking the treatment. Further subgroup analysis would be needed to confirm the cause of these findings

Part D   20

The NNT = 1/ARR

NNT = 1/0.05 = 20

22.40 and 22.41   Screening tests

Sensitivity is how good a test is at detecting patients with the condition. A highly sensitive test misses very few cases.

Specificity is how good a test is at excluding patients without the condition. A highly specific test has few false positives.

Expressing the results in a box table:

	DVT present	DVT not present
Test positive	75	25
Test negative	10	90

Part A   88%

Sensitivity = true positives/(true positives + false negatives)

Sensitivity = 75/(75+10)

Sensitivity = 75/85

Sensitivity = 88%

Part B   78%

Specificity = true negatives/(false positives + true negatives)

Specificity = 90/(25+90)

Specificity = 90/115

Specificity = 78%

Section 3

Chapter 23
Administration, ethical and regulatory frameworks

Single best answer questions

23.1   Caldicott principles
Which ONE of the following statements about the Caldicott principles is true? Select ONE option only.

○   A   The Caldicott principles apply only to clinicians

○   B   The Caldicott principles apply only where data are passed outside the NHS (eg insurance reports)

○   C   Every practice must have its own Caldicott guardian

○   D   Every primary care organisation must have a Caldicott guardian

○   E   The Caldicott principles are part of the Data Protection Act

23.2   Freedom of Information Act
Which ONE of the following statements about the Freedom of Information Act is correct? Select ONE option only.

○   A   General practices are covered by the Data Protection Act, so they are specifically excluded from the Freedom of Information Act

○   B   Individuals can seek information on individual salaries of doctors working in the practice

○   C   Practices are able to question the motive for a request before deciding whether to comply with a request

○   D   Practices have 20 working days to respond to a request

○   E   The Freedom of Information Act allows patients to gain access to their medical records

23.3 Exception reporting in QOF
Which ONE of the following situations with regard to the use of exception codes for the QOF would be appropriate? Select ONE option only.

○ A A 23-year-old woman with epilepsy has frequent fits despite apparently taking her medication. She is removed from the practice register as 'unsuitable'

○ B An 84-year-old woman with diabetes is housebound. She does not respond to three letters asking her to come into the surgery for a diabetic check. She is removed from the register as 'patient unsuitable'

○ C A 24-year-old woman with asthma has received three letters from the practice asking her to come in for an asthma check. She telephones the practice to say that she does not wish to be seen in the clinic. She is coded as 'informed dissent'

○ D A 73-year-old man with stable ischaemic heart disease cannot take aspirin. He is coded as 'patient unsuitable' for the ischaemic heart disease register

○ E A 79-year-old man with ischaemic heart disease is on warfarin for atrial fibrillation. To avoid adversely affecting the QOF performance for antiplatelet drugs, he is coded as 'H/O aspirin allergy'

23.4 Healthcare spending in the UK
Select the rank order of the options (1–4) that best fulfils the requirements given in the question. The following is a list of NHS areas of expenditure (options 1–4):

1 Community care
2 Elective hospital care
3 Mental health
4 Non-elective hospital care

The responses (A–E) rank the expenditure area options in various orders. Select the SINGLE response that places the options (1–4) in the order of expense, with the **lowest** NHS expenditure first to the **highest** NHS expenditure last. Select ONE rank order only.

○ A 1, 3, 2, 4

○ B 1, 3, 4, 3

○ C 3, 1, 2, 4

○ D 2, 1, 3, 4

○ E 3, 2, 4, 1

Multiple best answer questions

23.5 and 23.6   Insurance reports

You are asked to complete a medical report for life insurance for a patient on your list. Which TWO of the following statements are CORRECT regarding release of medical information to a third party.

○   A   Consent is implied when a patient applies for life insurance

○   B   Patients can ask to see a copy of a medical report only within 21 days of completion

○   C   Patients have a legal right to oblige the doctor to correct any information with which they disagree

○   D   Patients may request the completed report be retained for 21 days so that they may view the report

○   E   Patients who have requested to view the completed report can refuse the sending of the report

○   F   Where a patient has given consent to the completion of a medical report for life insurance, all material in the medical record may be released to the life insurance company

○   G   Where a patient requests to see a copy of a medical report, doctors cannot withhold any information present in that report

23.7 and 23.8   Notifiable deaths

A death should be referred to the coroner in which TWO of the following situations. Select TWO options only.

○   A   The death followed a medical termination of pregnancy

○   B   The death took place in hospital

○   C   The death was due to mesothelioma

○   D   The deceased patient was not seen by the certifying doctor in the last 28 days

○   E   The patient had a cardiac pacemaker *in situ*

Extended matching questions

Legislation affecting general practice

23.9–23.12

Options

A   Data Protection Act
B   Disability Discrimination Act
C   Employment Equality (Age) Regulations 2006
D   Equality Act
E   Freedom of Information Act
F   Human Rights Act
G   Mental Capacity Act 2005
H   Race Relations Act (RRA) 1976
I   Sex Discrimination (Amendment of Legislation) Regulations 2008
J   None of the above

For each of the statements below, select the SINGLE MOST relevant piece of legislation from the list above. Each option can be used once, more than once or not at all.

23.9   Outlaws discrimination on the basis of sexual orientation.
23.10   Allows adults to make decisions on behalf of learning disabled children.
23.11   Prevents discrimination on the basis of pregnancy.
23.12   Allows access to medical reports.

Sickness certification

23.13–23.17

Options

A   Cannot issue statement
B   Med 3
C   Med 4
D   Med 4 and Med 5
E   Med 5
F   Med 6 and Med 5
G   SC2

For each of the following patients select the SINGLE MOST appropriate certificate from the options above. Each option can be used once, more than once or not at all.

23.13   A 36-year-old banker who is known to be HIV positive has recently had a 2-week stay in hospital for treatment related to his HIV. He does not want his employer to know that he is HIV positive.

23.14   Mr Chester has been off work for 5 weeks after surgery; he is now fit to return to work and his employer requests a certificate to confirm that he is fit to return.

23.15   Mr West has not been to work today (Monday). He has been unwell since Friday evening and you diagnose viral gastroenteritis and recommend that he does not return to work until 48 hours after he is better. In the past his boss has not been happy with absences for sickness so Mr West requests a certificate.

23.16   Mrs Shand is a flight attendant. She broke her leg skiing 3 weeks ago. Yesterday you saw a letter from the orthopaedic consultant, dictated 3 weeks ago, saying that her leg had been pinned and she was to be in plaster for the next 6 weeks. Mrs Shand phones to request a certificate to cover this 6-week period.

23.17   Mrs Ward is going through a relationship break-up and has financial problems. She is low and tearful and not coping at work. You decide that she would benefit from 2 weeks off work.

NHS screening programmes

23.18-23.20

Options

A   Abdominal aortic aneurysm screening
B   Bowel cancer screening
C   Cervical screening
D   Mammography
E   Retinal screening

For each of the descriptions below, select the SINGLE MOST APPROPRIATE option from the list above.

23.18   Offered to women aged 50-70 every 3 years
23.19   Offered to women aged 50-64 every 5 years
23.20   Offered to all men in their 65th year

Antenatal and newborn screening

23.21-23.23

Options

A   Fetal anomaly screening programme
B   Infectious diseases in pregnancy screening programme
C   Newborn blood spot screening programme
D   Newborn hearing screening programme
E   NHS screening programme for sickle cell and thalassaemia

For each of the descriptions below, select the SINGLE MOST APPROPRIATE option from the list above.

23.21   Requires an initial dating scan between 8 and 14 weeks
23.22   Tests for phenylketonuria, congenital hypothyroidism and cystic fibrosis
23.23   In high prevalence areas should be routinely offered to all mothers

Complaints

23.24–23.27

The flowchart below describes the processes involved in management of complaints at a practice level, as recommended by NHS England. Complete the flowchart from the list of options below. Each option may be used once, more than once or not at all.

Options

A	1	E	24
B	2	F	36
C	10	G	48
D	12	H	72

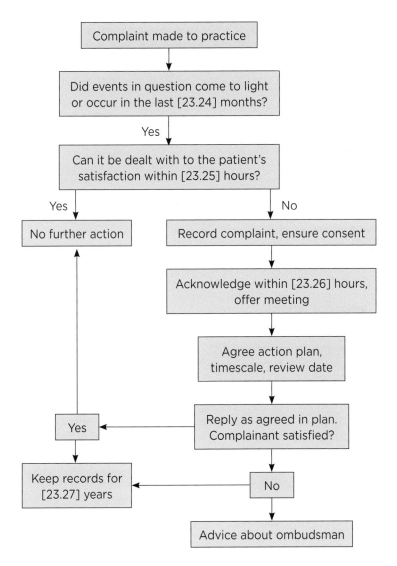

23.1   D: Every primary care organisation must have a Caldicott guardian

The Caldicott principles suggest the following: all uses of patient data should be justified; identifiable data should be used only when absolutely necessary, including when data are sent between different parts of the NHS; and each practice should have a responsible individual who ensures compliance with good practice and the law, including the Data Protection Act.

23.2   D: Practices have 20 working days to respond to a request

The Freedom of Information Act specifically includes general practices, which are expected to maintain a publication scheme containing policies and practice income. However, individual salaries are covered by the Data Protection Act. Practices cannot question motives, but a charge can be made. Failure to comply with a request will result in the practice being held in contempt of court.

23.3   C: A 24-year-old woman with asthma has received three letters from the practice asking her to come in for an asthma check. She telephones the practice to say that she does not wish to be seen in the clinic. She is coded as 'informed dissent'

The use of exception codes is an area of misreporting in many areas. Valid reasons for exception reporting include informed dissent or inappropriateness (eg people who are terminally ill), but being housebound or poorly controlled is not generally considered to be a valid reason. Caution should be taken when choosing the code to make sure that these are accurate. Individual indicator exception codes should be used wherever possible, rather than exclusion from the whole disease area.

23.4   C: 3, 1, 2, 4

3 Mental health; 1 Community care; 2 Elective hospital care; 4 Non-elective hospital care

Mental health accounts for 10%, community care 12.5%, and inpatient elective and non-elective care for 17.5% and 27.5%, respectively. Primary care and prescribing each account for 10% of funds.

23.5 and 23.6   Insurance reports

D: Patients may request the completed report be retained for 21 days so that they may view the report;
E: Patients who have requested to view the completed report can refuse the sending of the report

Patients may request that a report be retained for 21 days before sending, so that they have the opportunity to read and discuss the contents. Patients can add a codicil but cannot compel the GP to change his or her report. They can, however, refuse permission for the report to be sent. The GP must provide a copy on request within the 6 months after completion, but may withhold information, the release of which may cause serious harm to the mental or physical health of the patient. Consent must be explicit, and only relevant information from the medical record, about the patient (ie no third party references) should be released.

23.7 and 23.8   Notifiable deaths

> A: The death followed a medical termination of pregnancy;
> C: The death was due to mesothelioma

Deaths should be notified to the coroner if: the patient has not been seen in the last 14 days; the cause of death was unknown; followed an abortion or other surgical procedure; occurred during or shortly after police detention; it was due to suicide, self-neglect or accident; or it was due to industrial or occupational disease.

Legislation affecting general practice

23.9   D: Equality Act

Since 2007 the Equality Act outlaws discrimination on the basis of sexual orientation.

23.10   G: Mental Capacity Act 2005

The Mental Capacity Act governs decision-making on behalf of adults, where either they lose mental capacity at some point in their lives or the incapacitating condition has been present since birth.

23.11   I: Sex Discrimination (Amendment of Legislation) Regulations 2008

This amendment prevents direct or indirect discrimination on the basis of pregnancy now or in the last 26 weeks.

23.12   J: None of the above

The Access to Medical Reports Act allows access for patients to medical reports about them.

Sickness certification

23.13   F: Med 6 and Med 5

23.14   B: Med 3

23.15   G: SC2

23.16   E: Med 5

23.17   B: Med 3

An SC2 is used by employees to certify themselves as sick for the first 7 days of sickness for statutory sick pay purposes. For absences of more than 7 days: a Med 3 is used if the doctor signing saw the patient on the day or the day before issue; a Med 5 is used either to supply evidence of incapacity for a backdated period where you examined the patient on a previous occasion or to provide medical evidence without having seen the patient, based on a report written in the previous 4 weeks by another doctor covering a forward period of not more than 4 weeks; a Med 6 can be used to provide an accurate diagnosis where a vague diagnosis is used on a Med 3, 4 or 5, if you do not want the patient/employer to know the true diagnosis.

NHS screening programmes

23.18   **D:**   Mammography is offered to women between 50 and 70 every 3 years, and women over 70 may self-refer

23.19   **C:**   Cervical screening is offered to women aged 25–49 every 3 years, and to women aged 50–64 every 5 years

23.20   **A:**   Abdominal aortic aneurysm screening is offered to all men in the 65th year. Men over that age may self-refer.

Retinal screening is offered annually to all people with diabetes aged >12 years, and bowel cancer screening is offered to men and women aged 60–69 every 2 years, whereas those >70 can self-refer.

Antenatal and newborn screening

23.21   **A:**   Fetal anomaly screening programme

Down syndrome screening is incorporated into the fetal anomaly screening programme and comprises a dating scan, blood tests, nuchal translucency, and a detailed anatomical scan between 18 and 20 weeks. Screening for Down syndrome should be completed before the end of the first trimester.

23.22   **C:**   Newborn blood spot screening programme

This is carried out between 5 and 8 days after birth and tests for phenylketonuria, congenital hypothyroidism, sickle cell disorders, cystic fibrosis and medium-chain acyl-CoA dehydrogenase deficiency.

23.23   **E:**   NHS screening programme for sickle cell and thalassaemia

In low prevalence areas patients identified as low risk on a family origin questionnaire need have screening only for thalassaemia, whereas in high prevalence areas or where they are identified as at high risk on the questionnaire, screening is also carried out for sickle cell disease.

All women should be offered screening in the first trimester for HIV, HBV, syphilis and rubella, with further opportunities available for those who decline the initial offer. The newborn hearing screening programme is carried out on all babies between 0 and 5 weeks, usually in hospital before discharge.

Complaints

23.24–23.27

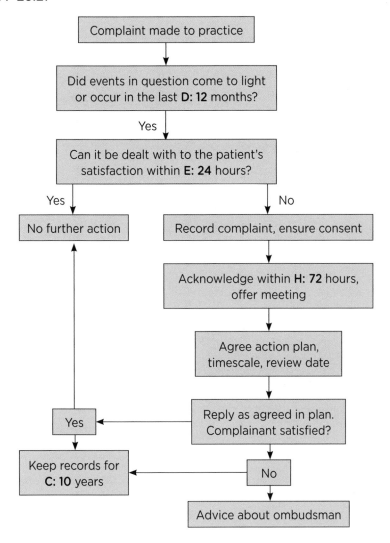

Section 4
Practice Papers

Paper 1 Questions

Total time allowed is three hours and ten minutes.

P1.1 **Shoulder problems**
Which ONE of the following statements regarding frozen shoulder is correct? Select ONE option only.

- O A Ninety per cent of patients make a complete recovery
- O B Frozen shoulder is more common in patients with diabetes mellitus
- O C Frozen shoulder is usually directly attributable to injury
- O D The mean age of onset is 20–30 years
- O E X-rays are necessary to make a diagnosis

P1.2 **Contraception**
A 22-year-old woman is going travelling around the world for 18 months and comes to see you to discuss using implants for contraception. Which ONE of the following statements about this contraceptive method is true? Select ONE option only.

- O A Progestogen implants cause weight gain in 50% of patients
- O B Progestogen implants are intrauterine contraceptive devices that release progesterone into the lining of the womb
- O C Progestogen implants need to be changed every 5 years
- O D Irregular bleeding is the most common side effect of progestogen implants
- O E Normal fertility returns in 3–6 months in 90% of women after removal of progestogen implants

Bleeding in end-of-life care

P1.3–P1.5

Options

A   Embolisation
B   Kaltostat dressing
C   Packing and cautery
D   Radiotherapy
E   Thalidomide
F   Tranexamic acid

Bleeding is common in end-of-life care and can be very distressing. For each of the sites of bleeding below, select the SINGLE MOST APPROPRIATE treatment option from the list above. Each option may be used once, more than once or not at all.

P1.3   **Bleeding from the mouth in a patient with a fungating tongue cancer**
P1.4   **Haemoptysis in a patient with lung metastases**
P1.5   **Nosebleeds in a patient with thrombocytopenia**

P1.6   **Screening for alcohol misuse**
        You are rewriting your practice protocol for new patient registrations and wish to incorporate an alcohol misuse screening tool into this.

        Which ONE of the following statements is true about this process? Select ONE option only.

    O   A   A CAGE score of ≥2 is suggestive of problem drinking

    O   B   Screening for alcohol abuse requires face-to-face consultation

    O   C   The Alcohol Use Disorders Identification Test C (AUDIT C) test identifies alcohol dependence

    O   D   The CAGE test identifies patients who drink excessively

    O   E   The Michigan Alcoholism Screening Test (MAST) questionnaire is suitable for brief screening in primary care

P1.7   **Antibiotic therapy**
        A 65-year-old patient with diabetes, who takes aspirin, atenolol, simvastatin, allopurinol and warfarin, develops cellulitis. You decide to treat with antibiotics. He is allergic to penicillin and tetracycline so you decide to use erythromycin. Which ONE of his medications should be stopped while taking the antibiotics? Write the answer, in words, in the box below.

P1.8　Blood pressure measurement

A 67-year-old man complains of pains in his legs when walking. You ask the nurses to do ankle and brachial blood pressures. These results are shown below:

Right brachial systolic pressure 150 mmHg

Left brachial systolic pressure 150 mmHg

Right dorsalis pedis systolic pressure 120 mmHg

Left dorsalis pedis systolic pressure 150 mmHg

Which ONE of the following statements is correct regarding this patient? Select ONE option only.

- ○　A　The readings are inaccurate and should be repeated
- ○　B　The readings show an ankle–brachial pressure index (ABPI) of 0.8 on the left side
- ○　C　The readings show an ABPI of 1.25 on the right side
- ○　D　The readings suggest the presence of significant peripheral vascular disease affecting the left side only
- ○　E　The readings suggest the presence of significant peripheral vascular disease affecting the right side only

P1.9　Neuralgia

Which ONE of the following statements regarding post-herpetic neuralgia is correct? Select ONE option only.

- ○　A　No treatments have been shown to be effective in preventing post-herpetic neuralgia
- ○　B　Pregabalin has been shown to be the most effective treatment for post-herpetic neuralgia
- ○　C　Prodromal dermatomal pain is a risk factor for post-herpetic neuralgia
- ○　D　The presence of paraesthesia suggests an alternative diagnosis
- ○　E　The side-effect profile of amitriptyline outweighs its benefits

P1.10   **Abdominal swelling**
A 15-month-old girl is brought in by her father, who has noticed that her umbilicus looks 'lumpy'. He tells you that it gets bigger when she cries or strains and is smaller when she is asleep. Her abdomen is shown below.

What is the SINGLE MOST appropriate management at this stage? Select ONE option only.

○   A   Admit under the on-call surgeons

○   B   Refer urgently to surgical outpatients

○   C   Reassure the parents that it will usually resolve spontaneously in time

○   D   Reassurance that this is normal at her age

○   E   Treat with a surgical support

Drug management of asthma

P1.11–P1.15

Options

A   Combination of inhaled corticosteroid and long-acting β_2 agonist
B   Inhaled anticholinergic
C   Inhaled β_2 agonist
D   Inhaled long-acting β_2 agonist
E   Inhaled low-dose corticosteroid
F   Oral β_2 agonist
G   Oral corticosteroids
H   Oral leukotriene receptor antagonist
I   Oral theophylline

For each of the statements below regarding the drug management of asthma, select the most appropriate option from the list above. Each option may be used once, more than once or not at all.

P1.11   **Indicated for the maintenance of asthma and relief of seasonal allergic symptoms.**

P1.12   **The SMART regimen allows patients to safely tailor their treatment with these drugs according to their symptoms.**

P1.13   **This drug has a narrow therapeutic window and toxicity is increased by concurrent use of erythromycin, quinolones and cimetidine.**

P1.14   **Inhibits bronchoconstriction and reduces mucus secretion in the lungs.**

P1.15   **If used for more than 10 days consideration should be given to coprescription of bisphosphonates.**

P1.16   Knee pain
A 28-year-old man complains of knee pain after being hit below the knee by an outstretched boot in a football match. On examination there is a small effusion but no laceration and the knee is fully mobile but seems to have excessive backward movement on pushing the lower leg back. What is the SINGLE MOST likely diagnosis? Select ONE option only.

    O   A   Anterior cruciate tear

    O   B   Medial collateral tear

    O   C   Meniscal tear

    O   D   Patellar tendon tear

    O   E   Posterior cruciate tear

P1.17   Neck lumps

You see an 82-year-old woman for a medication review and notice the appearance of her neck, shown below. She tells you it has been like that for many years. The lump moves on swallowing and is asymmetrical. You check her thyroid function and both TSH and T_4 are reported as normal.

What is the SINGLE MOST likely diagnosis? Select ONE option only.

O   A   Endemic goitre

O   B   Multinodular goitre

O   C   Thyroid cancer

O   D   Thyrotoxicosis

O   E   None of the above

P1.18 **Developmental delay**

A 5-year-old boy has been noted to have less vocabulary than his siblings and has rather monotonous repetitive speech. He finds it difficult to play with his peers, and does not respond to his mother arriving to pick him up from school. His mother describes him as a picky eater and obsessed with his model trains.

Which ONE of the following is the SINGLE MOST LIKELY diagnosis? Select ONE option only.

- A Attention deficit hyperactivity disorder
- B Asperger's syndrome
- C Autism
- D Developmental language disorder
- E Hearing loss

P1.19 **Catheter care**

An elderly man living in a nursing home has had a catheter fitted for the last 5 weeks. One of the staff in the home has sent a routine urine specimen, which has been reported as showing a pure growth of *Proteus* sp. sensitive to trimethoprim and ciprofloxacin. He is afebrile, with no urinary symptoms. Which one of the following would be the SINGLE MOST appropriate management of this patient? Select ONE option only.

- A Flush the catheter with citrate solution
- B No action required
- C Prescribe ciprofloxacin for 5 days
- D Prescribe trimethoprim for 3 days
- E Replace the catheter

Death certification

P1.20–P1.25

Options

A   Contact the police
B   Discuss the case with a doctor from a neighbouring practice
C   Discuss the case with the coroner
D   Discuss the case with the crematorium referee
E   Issue Certificate of Stillbirth
F   Issue Medical Certificate of Cause of Death
G   Issue Neonatal Death Certificate
H   None of the above

For each of the situations below select the SINGLE MOST appropriate action from the list of options above. Each option may be used once, more than once, or not at all.

P1.20   A 78-year-old woman diagnosed with untreatable metastatic bowel cancer 3 months ago is found dead in bed by her daughter. She was last seen by you 16 days ago.

P1.21   An 83-year-old man who has not seen a doctor for 7 years is found dead in an armchair at home. He has no medical history of note and seems to have died in his sleep.

P1.22   A 69-year-old former boiler-maker dies after a long illness with mesothelioma. You saw him the day before he died.

P1.23   A 57-year-old woman with a long history of mental illness commits suicide 2 days after a review by her consultant psychiatrist. She was last seen by you 10 days ago.

P1.24   A 37-year-old woman living on a remote farm who is 22 weeks pregnant goes into premature labour and rapidly delivers a baby at home, before the paramedics can arrive. The baby did not show any sign of life and was not successfully resuscitated. You attend the woman before admission to hospital and are asked to certify the death of the baby.

P1.25   A 93-year-old woman dies of heart failure in a nursing home. She was seen the day before death by you but was confirmed dead by the out-of-hours service and has been taken to an undertaker 30 miles away. The family have made an appointment to register the death this afternoon and have asked you to issue a certificate.

P1.26 Panic attacks
A 17-year-old student requests a note for school regarding her absences from lectures. She tells you that for several months she has been finding it increasingly difficult to cope with being in public places. She admits to having been shy since childhood but is now increasingly panicky in groups and feels inadequate around others, although she copes at home. Things have escalated to the point where she has vomited on several occasions. She has no other symptoms of note. Which ONE of the following statements regarding her management is correct? Select ONE option only.

- ○ A Cognitive-behavioural therapy is ineffective
- ○ B Reassurance that there is no organic disease is usually sufficient
- ○ C She should be treated with lithium
- ○ D She should be treated with olanzapine
- ○ E SSRIs should be used as first-line treatment

P1.27 Diarrhoea
A 4-year-old girl who returned from a camping holiday at a farm in Wales 2 days ago is brought in by her parents complaining of abdominal pain, vomiting and diarrhoea. This has been going on for 3 days but the diarrhoea has now become bloody. On examination she looks listless and has a capillary refill time of 3 seconds, a temperature of 37.6°C and generalised abdominal tenderness but no peritonism. A urine specimen shows microscopic haematuria. What is the SINGLE MOST appropriate management of this patient? Select ONE option only.

- ○ A Admit under paediatrics
- ○ B Advise parents regarding oral rehydration and review if no better
- ○ C Send urine for culture and treat if positive
- ○ D Send stool for culture and review with results
- ○ E Treat with oral trimethoprim and review in 3 days

P1.28 Chronic fatigue
Which ONE of the following statements regarding chronic fatigue syndrome is correct? Select ONE option only.

- ○ A Cognitive difficulties are unusual
- ○ B Exacerbations of fatigue are triggered by exertion and usually start during exertion, forcing patients to abandon the activity
- ○ C NICE guidelines suggest that the diagnosis should be considered in patients with unexplained fatigue of more than 6 weeks' duration
- ○ D The presence of chronic pain suggests an alternative diagnosis
- ○ E Cognitive-behavioural therapy (CBT) should be offered to all patients with this condition

P1.29 Eye pain

A 35-year-old man complains of a tender lump on the side of his eyeball. He says that it has been there for several days and came on acutely. He has no other symptoms and his vision is normal. On examination his cornea looks clear, with a reactive pupil and no conjunctival injection. There is no foreign body and no fluorescein staining, but he has an injected nodular area close to the corneal limbus on the white of the eye. The eyeball is tender over the nodule but otherwise is soft. What is the SINGLE MOST likely diagnosis? Select ONE option only.

○ A Acute angle-closure glaucoma

○ B Episcleritis

○ C Herpes simplex keratitis

○ D Iritis

○ E Scleritis

P1.30 Genetic counselling

A 34-year-old woman comes to see you for advice on genetic testing. Her mother and aunt have both had breast cancer in the late 40s and her mother has just told her that she has tested positive for the *BRCA-1* gene. She asks what her risk of inheriting the gene is. What is the risk in per cent? Type your answer in the box.

Childhood infections

P1.31–P1.35

Options

A   Group A streptococci
B   *Escherichia coli* O157
C   *Mycoplasma pneumoniae*
D   Parainfluenza virus
E   Paramyxovirus
F   Parvovirus B19
G   Poxvirus
H   Respiratory syncytial virus (RSV)
I   Rotavirus
J   Rubella
K   *Staphylococcus aureus*
L   Varicella

For each of the statements below, select the SINGLE MOST appropriate option from the list above. Each option may be used once, more than once or not at all.

P1.31   Causes crops of pinky-white shiny papules with a central pit.
P1.32   Causes epidemics of respiratory illness in approximately 3-year cycles, often associated with target-like skin lesions.
P1.33   After a prodromal fever this causes a macular rash to appear on the cheek that spreads to the trunk over several days.
P1.34   Around 24 hours after the development of tonsillitis this causes a macular rash to appear over the whole body; 2–3 days later the skin is shed, particularly on the hands and soles.
P1.35   After an incubation period of 14 days crops of vesicular lesions appear over the body. These heal over 2–3 days with new lesions appearing for 7–10 days.

P1.36   Bloody diarrhoea
A 27-year-old man complains of 3 weeks of diarrhoea and abdominal pain, with weight loss and fever. The stools are bloody on occasion. He has no recent history of travel and takes no regular medications. He reports recently being under a great deal of stress at work. On examination he is tender in the left iliac fossa with no peritonism and no perineal abnormalities. A stool sample is sent which is reported as negative for viral, bacterial and parasitic infections. What is the SINGLE MOST likely diagnosis? Select ONE option only.

O   A   *Campylobacter* sp.

O   B   Crohn's disease

O   C   Diverticulitis

O   D   Irritable bowel syndrome

O   E   Ulcerative colitis

P1.37   **Unwanted pregnancy**
       Which ONE of the following statements regarding termination of pregnancy is correct? Select ONE option only.

- ○   A   Girls under the age of 16 cannot have a termination without the consent of their parents

- ○   B   Medical termination is only suitable in patients up to 9 weeks' gestation

- ○   C   RU-486 (mifepristone) is safe to use in patients who are not fit for general anaesthesia

- ○   D   Suction termination can be carried out under local anaesthesia

- ○   E   The legal limit for abortion is 22 weeks

Personality disorders

P1.38–P1.42

Options

A   Anankastic personality disorder
B   Antisocial personality disorder
C   Borderline personality disorder
D   Histrionic personality disorder
E   Hyperthymic personality disorder
F   Narcissistic personality disorder
G   Paranoid personality disorder
H   Schizoid personality disorder

For each of the descriptions below, select the SINGLE MOST appropriate option from the list above. Each option may be used once, more than once or not at all.

P1.38   Always happy and optimistic, but tend to make rash decisions without fully considering the consequences.

P1.39   Characterised by impulsivity, outbursts of anger and unpredictable behaviour, often with episodes of deliberate self-harm or violence.

P1.40   A lack of adaptability to new situations, eg failing to take advantage of new opportunities, disabling perfectionism in even the most mundane tasks and lack of imagination.

P1.41   Typified by an excessive sense of self-importance and power without warmth or empathy.

P1.42   Solitary, humourless people who tend to avoid situations where they will have to socialise.

P1.43   Bladder problems
A 76-year-old man who is currently awaiting investigation for alternating diarrhoea and constipation presents with an episode of frank haematuria. He presents you with a specimen that is heavily blood stained with some sediment. On closer questioning he reports passing small lumps and bubbles in his urine. What is the SINGLE MOST likely diagnosis? Select ONE option only.

O   A   Bladder cancer

O   B   Glomerulonephritis

O   C   Renal calculus

O   D   Urinary tract infection

O   E   Vesicocolic fistula

P1.44   Swollen arm
A 53-year-old man had a pacemaker fitted for heart block last week. He complains that his left arm is swollen. On examination the left arm is red and swollen from the humerus down, with engorged veins that do not empty on elevating the arm. He is afebrile. What is the SINGLE MOST likely diagnosis? Select ONE option only.

O   A   Cellulitis

O   B   Compartment syndrome

O   C   Deep vein thrombosis

O   D   Postoperative wound infection

O   E   Subclavian arterial embolism

P1.45   Haemochromatosis
Mrs Jones comes to see you after her brother, who lives in New Zealand, is diagnosed with haemochromatosis. She asks for a screening test to see if she has the disease. She does not have any additional information about his diagnosis. You do some routine blood tests, including iron studies. Which ONE of the following is most indicative of haemochromatosis in this situation? Select ONE option only.

O   A   Raised mean corpuscular haemoglobin and raised mean corpuscular volume

O   B   Raised serum ferritin and raised total iron-binding capacity

O   C   Raised serum ferritin with reduced total iron-binding capacity

O   D   Reduced mean corpuscular haemoglobin and reduced mean corpuscular volume

O   E   Reduced serum ferritin with raised total iron-binding capacity

P1.46 Cough

A 23-year-old man complains that for the last 7 weeks he has had outbreaks of violent coughing, which last for minutes at a time, during which he feels he cannot breathe. He feels relatively well in between attacks. He has no previous medical history of note and takes no regular medications. He has been seen in accident and emergency twice and in the practice twice with no adverse findings. Which ONE of the following is the SINGLE MOST likely diagnosis? Select ONE option only.

○ A   Asthma

○ B   Diphtheria

○ C   *Mycoplasma pneumoniae* infection

○ D   Pertussis

○ E   Pneumococcal chest infection

Biological therapies

P1.47–P1.51

Options

A   Infliximab (Remicade)
B   Natalizumab (Tysabri)
C   Omalizumab (Xolair)
D   Ranibizumab (Lucentis)
E   Rituximab (Rituxan)
F   Trastuzumab (Herceptin)

For each of the diseases below, select the most appropriate treatment agent from the list above. Each option may be used once, more than once or not at all.

P1.47   Allergy-mediated asthma
P1.48   Multiple sclerosis
P1.49   Severe psoriasis resistant to PUVA and standard systemic treatment
P1.50   Breast cancer
P1.51   Macular degeneration

P1.52   Indigestion
A 39-year-old man with longstanding gastro-oesophageal reflux comes to see you about his condition. In spite of treatment with high-dose proton-pump inhibitors and alginates he is troubled by symptoms on a daily basis. He has tried lifestyle measures but feels that he cannot go on. He begs you to refer him for surgery. Which ONE of the following statements is true regarding this treatment option? Select ONE option only.

O   A   Nissen fundoplication requires a laparotomy

O   B   Patients who have had a fundoplication have a reduced gastric capacity and have to eat regular small meals

O   C   Surgery is indicated in patients who do not wish to take long-term medication

O   D   Surgery is suitable only for patients with a sliding hiatus hernia

O   E   Surgery will control symptoms and eliminate the need for maintenance medication

P1.53   Backache
A 27-year-old man asks for stronger painkillers for his back. He has always had backache, but is now finding it increasingly difficult to work. He is particularly stiff in the morning, although finds this improves somewhat during the day, and has been present for several years. He also suffers from intermittent iritis, but is on no regular medication. He frequently wakes in the early hours and on examination he has limited flexion and extension in his back. What is the SINGLE MOST likely diagnosis? Select ONE option only.

O   A   Ankylosing spondylitis

O   B   Mechanical backache

O   C   Polymyalgia rheumatica

O   D   Prolapsed intervertebral disc

O   E   Spinal stenosis

P1.54 Management of arthritis

A 36-year-old woman with severe rheumatoid arthritis has been advised to start methotrexate by her rheumatologist. She comes to see you to discuss this, having read about this treatment on the internet. Which ONE of the following statements about this treatment is correct? Select ONE option only.

○ A If a full blood count is normal initially and 1 month after starting treatment, no further testing is required

○ B If LFTs increase by 10% after starting treatment the drug should be stopped

○ C Methotrexate can be safely used in pregnancy

○ D Methotrexate frequently causes menstrual disturbances

○ E Methotrexate should not be used in patients taking folic acid supplements

P1.55 Behavioural problems

A 7-year-old boy is brought in to see you by his parents at the request of his schoolteachers. He has no friends in his class, is aloof and seems to find it very difficult to interact with others. He likes to play on his own and seldom shares his experiences in the classroom. His only interest is in Thomas the Tank Engine and he plays with these toys in a repetitive manner. He also flaps his hands many times through the day. He was born at term after an uneventful delivery and showed normal speech and language development up to the age of 3 years. What is the SINGLE MOST likely diagnosis? Select ONE option only.

○ A Asperger syndrome

○ B Attention deficit hyperactivity disorder

○ C Cerebral palsy

○ D Normal variant

○ E Temporal lobe epilepsy

Sleep disturbance

P1.56–P1.59

Options

A   Bed-time restriction
B   Cognitive–behavioural therapy
C   Intermittent short-term hypnotics
D   Light therapy
E   Melatonin
F   Mirtazapine
G   Regular hypnotics
H   Tricyclic antidepressant

Complete the algorithm below detailing the management of sleep disturbance in primary care from the list of options above. Each option may be used once, more than once or not at all.

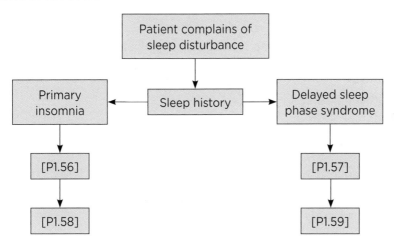

P1.60 Fibroids

A 38-year-old woman with a history of heavy periods has tried using the combined oral contraceptive pill, anti-inflammatories, progesterone-only pill and tranexamic acid without success. She has an ultrasound scan which confirms large fibroids. You refer her for a specialist opinion and she is listed for surgery, but asks if there is anything that she can try in the meantime as her daughter is getting married next month and she is worried about flooding. Which ONE of the following would be the SINGLE MOST appropriate management option? Select ONE option only.

O A Cerazette

O B Danazol

O C Hormone replacement therapy

O D Mefenamic acid

O E Ulipristal acetate

P1.61 Sea sickness

A 67-year-old woman, who is about to embark on a cruise, requests a prescription for some sea-sickness tablets. Which ONE of the following statements is correct about this condition? Select ONE option only.

O A Cinnarazine is an effective treatment

O B Drug treatment has a placebo effect only

O C Hyoscine should not be used because it exacerbates motion sickness

O D Patients suffering sea-sickness should be advised to avoid standing on deck because the view of the moving sea can exacerbate symptoms

O E Promethazine is effective, with minimal side effects, making it the first-line treatment for most patients

P1.62 Tuberculosis

One of your patients has recently been diagnosed with tuberculosis. He has spent several weeks in the last 3 months in a community hospital and was a frequent visitor to the surgery. You attend a public health meeting to discuss contact tracing. Which ONE of the following statements about contact tracing is correct? Select ONE option only.

O A All contacts should be removed from patient care until they have been screened

O B Heaf testing has high sensitivity and specificity

O C Presence of a BCG scar implies immunity and these patients do not need to be screened

O D Quantiferon testing is the investigation of choice in screening contacts

O E An X-ray is the most appropriate investigation in TB outbreaks

P1.63 **Sore eyes**

A 39-year-old man with no history of note complains that his eyes are constantly sore. He has been seen several times both in the surgery and by his optician and has been found to have blepharitis. In spite of good eyelid hygiene and short courses of topical antibiotics he still has daily troublesome symptoms. Which ONE of the following would be an appropriate management option at this stage? Select ONE option only.

- O   A   Encourage to persevere with lid cleaning
- O   B   Oral doxycycline 100 mg once daily for 6 weeks
- O   C   Prednisolone eye drops for 1 week
- O   D   Refer to outpatients
- O   E   Topical Fucithalmic for 6 weeks

P1.64 **Ankle pain**

A 27-year-old man complains of pain above his right ankle after a dry ski slope session in preparation for his skiing holiday. He reports falling awkwardly and was unable to continue, but he can weight bear. On examination he has tenderness and bruising 4 inches (10 cm) above his lateral malleolus, with numbness over the lateral border of the foot. What is the SINGLE MOST appropriate management? Select ONE option only.

- O   A   Advise him to return if he is still in pain when the swelling has subsided
- O   B   Advise rest, ice, compression and elevation (RICE)
- O   C   Apply a backslab cast for support
- O   D   Reassure him that he can weight bear, making a fracture unlikely
- O   E   Refer immediately to the emergency department for X-ray

Abdominal pain

P1.65–P1.69

Options

A   Abdominal aortic aneurysm
B   Acute appendicitis
C   Acute cholecystitis
D   Acute pancreatitis
E   Crohn's disease
F   Colonic carcinoma
G   Diverticulitis
H   Gastric carcinoma
I   Irritable bowel syndrome
J   Peptic ulcer
K   Renal colic
L   Ruptured ectopic pregnancy

For each of the clinical scenarios described below, select the SINGLE MOST appropriate diagnosis from the list of options above. Each option may be used once, more than once or not at all.

P1.65   A 76-year-old man complains of recurrent attacks of colicky left iliac fossa pain. On examination he has left iliac fossa tenderness but no peritonism.

P1.66   A 39-year-old man complains of acute colicky pains radiating from his back to his groin and coming in waves.

P1.67   A 33-year-old woman complains of 3 months of diarrhoea, weight loss and abdominal pain. On examination she has a right iliac fossa swelling and fleshy skin tags around her anus.

P1.68   A 44-year-old woman complains of fever, vomiting and pain in her shoulder. On examination she is tender in the right upper quadrant.

P1.69   A 67-year-old man complains of several weeks of dysphagia, weight loss and, more recently, epigastric pain. On examination he is cachectic with generalised abdominal tenderness.

P1.70 **Drug side effects**

A 56-year-old diabetic woman who takes simvastatin has come to see you after reading an article in her daily newspaper about the dangers of taking statins. She would like your advice on whether to continue. Which ONE of the following statements about the side effects of cholesterol-lowering treatment is true? Select ONE option only.

- ○ A   Ezetimibe has been reported to be associated with an increased risk of cancer

- ○ B   Patients with familial hypercholesterolaemia should all be treated with 40 mg simvastatin

- ○ C   Patients with mixed hyperlipidaemias should be treated with a statin and a fibrate

- ○ D   Simvastatin is the only statin that interacts significantly with other drugs

- ○ E   Sleep disturbance is rare

P1.71 **Hair problems**

A 7-year-old girl is brought to see you by her mother who has noticed that her hairs have the appearance below. Examination of her hair is otherwise normal, although there are several other similar hairs. Her mother admits to having treated her for nits some months ago.

Which ONE of the following would be appropriate management in this situation? Select ONE option only.

- ○ A   Malathion used twice 7 days apart

- ○ B   Permethrin used twice 7 days apart

- ○ C   Simethicone used twice 7 days apart

- ○ D   Wet combing with conditioner

- ○ E   No treatment needed

P1.72 Data interpretation

The figures below show changes in the incidence of prostate cancer and death rates over the last 10 years.

Figure (a) Percentage change in new cases of prostate cancer diagnosed per year.

Figure (b) Percentage change in deaths from prostate cancer per year.

Which ONE of the following is the most likely explanation for these data? Select ONE option only.

○ A   Advances in treatment have led to improved survival rates

○ B   Changes in lifestyle have increased the risk of developing cancer

○ C   Clinically asymptomatic cancers are being diagnosed earlier

○ D   New cases are being diagnosed at the same rate but survival is increasing

○ E   Newer treatments do not improve life expectancy

P1.73 **Laxatives in palliative care**
Several different drug classes are available to treat constipation in palliative care.

A   Bisacodyl
B   Co-danthramer
C   Docusate sodium
D   Macrogols
E   Methylnaltrexone

MATCH each drug to its action group. All FIVE must be correctly matched to score ONE mark.

Action group	Drug
μ-Opioid receptor antagonist	
Stimulants	
Osmotics	
Softeners	
Combined preparation	

P1.74 **Throat pain**
A 47-year-old man complains of recurrent episodes of fleeting pain radiating from his tonsils to his right ear. He describes the pain as like an electric shock, typically lasting a few seconds. The only obvious trigger that he can identify is eating certain foods. Examination of the head and neck is unremarkable, with no skin lesions or lymphadenopathy. He has no associated vertigo, deafness or tinnitus.

What is the SINGLE MOST likely diagnosis? Select ONE option only.

○   A   Glossopharyngeal neuralgia

○   B   Ménière syndrome

○   C   Ramsay Hunt syndrome

○   D   Tonsillar carcinoma

○   E   Trigeminal neuralgia

P1.75 Fatigue

A 57-year-old woman complains of fatigue. She rarely attends the practice and takes no regular medication. She denies depression. You arrange some blood tests, the results of which are shown below:

Hb	141 (120.0-160.0) g/l
WBC	8.9×10^9 ($3.6-11.0 \times 10^9$)
Platelets	232×10^9 ($150.0-400.0 \times 10^9$)
MCV	100.9 (82.0-98.0) fl
MCH	33.2 (27.0-33.0) pg
ALT	37 (10.0-33.0) IU/l
Bilirubin	14 (<21.0) µmol/l
Alkaline phosphatase	345 (30.0-130.0) IU/l
GGT	1539 (5.0-35.0) IU/l
Total protein	69 (60.0-80.0) g/l
Albumin	44 (35.0-50.0) g/l
Na^+	136 (137-145) mmol/l
K^+	5.3 (3.5-5.5) mmol/l
Creatinine	76 (46-92) µmol/l
HbA1c	41 (20-42) mmol/mol
Vitamin B_{12}	500 (>180.0) ng/l
Folate	8.9 (4.6-34.8) µg/l

What is the SINGLE most likely underlying cause for these results? Write your result in the box below.

P1.76   Epidemiology
Comparing retrospective with prospective studies, which ONE of the
following statements is true? Select ONE option only.

O   A   Retrospective studies are less prone to bias than prospective studies

O   B   Retrospective studies are more expensive to conduct than prospective
studies

O   C   Retrospective studies are quicker to conduct than prospective studies

O   D   Results from retrospective studies carry more statistical significance
than prospective studies

O   E   Prospective studies are designed to detect differences in populations
and therefore always produce statistically significant data

End-of-life care in patients with renal failure

P1.77–P1.80

Options

A   Clonazepam
B   Cyclizine
C   Levomepromazine
D   Loratadine
E   Metoclopramide
F   Morphine
G   Naproxen
H   Ondansetron
I   Oxycodone

For each of the symptoms below seen in patients with end-stage renal failure,
select the SINGLE MOST APPROPRIATE treatment from the list above.

P1.77   Itching
P1.78   Hiccups
P1.79   Restless legs
P1.80   Pain

P1.81   Skin lesion
A 77-year-old woman comes to see you for her annual blood pressure
review. While there she mentions a lump on her cheek that has been there
for several years. This is shown below.

Which ONE of the following is the SINGLE MOST LIKELY diagnosis? Select
ONE option only.

○   A   Basal cell carcinoma

○   B   Dermatofibroma

○   C   Keratoacanthoma

○   D   Seborrhoeic keratosis

○   E   Squamous cell carcinoma

P1.82 **Antenatal care**

A 33-year-old woman who is 33 weeks into her second pregnancy presents with reduced fetal movements. She has no abdominal pain or bleeding but has not felt the baby move since the previous evening. On examination her abdomen is soft, with fundal height consistent with dates. Which ONE of the following is the SINGLE MOST appropriate management of this situation?

- A   Admit under on-call obstetric team

- B   Ask her to contact the midwife if she has not felt 10 movements by 17:00 the following day

- C   Do cervical examination to assess for pre-term labour

- D   Reassure her that this is normal in the last trimester

- E   Refer directly to the antenatal unit for biophysical profile

P1.83 **Agoraphobia**

You are asked to visit a 20-year-old man at home. His mother is at the end of her tether, and tells you that he has not left the house for 3 years. He reports feelings of panic, dizziness and depersonalisation at the thought of going out, which get much worse when he is out. He presents as a rather shy, introvert character but denies any other symptoms of mental illness. Which ONE of the following is the SINGLE MOST appropriate management for this patient? Select ONE option only.

- A   Diazepam used as needed

- B   Fluoxetine

- C   Hypnotherapy

- D   Risperidone

- E   Systematic desensitisation therapy

P1.84   Nail changes
A 27-year-old marketing executive asks for advice about her nails. She has recently been through a stressful relationship break-up and is applying for new jobs. She is self-conscious about the appearance of her thumbnails, shown below.

Which ONE of the following would be the SINGLE MOST appropriate management of this condition? Select ONE option only.

○   A   Amorolfine nail lacquer

○   B   Avoidance of nail rubbing

○   C   Calcium supplementation

○   D   Reassurance

○   E   Terbinafine tablets

P1.85   Swollen arm
A 56-year-old woman who had a wide local excision of a breast cancer and axillary clearance 5 years ago presents with a 6-month history of an increasingly swollen arm on the side of her previous surgery. On examination the oedema is non-pitting, with no erythema and minimal tenderness. Which ONE of the following is the SINGLE MOST likely diagnosis? Select ONE option only.

○   A   Cellulitis

○   B   Deep vein thrombosis

○   C   Lymphoma

○   D   Lymphoedema

○   E   Recurrent breast cancer

P1.86 Data Interpretation

A 56-year-old man attends for routine blood tests in the surgery. He has a history of chronic obstructive pulmonary disease (COPD), with an FEV_1 of 75% predicted, and also suffers from essential hypertension. Unfortunately he continues to smoke 10–20 cigarettes a day. A full blood count is taken and the results are shown below.

Haemoglobin	19.6 g/dl (NR 13.5–18.0 mg/dl)
WCC	$6.7 \times 10^9/l$ (4.0–$11.0 \times 10^9/l$)
Platelets	$276 \times 10^9/l$ (150–$400 \times 10^9/l$)

What would be the SINGLE MOST appropriate initial management step in this case? Select ONE option only.

○ A Prescribe aspirin 300 mg once daily

○ B Reassure him that these results are normal

○ C Refer under 2-week rule to haematology

○ D Start a smoking cessation programme and repeat the blood tests in 4 weeks

○ E Venesect until the haemoglobin is in the normal range

P1.87 Moles

While visiting your parents your mother asks you if you can have a look at a mole that she is worried about. She tells you that she doesn't particularly like her own GP due to his rudeness and is too busy to see one of the other doctors at the surgery. Which ONE of the following would be the SINGLE MOST appropriate response in this situation, according to General Medical Council guidelines?

○ A Encourage her to complain to the practice manager about the doctor's rudeness

○ B Examine the mole and advise her on management accordingly

○ C Suggest that she sees another doctor at the practice

○ D Refer her to a local dermatologist

○ E Telephone her GP and explain the situation

Upper gastrointestinal disorders

P1.88–P1.92

Options

A   Achalasia
B   Barrett's oesophagus
C   Coeliac disease
D   Hiatus hernia
E   MALToma
F   Oesophageal cancer
G   Oesophageal dysmotility
H   Oesophageal stricture
I   Plummer–Vinson syndrome
J   Reflux oesophagitis

For each of the statements below, select the option from the list above that is the SINGLE MOST appropriate. Each option may be used once, more than once or not at all.

P1.88   Associated with *Helicobacter pylori* infection.
P1.89   Causes a slowly progressive, intermittent dysphagia, often causing chest infections.
P1.90   Associated with a 1% annual risk of developing oesophageal cancer.
P1.91   Usually presents with bolus obstruction.
P1.92   Causes dysphagia in association with glossitis, koilonychia and angular stomatitis.

P1.93   PSA screening
        A 44-year-old man asks for a PSA test to make sure that he doesn't have prostate cancer. He has no urinary symptoms and no family history of note. Which ONE of the following statements is true about screening for prostate cancer? Select ONE option only.

   O   A   PSA screening has been shown to increase diagnosis of early prostate cancer

   O   B   PSA screening has been shown to increase quality of life

   O   C   PSA screening has been shown to reduce mortality

   O   D   PSA screening is cost-effective

   O   E   Surgical treatment of asymptomatic prostate cancer detected on routine screening improves long-term morbidity and mortality

P1.94 Genetic disease
A 43-year-old man has recently discovered that his father has Huntington's disease. He has been tested and does not have the disease. He has two small children and would like to know their risk of developing the disease. There is no family history of Huntington's disease in the mother's pedigree. Which ONE of the following statements is true about this situation? Select ONE option only.

○ A   Each child has a 25% chance of being affected

○ B   Each child has a 25% chance of being a carrier

○ C   Each child has a 0% chance of being affected

○ D   He has a 25% chance of being a carrier

○ E   He has a 50% chance of being a carrier

P1.95 Cold sores
A 29-year-old woman comes to see you for advice. She is due to get married in 3 weeks and is concerned that she will have a flare of her cold sores, which always seems to occur when she is stressed. She asks if anything can be done to prevent this. Which ONE of the following statements is correct about this scenario? Select ONE option only.

○ A   Cold sores are caused by infection with *Staphylococcus aureus* and using flucloxacillin will usually prevent an exacerbation

○ B   Cold sores are caused by primary infection with herpes simplex virus and can be prevented by taking oral aciclovir

○ C   Exacerbations are more common in the winter

○ D   Topical aciclovir is an effective prophylactic treatment

○ E   Ultraviolet light used at the onset of symptoms may abort the attack

P1.96 Wrist pain
A 45-year-old woman complains of pain on the radial side of her wrist, which came on after a weekend trimming flowers for a wedding display. On examination she has tenderness and swelling along the radial border of the thumb, with maximal tenderness over the head of the radius. Resisted abduction exacerbates the pain. What is the SINGLE MOST likely diagnosis? Select ONE option only.

○ A   Carpal tunnel syndrome

○ B   De Quervain's tenosynovitis

○ C   Lateral epicondylitis

○ D   Medial epicondylitis

○ E   Osteoarthritis of the first metacarpophalangeal joint

P1.97   Renal problems

A 34-year-old man has a renal ultrasound scan carried out to investigate renal colic. He is shocked to be told he that has a duplex ureter on the right and comes to see you to discuss the significance of this. Which ONE of the following statements about this condition is true? Select ONE option only.

○   A   Duplex ureters are of no clinical significance

○   B   Pelviureteric junction (PUJ) obstruction is more common in patients with duplex ureters

○   C   Surgery is indicated in all cases

○   D   This condition is extremely rare

○   E   Treatment with an ACE inhibitor is indicated to prevent nephropathy

P1.98   Squint

A 2-year-old boy is brought to see you by his mother, who is concerned that he is developing a squint. On examination he appears to have a right-sided squint, and also when you look at his eyes with an ophthalmoscope you see that he has a white pupillary reflex on that side. He was adopted at birth and his parents have no knowledge of his family or antenatal history. Which ONE of the following would be the most appropriate management for this child? Select ONE option only.

○   A   Reassure the mother and arrange to review him in 4 weeks

○   B   Refer to ophthalmology for assessment of vision

○   C   Refer to optician for glasses

○   D   Refer to the orthoptic department for patching

○   E   Refer under the 2-week rule

P1.99   Weight gain

A 53-year-old woman complains of increasing difficulties with her figure. She tells you that she has always had a slim figure but that over the last 6 months she has noticed that her waist is getting bigger in spite of regular exercise and dieting. She also reports new onset of urinary frequency and constipation. On examination she has some dullness in her flanks but no other obvious abnormalities on abdominal palpation. Which ONE of the following would be the most appropriate next step in her assessment? Select ONE option only.

○   A   Bimanual examination

○   B   Check thyroid function

○   C   Refer for colonoscopy in view of change in bowel habit

○   D   Refer for ultrasound scan

○   E   Trial of anticholinergic

P1.100 Haematuria
A 9-year-old boy is brought into the surgery by his mother after an episode of frank haematuria. This seems to have started after a viral infection and he has complained of loin pain over the last 24 hours. On examination he appears well with no fever or oedema and no masses in his abdomen. Urinalysis is positive for blood but negative for nitrites and leukocytes, with protein 1+. Reviewing his notes you discover that he was treated last year for a suspected urinary tract infection by a locum after presenting with macroscopic haematuria. What is the SINGLE MOST likely diagnosis? Select ONE option only.

○ A Beetroot consumption

○ B IgA nephropathy

○ C Polycystic kidneys

○ D Urinary tract infection

○ E Wilms' tumour

P1.101 Drug dose calculation
An elderly woman attends your local minor injury unit after a fall. She has several superficial lacerations on her scalp and leg. You plan to suture these using 1% lidocaine as a local anaesthetic. She weighs 50 kg. The maximum safe dose of lidocaine is 3 mg/kg.

What is the maximum number of millilitres of 1% lidocaine that can be safely used in this patient?

Write your answer in the following text box. Use figures NOT words. Percentages, equations and fractions are NOT acceptable.

P1.102 Child health surveillance

Which ONE of the following should be part of a routine 8-week check for newborn infants? Select ONE option only.

O   A   Coordination

O   B   Cover test for squint

O   C   The Guthrie test

O   D   Hearing

O   E   Presence of cataracts

P1.103 Visual loss

A 41-year-old woman complains of sudden onset of visual loss in her right eye, which she noticed on waking. She also complains of discomfort in the eye, which is worse when looking upwards. On examination she has a central defect on field testing and a relative afferent pupillary defect, although her fundus looks normal. The contralateral eye is normal. What is the SINGLE MOST likely diagnosis? Select ONE option only.

O   A   Acute glaucoma

O   B   Amaurosis fugax

O   C   Central retinal vein occlusion (CRVO)

O   D   Optic neuritis

O   E   Papilloedema

P1.104 Unwell adult

A 78-year-old woman with a previous history of hypertension presents with a 24-hour history of fever and malaise. On examination she has a temperature of 39.0C, pulse 97 beats/min, respiratory rate of 23/min with faint basal crepitations and blood sugar of 9.1 mmol/l, and she seems confused. Urine dipstick is positive for leukocytes.

Which ONE of the following is the single MOST LIKELY diagnosis?

O   A   Lower respiratory tract infection (LRTI)

O   B   Meningitis

O   C   Sepsis

O   D   Upper respiratory tract infection (URTI)

O   E   Urinary tract infection (UTI)

Childhood vaccinations

P1.105–P1.108

Options

A   Bacillus Calmette–Guérin (BCG) vaccine
B   *Haemophilus influenzae* type B vaccine
C   Hepatitis B vaccination
D   Human papillomavirus (HPV) vaccine
E   Influenza vaccine
F   Meningitis B vaccine
G   Meningitis ACWY vaccine
H   Pneumococcal conjugate vaccine
I   Rotavirus vaccine

For each of the statements below, select the SINGLE best matching option from the list above.

P1.105   In the UK given to girls aged 12 and 13 years
P1.106   Offered to infants whose parents were born in India
P1.107   Given as a live attenuated nasal vaccine to children from 2 years
P1.108   An oral vaccine given at 8 weeks

P1.109 Fitness to practice
You work in small town with two practices. The other practice is run by a single-handed GP with a part-time nurse. Several patients have expressed concerns about his drinking. You arrange to meet him at lunchtime but when you arrive he is drunk and abusive, even though he has a surgery booked for the afternoon. The following day you telephone him to discuss this but he refuses to do so. Which ONE of the following is the SINGLE MOST IMPORTANT action in this situation? Select ONE option only.

O   A   Contact his GP to express your concerns

O   B   Contact other doctors in the area to enquire if anyone else has concerns

O   C   Contact the Local Medical Committee to provide support

O   D   Contact the regional Responsible Officer to report your concerns

O   E   Contact the Sick Doctors Trust to support him with his addiction

P1.110 Barrett's oesophagus
One of your patients has recently had an upper gastrointestinal endoscopy that has shown Barrett's oesophagus. He is concerned that this means that he will get cancer and comes to see you to discuss this diagnosis. Which ONE of the following statements regarding this condition is true? Select ONE option only.

- A   Barrett's oesophagus is a benign condition with no long-term complications
- B   Barrett's oesophagus will often resolve if *Helicobacter pylori* infection is treated
- C   Patients with Barrett's oesophagus should be referred for oesophagectomy
- D   There is a 1% annual risk of developing malignancy in patients with Barrett's oesophagus
- E   There is no treatment for Barrett's oesophagus other than surveillance

P1.111 Chronic obstructive pulmonary disease
Which ONE of the following statements is correct with regard to current management of COPD? Select ONE option only.

- A   β Blockers are contraindicated in COPD
- B   Long-acting β agonists need to be given twice daily in patients with COPD
- C   Patients who wish to fly should be reassured that, if their oxygen saturation at rest is >90%, they can fly without supplemental oxygen
- D   Self-management of COPD has been shown to significantly reduce hospital admission
- E   Tiotropium should be considered at step 2 in COPD management

P1.112 Headache
A 47-year-old woman with a history of focal migraine comes to see you with 3-hour history of severe headache centred around her right eye, with loss of vision in that eye and nausea and vomiting. On examination her conjunctiva is injected and her pupil does not constrict to light. What is the SINGLE MOST likely diagnosis? Select ONE option only.

- A   Acute angle-closure glaucoma
- B   Cluster headache
- C   Giant-cell arteritis
- D   Focal migraine
- E   Subarachnoid haemorrhage

P1.113 Data interpretation
The local prescribing officer has generated the Cates' plot below to help explain to patients the benefits of an exercise programme for osteoarthritis, as part of a drive for greater patient involvement in clinical decisions.

Which ONE of the following statements is correct about interpretation of this data? Select ONE option only.

O   A   Although there are no side effects from the intervention, 30% of patients will not benefit from the intervention

O   B   Each patient has a 70% chance of improving after the intervention

O   C   Individual patients will experience an average improvement of 70% in their symptom score

O   D   The intervention is as likely to produce harm as benefit

O   E   The intervention is cost-effective

P1.114 Ankle pain
A 52-year-old woman who enjoys recreational jogging is diagnosed with a chest infection and treated with levofloxacin. One week later she complains of pain in both ankles, with stiffness in her Achilles tendon, worse on waking. On examination there is diffuse tenderness but no palpable defect and she is able to plantarflex her feet against resistance. What is the SINGLE MOST likely diagnosis? Select ONE option only.

O   A   Achilles tendon rupture

O   B   Achilles tendinopathy

O   C   Overuse injury

O   D   Polymyalgia rheumatica

O   E   Rhabdomyolysis

P1.115 Chest symptoms

A 33-year-old farm labourer complains that he has developed a cough, chest tightness and breathlessness, with myalgia. He has had this in the past and has been treated with a salbutamol inhaler with slight benefit. He is well most of the year but reports getting these symptoms at certain times of the year when he is working indoors. On examination he is afebrile and has a respiratory rate of 30/min with fine crepitations in both lung fields. He has no wheeze or finger clubbing. Which ONE of the following is the most likely diagnosis? Select ONE option only.

- ○ A   Asthma
- ○ B   Atypical pneumonia
- ○ C   Bronchiectasis
- ○ D   Extrinsic allergic alveolitis
- ○ E   Pulmonary fibrosis

P1.116 Period pains

Which ONE of the following statements about evidence-based management of dysmenorrhoea is correct? Select ONE option only.

- ○ A   Aspirin is the most effective NSAID in the management of primary dysmenorrhoea
- ○ B   The combined oral contraceptive has a number needed to treat of 5 for management of primary dysmenorrhoea
- ○ C   COX-2 inhibitors have been shown to have no additional efficacy compared with placebo
- ○ D   Paracetamol is as effective as ibuprofen, with fewer side effects
- ○ E   Spinal manipulation has been proved to be of benefit in primary dysmenorrhoea

P1.117 **Partnership agreements**
Which ONE of the following statements regarding partnership agreements is correct? Select ONE option only.

O A A partnership agreement does not need to be updated to reflect partnership changes, as long as new partners agree to the terms of the old agreement

O B A partnership without a formal partnership agreement is not considered to be a legal partnership

O C Only qualified general practitioners can legally be partners in a medical practice

O D Under the Partnership Act 1890 all financial decisions made by a partnership must be unanimous

O E Where a partnership agreement does not exist, the partnership can be terminated at any time by one of the partners

Bowel symptoms

P1.118–P1.121

Options

A Check CA-125
B Gluten-free diet
C Mebeverine
D Refer for colonoscopy
E Refer for gastroscopy
F Refer for ultrasound
G Stool culture
H None of the above

For each of the patients described below, select the SINGLE MOST APPROPRIATE initial management from the list above.

P1.118 A 53-year-old woman with no previous history of note is currently going through a divorce. She complains of bloating and wind, worse towards the end of the day.

P1.119 A 19-year-old student who has recently returned from a gap year complains of bloody diarrhoea for 6 weeks with urgency and tenesmus.

P1.120 A 27-year-old store manager with no previous history of note complains of 12 months of abdominal pain relieved by defecation, bloating and loose bowels. She has no other symptoms. Blood tests are normal.

P1.121 A 47-year-old man complains of upper abdominal discomfort. He is tender in the epigastrium and right upper quadrant. Blood tests show a Hb of 11.9 and a platelet count of 531×10^9.

P1.122 Toe pain

A 23-year-old keen runner comes to see you a few hours after completing a fell running competition complaining of pain in his toes. The appearance is shown below.

In the box below, write the SINGLE MOST appropriate intervention if any, for this condition.

P1.123 Contraceptive choices

A 23-year-old woman comes to see you for her 6-week check after delivering a boy by caesarean section. She is breastfeeding and has not had a period yet, but would like to discuss contraception. Which ONE of the following statements is true? Select ONE option only.

- O A A negative pregnancy test is required before starting the contraceptive pill if periods have not yet returned
- O B A combined oral contraceptive pill (COCP) can be started at any time from 1 week after the birth onwards
- O C The earliest possible fertile ovulation is around 28 days postpartum
- O D Ovulation does not occur until after the return of periods
- O E Progesterone-only pills interfere with breastfeeding and should be avoided in lactating mothers

Management of back pain

P1.124–P1.128

Options

A   Discharge
B   GP management
C   NSAIDs
D   Physiotherapy
E   Red flag symptoms
F   Refer to back school
G   Refer to secondary care
H   Review in 2 weeks
I   Review in 4 weeks
J   Strong opioids

Your local physiotherapy department have developed a new spinal triage system to simplify the management of mechanical back pain. They wish to simplify this with a flowchart. Complete the figure below from the list of options above. Each option may be used once, more than once or not at all.

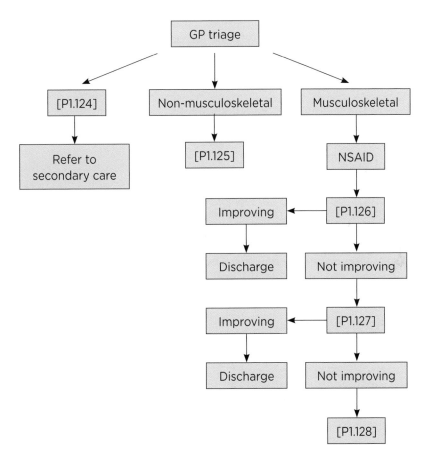

P1.129 MMR vaccination

You receive a telephone call from a concerned mother. Her 17-month-old son had his MMR vaccination at 14 months. There have been six confirmed cases of measles at her son's crèche and she asks your advice as to what precautions she should take. Which ONE of the following is the SINGLE MOST appropriate advice in this case?

- A He should have a MMR booster at 4$\frac{1}{2}$ years of age
- B He should have a measles booster vaccine
- C He should have an MMR booster immediately
- D He should have blood sent to assess if he is immune
- E She should be reassured that no further vaccinations are required

P1.130 Heart murmurs

A 35-year-old woman is diagnosed with a heart murmur at a routine employment medical. A subsequent echocardiogram shows mitral valve prolapse. She comes to see you to discuss the implications of this. Which ONE of the following statements is correct regarding this condition? Select ONE option only.

- A All patients should be referred for valve replacement
- B It commonly causes congestive cardiac failure
- C It is usually caused by streptococcal infection
- D It can be associated with palpitations
- E Patients should be anticoagulated with warfarin

P1.131 Loss of smell

A 48-year-old man complains of 6 months of loss of smell and reduced taste. He reports that his symptoms are constant and seemed to have started for no obvious reason. He is a lifelong hayfever sufferer but says he can breathe through his nose. You do not have a Thudichum's nasal speculum in the surgery but limited examination of the nose with an otoscope does not show any obvious pathology. Which ONE of the following is the SINGLE MOST likely diagnosis?

- A Deviated nasal septum
- B Frontal lobe tumour
- C Head injury
- D Nasal polyps
- E Overuse of decongestant

Causes of pneumonia

P1.132–P1.136

Options

A   Aspergillosis
B   Actinomycosis
C   *Coxiella burnetii* pneumonia
D   Cytomelagovirus
E   Legionnaires' disease
F   Measles
G   *Mycoplasma pneumoniae*
H   *Pneumocystis jiroveci* pneumonia
I   Psittacosis
J   Q fever
K   Tuberculosis
L   Varicella

For each of the descriptions below, select the SINGLE MOST appropriate option from the list above. Each option may be used once, more than once or not at all.

P1.132   Epidemics occur in 3- to 4-year cycles, predominantly affecting children.
P1.133   Causes a prodromal illness with fever, coryza, conjunctivitis and cough, followed by the development of a rash starting on the neck.
P1.134   Affects immunocompromised individuals, causing a suppurative pneumonia; it has a poor prognosis.
P1.135   Causes a primary viral pneumonia in adults.
P1.136   Causes a prodromal illness with fever, diarrhoea, headache and myalgia, followed by the development of respiratory symptoms; hyponatraemia is often found.

P1.137   Rash
A 65-year-old woman develops a painful rash on her back. On examination she has numerous circular target lesions over her back and torso. These have a central blister. Which ONE of the following statements is correct regarding this scenario? Select ONE option only.

O   A   These lesions are never seen in the mouth

O   B   This condition is always iatrogenic and a full drug history should be taken

O   C   This condition often has an infectious cause

O   D   This condition usually resolves spontaneously in 3–5 days

O   E   This patient has erythema nodosum and should have a chest X-ray to exclude sarcoidosis

P1.138 Suspected female genital mutilation
        A 17-year-old girl originally from Somalia is seen in the antenatal clinic
        at 36 weeks' gestation. During the course of the consultation the patient
        tells you that 3 years earlier her mother took her to Somalia, where she
        underwent cutting. Which ONE of the following is required at this point?
        Select ONE option only.

    ○   A   Encourage the patient to make a complaint to the police

    ○   B   Ensure that the obstetric team are aware

    ○   C   Refer the patient for reconstructive surgery post-partum

    ○   D   Report the incident to social services

    ○   E   Report the incident to the police

P1.139 Palpitations
        A 78-year-old man is thought to have an irregular heartbeat at a blood
        pressure check. The nurse who sees him takes an electrocardiogram, which
        is shown below.

        Which ONE of the following is the correct diagnosis of this ECG trace?
        Select ONE option only.

    ○   A   Atrioventricular dissociation

    ○   B   Paroxysmal atrial fibrillation

    ○   C   Ventricular bigeminy

    ○   D   Wenckebach's phenomenon

    ○   E   2:1 heart block

P1.140 Erectile dysfunction
Which ONE of the following drugs for erectile dysfunction can be prescribed on the NHS without restriction? Select ONE option only.

○ A   Alprostadil

○ B   Avanafil

○ C   Sildenafil

○ D   Tadalafil

○ E   Vardenafil

Difficult patients

P1.141–P1.145

Options

A   Dependent clingers
B   Entitled demanders
C   Frequent attenders
D   Heartsink patient
E   Manipulative help rejector
F   Self-destructive denier
G   None of the above

For each of the descriptions below, select the SINGLE MOST appropriate option from the list above. Each option may be used once, more than once or not at all.

P1.141   Often try to take control of the doctor–patient relationship.
P1.142   More commonly identified by male rather than by female GPs.
P1.143   Unconsciously engages in behaviour that is likely to be detrimental to the patient's own health.
P1.144   Seem to derive satisfaction from the physician's inability to treat their symptoms.
P1.145   An objective description that is medicolegally appropriate.

P1.146 Eye symptoms
A 39-year-old schoolteacher complains that her right eye seems to be protruding more than the left. She has no visual symptoms or pain. Previous history is unremarkable other than chronic rhinosinusitis, for which she takes nasal steroids. On examination she does appear to have some asymmetry and proptosis. She saw her optician before this visit and has normal visual acuity, colour vision, fundoscopy and visual fields. She has no headache or any symptoms of hypothyroidism or hyperthyroidism. Blood tests, including thyroid function, are normal. What is the SINGLE MOST appropriate next step in her management? Select ONE option only.

○ A   Check thyroid autoantibodies

○ B   Check for anti-acetylcholine receptor antibodies

○ C   Reassure her that this is normal

○ D   Refer under the 2-week rule for suspected brain tumour

○ E   Treat with broad-spectrum antibiotics

P1.147 Water-borne disease
Your local water supply has been temporarily suspended due to the discovery of *Cryptosporidium* sp. in a reservoir. A number of your patients have come to see you, concerned that they might have been exposed before the shutdown. Which ONE of the following statements is true with regard to this situation? Select ONE option only.

○ A   Cryptosporidia affect all age groups, causing severe diarrhoea and vomiting

○ B   Cryptosporidia can be resistant to chlorination of water

○ C   Cryptosporidia in children cause a mild diarrhoea that lasts less than 48 hours

○ D   Cryptosporidia can cause haemoytic uraemic syndrome

○ E   Humans are a secondary host and do not transmit the infection to others

Driving and neurological disorders

P1.148–P1.152

Options

A   May drive and need not inform Driver and Vehicle Licensing Authority (DVLA)
B   Must not drive and must notify DVLA
C   Must not drive for 1 month and must inform DVLA
D   Must not drive for 3 month and must inform DVLA
E   Must not drive for 1 month but need not inform the DVLA
F   Must notify DVLA but may continue to drive

For each of the medical conditions below, select the SINGLE MOST APPROPRIATE option from the list of actions above. Each option may be used once, more than once or not at all.

P1.148   A Group 1 licence holder has a solitary episode of vasovagal syncope with prodrome while sitting. All neurological and cardiovascular investigations are normal.

P1.149   A Group 2 licence holder with mild Parkinson's disease, not treated with medication.

P1.150   A Group 2 licence holder is diagnosed with a single transient ischaemic attack.

P1.151   A Group 1 licence holder has an unprovoked grand mal seizure. Brain imaging, EEG and blood tests are all normal.

P1.152   A Group 1 licence holder suffers a stroke; 4 weeks later he has very minor right arm weakness but has full function.

P1.153   Cardiomyopathy
Which ONE of the following statements with regard to hypertrophic obstructive cardiomyopathy (HOCM) is true? Select ONE option only.

O   A   The cause is usually viral

O   B   It is a cause of sudden death in young athletes

O   C   It is a benign condition

O   D   Treatment with β blockers will increase life expectancy

O   E   It usually presents with signs of congestive cardiac failure

P1.154 Hand symptoms

A 62-year-old man asks you to look at his hand. He is unable to fully straighten his fingers. Examining the hand nodular thickening is palpable proximal to the fourth and fifth metacarpophalangeal joints. The hand is shown below.

What is the SINGLE MOST LIKELY diagnosis? Write your answer in words in the box below.

P1.155 Irregular bleeding

A 25-year-old nulliparous woman complains of breakthrough bleeding most months on her 30-mcg COCP. She has been taking this for 12 months now, takes no other medications and does not miss pills. Examination is unremarkable and she recently had a cervical smear that was reported as negative. She does not get any post-coital bleeding and high vaginal swabs and chlamydial swabs were recently negative. Which ONE of the following is the most appropriate management? Select ONE option only.

- ○ A   Advise her to take two pills a day
- ○ B   Change to a triphasic pill
- ○ C   Change to the mini-pill for better cycle control
- ○ D   Suggest a Mirena intrauterine system (IUS)
- ○ E   Reassure her that this is normal and no action is needed

P1.156 Headache

A 19-year-old student who lives in private rented accommodation is brought in by his mother who found him complaining of weakness, nausea and vomiting, sleepiness and severe headache for several days. Which ONE of the following is a possible cause if his symptoms? Select ONE option only.

- ○ A   Carbon monoxide poisoning
- ○ B   Haemolytic–uraemic syndrome
- ○ C   Influenza
- ○ D   Meningitis
- ○ E   Migraine

Treatment of prostate cancer

P1.157–P1.161

Options

A   Brachytherapy
B   Cryotherapy
C   Cyproterone acetate
D   Docetaxel
E   External-beam radiotherapy
F   LHRH analogue
G   Orchidectomy
H   Radical prostatectomy
I   Watchful waiting

For each of the statements below regarding the management of prostate cancer, select the SINGLE MOST appropriate option from the list above. Each option may be used once, more than once or not at all.

P1.157   Associated with a >10% risk of proctitis.
P1.158   Shown in the Scandinavian Prostate Cancer Group Study to be as effective as radical prostatectomy in terms of its effect on overall mortality.
P1.159   Indicated for non-hormone-sensitive recurrent disease in patients who have previously been treated with radiotherapy.
P1.160   Useful in patients with metastatic disease who cannot tolerate LHRH agonist treatment.
P1.161   Causes an initial increase in testosterone production.

P1.162   Gout
Which ONE of the following statements about gout is true? Select ONE option only.

○   A   Colchicine should be prescribed as one tablet every hour until the pain resolves or diarrhoea develops

○   B   Dietary factors are the most common triggers for an acute attack of gout

○   C   Joint aspiration typically reveals cloudy fluid and this is diagnostic in larger joints

○   D   Normal serum uric acid during an acute attack of arthritis excludes gout

○   E   Patients who are intolerant of colchicine or NSAIDs should be treated with prednisolone

P1.163 Skin disease

A 63-year-old woman has noticed an itchy rash in her cleavage.

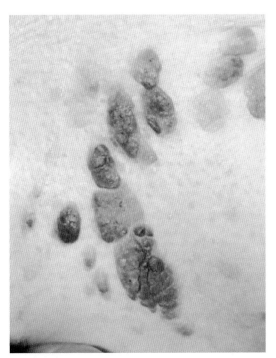

What is the SINGLE MOST likely diagnosis? Select ONE option only.

- ○ A Basal cell carcinoma
- ○ B Dermatofibroma
- ○ C Malignant melanoma
- ○ D Seborrhoeic keratosis
- ○ E Viral wart

P1.164 Vaginal discharge

Regarding vaginal infections, which ONE of the following statements is true? Select ONE option only.

- ○ A A fishy smell suggests candidal infection
- ○ B Bacterial vaginosis is always symptomatic
- ○ C Candidal infection is more common in pregnancy
- ○ D *Trichomonas* sp. does not cause disease in men
- ○ E Where bacterial vaginosis is confirmed, the partner must also be treated to prevent re-infection

P1.165 Data interpretation

A pilot weight-loss clinic has been running for 12 months and the primary care trust would like to extend the service based on its results. The results are shown below (BMI, body mass index; CI, confidence interval; N/A, not applicable).

Time since start (months)	No. patients	Mean weight change (kg)	95% CI	Mean BMI (kg/m²)
0	1500	N/A	N/A	32
1	1200	-2.6	-4.1 to +1.3	31
2	1000	-3.1	-3.9 to +0.5	29
3	900	-3.3	-3.4 to -1.8	28
6	600	-3.4	-3.6 to -2.5	28
12	300	-2.9	-3.2 to -2.6	29

Which ONE of the following statements about these data is correct? Select ONE option only.

O A   On an intention-to-treat basis the data show a mean weight loss of -2.9 kg at 12 months

O B   The data show a statistically significant weight loss at 3 months

O C   The data show high levels of concordance

O D   Most patients who complete 12 months' treatment achieve a normal BMI

O E   Weight loss is maintained at 12 months in most patients

Viral infections

P1.166–P1.170

Options

A   Adenovirus
B   Coxsackievirus
C   Epstein–Barr virus
D   Herpes simplex
E   Human papillomavirus
F   Hepatitis D
G   Influenza A
H   Norovirus
I   Parvovirus B19

For each of the diseases below, select the SINGLE MOST likely causative agent from the list above. Each option may be used once, more than once or not at all.

P1.166   Oropharyngeal cancer
P1.167   Gastroenteritis
P1.168   Slapped cheek syndrome
P1.169   Hand, foot and mouth disease
P1.170   Burkitt's lymphoma

P1.171   Groin pain
A 6-year-old girl comes to see you with her mother. She has been complaining for 6 months of intermittent pain in the right side of her groin and she has a persistent limp. She is otherwise well but seems to be limping most of the time. On examination she has a full range of movement on the left side of her hip but movements on the right side are limited in all directions. Examination of the groin reveals no hernia and no lymphadenopathy. Blood tests are taken, which are normal. What is the SINGLE MOST likely diagnosis? Select ONE option only.

○   A   Congenital dislocation of the hip

○   B   Irritable hip

○   C   Perthes' disease

○   D   Septic arthritis

○   E   Slipped upper femoral epiphysis

P1.172 **Bone health**
Which ONE of the following statements with regard to the management of osteopenia and osteoporosis is correct? Select ONE option only.

- ○ A Bisphosphonates are available only in oral formulation
- ○ B Bisphosphonates have been shown to increase bone density but not to reduce fractures
- ○ C Patients diagnosed with osteoporosis should be investigated for coeliac disease
- ○ D Patients diagnosed with postmenopausal osteoporosis should be treated with bisphosphonates for life
- ○ E A T-score <1.5 is diagnostic of osteoporosis

P1.173 **Knee pain**
A 67-year-old man complains of increasing frequency of pain in both knees, worse on the right. He has is slightly overweight with a body mass index of 27 but has no previous medical history of note and takes no regular medication. Clinical examination reveals a mild varus deformity, some crepitus on both sides on flexion, but no erythema or effusion. Which ONE of the following statements about management is correct? Select ONE option only.

- ○ A All patients should be advised to exercise regularly
- ○ B All patients should have an initial X ray
- ○ C Referral to an orthopaedic surgeon is indicated if symptoms cannot be controlled with oral analgesia
- ○ D Weight-bearing exercise is contraindicated
- ○ E Weight loss is unlikely to be helpful in patients with a BMI <30

P1.174   Headache
A 34-year-old woman in week 12 of her first pregnancy complains of several weeks of increasing headaches. These are present mostly in the mornings and late at night, and seem to resolve once she gets up. She has no other previous history of note. Examination reveals a blood pressure of 128/72 mmHg, negative urinalysis and a BMI of 34. Her pupils are equal and reactive and she has no ophthalmoplegia or obvious visual field loss. Fundoscopy shows a hyperaemic disc with loss of cupping. What is the SINGLE MOST likely diagnosis? Select ONE option only.

- ○ A   Acute glaucoma
- ○ B   Benign intracranial hypertension
- ○ C   Brain tumour
- ○ D   Malignant hypertension
- ○ E   Pre-eclampsia

Management of abnormal smears

P1.175–P1.179

Options

A   Refer for colposcopy
B   Refer under 2-week rule
C   Repeat in 1 month
D   Repeat in 6 months
E   Repeat in 1 year
F   Repeat in 3 years
G   Repeat in 5 years
H   Smear no longer necessary

Regarding the management of cervical smear results, for each of the situations described below select the SINGLE MOST appropriate management option from the list above. Each option may be used once, more than once or not at all.

P1.175   A 34-year-old woman has had a smear reported as 'borderline, with endocervical changes'. She has not previously had abnormal smears.

P1.176   A 27-year-old woman with a history of previous chlamydial infection has had two consecutive inadequate smears.

P1.177   A 63-year-old woman who has not had any previous abnormal smears has a normal smear. She enquires about follow-up smears.

P1.178   A 36-year-old woman with no history of abnormal smears has a smear reported as showing mild dyskariosis.

P1.179   A 31-year-old woman has a smear that shows suspected carcinoma in situ.

P1.180 Rash

A 24-year-old girl attends for a new patient check. She asks if there is anything else that she can use for the rash on her arms. She has had this for most of her life and uses regular moisturisers, otherwise the skin becomes dry. She also reports that the rash improves when she is away from the stress of the office on holiday. The rash is shown below.

What would the SINGLE MOST appropriate management be in this instance? Select ONE option only.

- A   Prescribe topical steroids
- B   Prescribe topical tacrolimus
- C   Prescribe vitamin D analogues
- D   Refer for PUVA therapy
- E   Treat with antifungal treatment

P1.181 **Eye symptoms**

A 17-year-old girl has a lump in her lower eyelid, which has been present for 9 months and is slowly enlarging. She reports that this started after she developed a stye, but she is becoming increasingly self-conscious and would like your advice on management. Which ONE of the following is the SINGLE MOST appropriate action?

○ A She should be offered incision and curettage

○ B She should be told that it is unlikely to resolve spontaneously

○ C She should be referred immediately to ophthalmology outpatients for excision

○ D She should be treated with antibiotic ointment

○ E She should be treated with cryotherapy

P1.182 **Pre-pregnancy care**

You see a 31-year-old woman who is planning to start a family soon. Which ONE of the following statements is correct about pre-pregnancy counselling? Select ONE option only.

○ A All pregnant women should take vitamin D supplements

○ B Nicotine replacement therapy is contraindicated in pregnancy

○ C Patients should be advised to drink no more than 14 units of alcohol a week

○ D Patients taking anticonvulsants should take 400 μg folic acid a day

○ E Patients with pre-existing hypertension should be switched to an ACE inhibitor pre-conception

P1.183 **Diarrhoea**

A 36-year-old woman with no previous history of note complains of nausea and vomiting with fever, followed by watery diarrhoea and abdominal pain, which started 12 hours after attending a wedding with a buffet reception. Which ONE of the following is the SINGLE MOST likely organism responsible? Select ONE option only.

○ A *Campylobacter* sp.

○ B Cryptosporidia

○ C *Salmonella* sp.

○ D *Shigella* sp.

○ E Typhoid

P1.184 Eye problems

A 52-year-old man attends his optician for a routine eye test. His optician asks him to make an appointment to see you, and the letter from the optician states that he has normal intraocular pressure but has cupped discs. Which ONE of the following statements is correct regarding this situation? Select ONE option only.

O   A   Annual follow-up is indicated with onward referral if intraocular pressures exceed 21 mmHg

O   B   Cupping of the disc indicates damage to the eye despite normal intraocular pressure

O   C   Laser iridotomy is indicated to reverse the cupping

O   D   No action is required at this time but he should be asked to report any change in his vision

O   E   No further action is needed

P1.185 Backache

A 78-year-old man complains of mid-thoracic backache for the last 3 months. He looks pale and has lost weight. On examination he has some tenderness over his eighth thoracic vertebra, but there are no other obvious signs. You arrange for some blood tests, which show raised plasma viscosity, a normochromic/normocytic anaemia with normal WCC and platelets, a raised calcium and an eGFR of 42 ml/min. What is the SINGLE MOST likely diagnosis? Select ONE option only.

O   A   Chronic lymphocytic leukaemia (CLL)

O   B   Lung cancer

O   C   Multiple myeloma

O   D   Prostate cancer

O   E   Sarcoma

P1.186 Molar pregnancy

A 32-year-old woman has recently been discharged from hospital after having a molar pregnancy. She comes to see you to discuss the implications of this diagnosis. Which ONE of the following statements is true? Select ONE option only.

O   A   Ninety per cent of patients with a molar pregnancy will go on to develop neoplastic disease within 2 years

O   B   Prognosis is poor in patients who develop neoplastic disease

O   C   Patients should be monitored with regular bhCG levels for 2 years

O   D   Recurrence risk is high and patients should be advised to undergo sterilisation

O   E   The COCP is suitable contraception in the bhCG monitoring phase

The Mental Health Act

P1.187–P1.191

Options

A   Section 2
B   Section 3
C   Section 4
D   Section 7
E   Section 12
F   Section 17
G   Section 135
H   Section 136
I   None of the above

For each of the situations described below, select the SINGLE MOST appropriate option from the list above. Each option may be used once, more than once or not at all.

P1.187   A 23-year-old man who has been living with his mother has developed an addiction to heroin. He refuses treatment but his mother asks you to have him sectioned so that he can be treated.

P1.188   A 77-year-old man is found confused and wearing only his pyjamas in the street in the middle of the night in early February. He is unable to give his name to the police or explain why he is there, but refuses to go with them. They feel that he is at risk and would like to take him to a safe place.

P1.189   A 31-year-old paranoid schizophrenic has stopped taking his medication and is refusing to leave the house where he lives with his mother. He has started to self-harm and will not see his doctor, who he believes is the devil.

P1.190   A 52-year-old man with severe learning disabilities due to Down syndrome can no longer be looked after by his elderly mother, but refuses to go into a residential home. Social services have requested that he be admitted to one under the provisions of the Mental Health Act.

P1.191   The 31-year-old paranoid schizophrenic has been assessed and treated in hospital and it is felt that he needs a further period of supervised patient treatment, but that this can be given in the community. He has a history of non-compliance and subsequent relapse.

Management of heavy menstrual bleeding

P1.192–1.196

Options

A   Contraceptive pill
B   Danazol
C   Fibroids present on ultrasound
D   Luteal phase progestogens
E   Mirena
F   Normal ultrasound
G   Refer routinely
H   Refer under the 2-week rule
I   Tranexamic acid

The algorithm below describes the management of women with heavy menstrual bleeding. From the list of options above, select the SINGLE MOST appropriate management for each missing step. Each option may be used once, more than once or not at all.

P1.197 Snoring

A 37-year-old man comes to see you with his new wife. They have been married for only 3 months but already she has had to resort to sleeping in the spare room because of his snoring. He has no symptoms or signs of sleep apnoea, and is otherwise well. On examination he has a collar size of 15 inches, a BMI of 27 kg/m², and examination of his nose and throat are normal. He does not smoke and drinks 18 units of alcohol a week. Which ONE of the following is the most appropriate action in this situation? Select ONE option only.

- A Advise the patient that his snoring is harmless and no treatment is needed
- B Cessation of alcohol for at least 4 weeks
- C Prescribe sedatives for his wife
- D Refer for continuous positive airway pressure (CPAP) treatment
- E Refer for uvulopalatoplasty (UVPP)

P1.198 Hepatitis screening

Following a needlestick injury to one of your practice nurses and the subsequent significant-event audit, your practice decides to undertake an active approach to identifying patients who might have hepatitis C. This would have the benefit of treating early infection and reducing the risk of transmission. Which ONE of the following patients are at risk and would benefit from screening? Select ONE option only.

- A A 56-year-old man who worked as an oil worker in West Africa for many years
- B A 23-year-old man who has recently returned from a year travelling in south-east Asia with a new tattoo
- C A 38-year-old woman who had a 4 unit blood transfusion following a postpartum haemorrhage in 1988
- D A 31-year-old businessman who has had extensive dental treatment in a dental facility in Singapore
- E A 56-year-old man with a persistently raised GGT on his blood results

P1.199 Ear symptoms

A 35-year-old semi-professional surfer complains of recurrent episodes of water trapping in his ears after surfing. On examination you note the appearance below.

Which ONE of the following is the SINGLE MOST likely diagnosis Select ONE option only.

○ A   Cholesteatoma

○ B   Chronic otitis externa

○ C   Exostoses

○ D   Foreign body

○ E   Inflammatory polyp

P1.200 Depression

A 26-year-old woman is brought in by her mother concerned about her low mood. She has been unhappy for several months without any obvious triggers. A PHQ-9 questionnaire is completed and the result is 13. Which ONE of the following is a correct interpretation of this result? Select ONE option only.

○ A   Normal

○ B   Mild depression

○ C   Moderate depression

○ D   Moderately severe depression

○ E   Severe depression

Paper 1 Answers

P1.1   **B:**   **Frozen shoulder is more common in patients with diabetes mellitus**

Long-term studies suggest that only 39% of patients make a full recovery, although another 54% have no functional limitation despite a small reduction in mobility. Secondary frozen shoulder is generally rare, but diabetes increases the risk with prevalence up to 36% in this group. Mean age of onset is 40–60 years. The diagnosis is essentially a clinical one, although X-rays or blood tests might be necessary to exclude other pathology if clinically suspected.

P1.2   **D:**   **Irregular bleeding is the most common side effect of progestogen implant**

Implanon capsules are inserted in the skin above the elbow and consist of a single capsule changed every 3 years, unlike Norplant, which consisted of five rods that were changed every 5 years. Irregular bleeding is common in Implanon users, and can be treated with the combined contraceptive pill or tranexamic acid in the first 6 months, after which it usually settles down. Acne is common, but there is no evidence of an effect on mood, weight or libido. Around 50% of women become amenorrhoeic on Implanon. After removal, blood levels of etonogestrel are undetectable within 1 week and ovulation occurs in 90% of women within 3 weeks. The implants are changed after 3 years and the pregnancy rate in users is <0.1 in 100 women over 3 years.

Bleeding in end-of-life care

P1.3   F: Tranexamic acid

Tranexamic acid mouthwash and sucralfate suspension can both be used for oral bleeding.

P1.4   D: Radiotherapy

Radiotherapy is often helpful in haemoptysis, haematuria and skin bleeding.

P1.5   C: Packing and cautery

Nosebleeds can be treated with packing and cautery. Tranexamic acid may also be helpful, or adrenaline-soaked gaze.

Kaltostat, topical adrenaline soaks or topical tranexamic acid can be used for skin bleeding and, if it persists, radiotherapy may be considered. Tranexamic acid may help with haematuria but increases the risk of clot retention. Embolisation may help with recurrent upper GI bleeds or liver bleeds, whereas thalidomide may help with GI tumours.

P1.6   A: A CAGE score of ≥2 is suggestive of problem drinking

The AUDIT C test identifies heavy drinking, and measures frequency of drinking, binge drinking and total consumption. The CAGE test identifies alcohol dependence, and focuses on experiences of alcohol rather than consumption. A CAGE score of ≥2 has a sensitivity of 93% and a specificity of 76% for the identification of problem drinkers, and a score of 4 is virtually diagnostic. The MAST is a 24-item screening tool designed to detect severe alcohol dependence. It is used in research and treatment programmes but is too complex for brief interventions.

P1.7   Simvastatin

Macrolide antibiotics have numerous interactions and in particular should not be co-administered with simvastatin, amisulpiride, ergotamine, tolterodine or terfenadine. It may increase serum concentrations of carbamazepine, phenytoin, tacrolimus, theophylline valproate, warfarin and digoxin. Patients taking statins should stop these temporarily, whereas patients on warfarin should have their INR closely monitored and adjusted as necessary.

P1.8   E: The readings suggest the presence of significant peripheral vascular disease affecting the right side only

The ABPI is 0.8 on the right side and 1.0 on the left. An ABPI <0.9 suggests the presence of significant peripheral vascular disease, whereas an ABPI <0.8 suggests a risk of ulceration. Once the ABPI is <0.5 this indicates critical ischaemia. ABPI readings >1.0 can be seen where the patient is not supine or where there is reduced arterial compliance, as in atherosclerosis.

P1.9   C: Prodromal dermatomal pain is a risk factor for post-herpetic neuralgia

Risk factors for severe post-herpetic neuralgia include age >50, prodromal pain, and severe pain and rash during the attack. Prompt use of antivirals reduces the incidence of post-herpetic neuralgia by up to 50%. Systematic review suggests the best evidence is for tricyclic antidepressants, although there is also evidence for anticonvulsants, 5% lidocaine plasters, opiates and capsaicin. Severe intractable pain might be helped by ketamine injections.

P1.10   C: Reassure the parents that it will usually resolve spontaneously in time

This is an umbilical hernia. Spontaneous closure is the norm and surgery is indicated only if closure fails to occur. Such hernias are more common in African–Caribbean children and occur twice as commonly in boys as girls. Incarceration is uncommon below the age of 3 years, so there is usually no indication for surgical treatment below this age, and 93% close without any intervention. Some surgeons advocate taping the skin over the hernia to bring the edges of the hernia together in an attempt to hasten closure, but this is not usually necessary.

Drug management of asthma

P1.11   H: Oral leukotriene receptor antagonist

Leukotriene receptor antagonists are of no value in acute asthma but have a role in the maintenance treatment of asthma. They also have some benefits in allergic rhinitis. They are licensed in children and can be useful as a steroid-sparing agent.

P1.12   A: Combination of inhaled corticosteroid and long-acting β_2 agonist

The SMART (Symbicort as maintenance and reliever therapy) approach allows patients to self-manage their asthma according to their symptoms. It has been shown to reduce the use of oral steroids and the number of doctor consultations.

P1.13   I: Oral theophylline

Theophylline is rarely used due to the risk of adverse effects, including arrhythmias, nausea and diarrhoea. Particular care should be taken to ensure that patients are not using inhaled theophylline before starting oral treatment due to the risk of toxicity.

P1.14   B: Inhaled anticholinergic

Inhaled anticholinergics reduce vagal tone and have the benefit of reducing mucus secretion, which makes them useful in patients with chronic obstructive pulmonary disease.

P1.15   G: Oral corticosteroids

Long-term (>3 months) oral steroids at a dose >5 mg/day should prompt the use of bisphosphonates to prevent osteoporosis. The Royal College of Physicians further recommends that three separate short courses over a 12-month period should be considered to be equivalent to 3 months' prescribing.

P1.16   E: Posterior cruciate tear

The positive posterior draw test indicates a posterior cruciate tear. This injury is typically seen in patients who have received a blow to the proximal tibia with the knee flexed, eg in a road traffic accident or by falling on to a flexed knee. Management involves a splint initially, followed by physiotherapy. Anterior cruciate tears are associated with a positive anterior draw test. In younger patients, surgery is usually necessary, particularly in sportsmen and -women. Patellar tendon tears result in an inability to extend the knee. Medial and lateral collateral tears are associated with laxity when the knee is stressed laterally or medially.

P1.17   B: Multinodular goitre

This is a multinodular goitre. It may be associated with thyrotoxicosis or hypothyroidism. Multinodular goitre with abnormal thyroid function tests should be referred to endocrinology, whereas new presentations of non-toxic goitre should be referred to ENT for investigation to exclude a dominant nodule, associated with increased risk of malignancy. The overall rate of malignant transformation in a multinodular goitre is 5%.

P1.18   C: Autism

Autism should be suspected when there is a combination of delay in development in terms of social interaction and reciprocal communication behaviours (including non-verbal communication such as body language), unusual or restricted interests and/or repetitive behaviours, eg food fads, strong preference for exact routine. and an often unusual profile of skills and deficits, eg poor social skills combined with advanced reading skills. Asperger syndrome patients have specific difficulties with social skills but usually have normal language skills, although they may be literal and have difficulty with emotional context. Deafness should always be considered in children with speech delay. Developmental language disorder is usually primarily a language disorder.

P1.19   B: No action required

The presence of asymptomatic bacteriuria is common in catheterised patients and no action is necessary unless they are unwell. *Proteus* sp. is often associated with urinary stones or foreign bodies. Replacing the catheter would increase the risks of infection by causing local trauma, and irrigation would simply flush bacteria into the bladder.

Death certification

P1.20   C: Discuss the case with the coroner

Where a patient has not been seen in the last 14 days you cannot issue a death certificate without discussing the case with the coroner. In a situation such as this the coroner will often allow a death certificate to be issued.

P1.21   A: Contact the police

Sudden deaths should be referred to the police who will arrange appropriate investigation and a postmortem examination. You cannot issue a death certificate in this situation.

P1.22 C: Discuss the case with the coroner

Where industrial disease is implicated the employment box should be ticked on the death certificate and the coroner informed.

P1.23 C: Discuss the case with the coroner

Unnatural deaths should always be referred to the coroner.

P1.24 H: None of the above

A stillborn baby can be certified on a Certificate of Stillbirth only after 24 weeks of pregnancy. If the baby does breathe after birth, no matter what gestation, a neonatal death form should be used. This case should be referred to the obstetrics and gynaecology department to arrange investigation and appropriate counselling, and to liaise with the coroner.

P1.25 F: Issue Medical Certificate of Cause of Death

Death certificates do not require the doctor to have seen the body after death, as long as another medical practitioner has seen the body and confirmed death.

P1.26 E: SSRIs should be used as first-line treatment

Social phobia has a lifetime risk of 13% and is particularly common in women from lower social classes. Affected people experience feelings of panic in public situations and nausea and vomiting are common. Management comprises CBT where available and SSRIs in the short term. Benzodiazepines or β blockers can also help with crises.

P1.27 A: Admit under paediatrics

This patient has haemolytic uraemic syndrome, which may follow *Escherichia coli* O157 infection. Risk factors include extremes of age. Clinical suspicion should be raised in children with bloody diarrhoea. Oliguria and dehydration are common and thrombocytopenic purpura can be seen. Treatment is supportive, although some patients need short-term dialysis.

P1.28 E: CBT should be offered to all patients with chronic fatigue syndrome

The diagnosis of chronic fatigue syndrome should be considered in patients with unexplained fatigue lasting more than 3 months in a child or 4 months in an adult. Chronic pain, sleep disturbance and cognitive difficulties are common. Exacerbations usually start 24–48 hours after exertion. The treatment of this condition involves graded exercise and CBT. The prognosis is extremely variable, with some patients making a quick recovery and others developing chronic disease. The disease has been reported to follow infection with a number of viruses, and it is estimated that 10% of patients with clinical Epstein–Barr virus infection will develop chronic fatigue syndrome.

P1.29 B: Episcleritis

Episcleritis is a localised, self-limiting condition affecting the sclera. Iritis can be excluded on examination and scleritis is usually a severe boring pain rather than a dull ache. Scleritis is usually bilateral and associated with connective tissue disease. The inflammation in episcleritis is usually limited to a small sector and typically settles over 7–10 days. Topical non-steroidal drops might accelerate this process and steroid drops are also helpful, but should be given only after expert assessment to exclude keratitis. Keratitis is usually obvious on fluorescein staining but a slit lamp should be used. Acute angle-closure glaucoma usually causes stony-hard eyes and vomiting with severe pain.

P1.30   50%

The BRCA-1 and BRCA-2 genes are inherited as autosomal dominants with incomplete penetration, ie can be inherited from either father or mother. The risk of carrying the gene if you have a carrier parent is 50%. Carriers of the BRCA-1 gene have lifetime risk of breast cancer of 80% and of ovarian cancer of 40–60% whereas BRCA-2 has a lower rate of ovarian cancer, of 20–30%. Patients testing positive can be offered prophylactic surgery, although those with a carrier in the family who do not choose to be tested are offered annual mammograms from age 40.

Childhood infections

P1.31   G: Poxvirus

Molluscum contagiosum causes crops to appear and spread through autoinoculation. They are typically seen in the pre-school age group and individual lesions can last from 2–3 weeks to several months. No specific treatment is needed and they regress spontaneously.

P1.32   C: *Mycoplasma pneumoniae*

Mycoplasma pneumoniae causes respiratory symptoms in young children and can be associated with erythema multiforme. These patients usually respond to oral macrolides, eg erythromycin.

P1.33   F: Parvovirus B19

Parvovirus B19 (also called erythrovirus B19) causes a mild, self-limiting disease in children but unexposed pregnant women can develop fetal hydrops as a result of this infection.

P1.34   A: Group A streptococci

Scarlet fever follows infection with β-haemolytic streptococci and can cause rheumatic fever or glomerulonephritis. Children should be treated with at least 10 days of phenoxymethylpenicillin and excluded from school until the antibiotics are started.

P1.35   L: Varicella

Varicella need be treated only in adults, neonates or immunocompromised individuals.

P1.36   E: Ulcerative colitis

Ulcerative colitis often presents as an isolated proctitis and attacks can start after periods of stress. The diagnosis is usually made at proctoscopy, where a typical granular and ulcerated appearance is seen. Crohn's disease is the major differential in this age group but is often associated with piles or fistulae, and tends to cause more systemic features. Management usually consists of rectal steroids or aminosalicylates; loperamide should not be used because it does not work and can increase the risk of toxic megacolon. Long-term management is usually with aminosalicylates. Patients with ulcerative colitis are at increased risk of colorectal cancer and should be screened regularly.

P1.37   D: Suction termination can be carried out under local anaesthesia

Mifepristone can be used for late abortions (>15 weeks) with prostaglandin pessaries and is an alternative to surgical termination. It cannot be used in women with a history of cardiac or respiratory disease. Two doctors must sign the certificate before a termination can take place; if they feel that a patient is Gillick competent the parents need not be informed. The legal limit for termination is 24 weeks but there is some debate about lowering this to 22 weeks. At present <1% of abortions take place after 20 weeks.

Personality disorders

P1.38   E: Hyperthymic personality disorder

Hyperthymic personality is characterised by persistent enthusiasm and optimism which is associated with rash judgements (eg poor financial investments).

P1.39   C: Borderline personality disorder

Borderline personality disorders are typified by young men who frequently get drunk and are involved in fights or acts of vandalism. They are often lonely and crave company, but are unable to develop rewarding relationships.

P1.40   A: Anankastic personality disorder

Anankastic personality disorders show considerable overlap with obsessional neurosis, and these people are often ill at ease in company and very sensitive to criticism.

P1.41   F: Narcissistic personality disorder

Narcissistic personality types are also very sensitive to criticism, but are easily bored and have difficulty forming emotional attachments to others.

P1.42   H: Schizoid personality disorder

Schizoid personality types are typically seen as aloof or boring, and are happiest in their own company.

P1.43   E: Vesicocolic fistula

Recurrent or refractory symptoms of UTI with pneumaturia or faecaluria are hallmarks of vesicocolic fistula. These affect men more than women in the ratio 3:1 and are the most common of the abdominal fistulae. Diverticulosis is the most common cause, although bowel and bladder cancer should be excluded. Crohn's disease may also present as a vesicocolic fistula. Approximately 50% of fistulae close spontaneously once the underlying cause has been treated, but where they don't surgery is indicated

P1.44   C: Deep vein thrombosis

DVT is a complication of pacemaker placement and should be treated with low molecular weight heparin and warfarinisation, as for other thromboembolic disease. Cellulitis or wound infection should be considered in the differential but would be unusual in the absence of fever. Arterial embolism would normally cause pain, pulselessness and pallor.

P1.45   C: Raised serum ferritin with reduced total iron-binding capacity

Haemochromatosis is due to iron overload and commonly damages the heart, liver, pancreas and pituitary. It may be hereditary or acquired. Hereditary cases can be investigated with genotyping if this has been done on the index case. Siblings should be screened, and the characteristic findings on iron studies are raised ferritin with reduced total iron-binding capacity and raised iron-binding saturation. If liver function is abnormal a biopsy should be considered. Raised MCV and MCH are suggestive of vitamin B_{12}/folate deficiency whereas reduced MCV and MCH are suggestive of iron deficiency.

P1.46   D: Pertussis

Pertussis causes a prolonged cough characterised by paroxysms lasting minutes, during which the patient may feel unable to breathe. It lasts 4–8 weeks and can be associated with loud whoops at the end of the spasm of coughing. Antibiotics such as azithromycin will reduce infectivity but not shorten the duration of illness. Vaccination programmes offer 95% coverage but cases in children and adults do occur, with significant morbidity and mortality for infants.

Biological therapies

P1.47   C: Omalizumab (Xolair)

Omalizumab is useful in allergy-mediated asthma. Patients need to have elevated IgE levels, and it is not suitable for other forms of asthma. It is given by regular injection.

P1.48   B: Natalizumab (Tysabri)

Natalizumab acts on T cells to reduce severity of symptoms in multiple sclerosis. It is licensed as monotherapy for relapsing MS and is given by injection. It can reduce the frequency of attacks and slow down the accumulation of disability. It might also be helpful in Crohn's disease.

P1.49   A: Infliximab (Remicade)

NICE guidance recommends the use of infliximab for severe psoriasis (a psoriasis area severity index >20) in patients not responding to or not suitable for PUVA or ciclosporin and other systemic treatments. It also has a role in acute Crohn's disease and rheumatoid arthritis.

P1.50   F: Trastuzumab (Herceptin)

Trastuzumab acts on the HER2 receptors on malignant cells, and is accordingly licensed for HER2-positive patients. It reduces the risk of early recurrence by 50%. NICE recommends its use after surgery, chemotherapy and radiotherapy if appropriate. It can cause congestive cardiac failure and cardiac work-up is required.

P1.51   D: Ranibizumab (Lucentis)

Ranibizumab is licensed for wet macular degeneration and is given as an injection into the eye. It has been shown to stabilise eyesight in most patients and 30–40% of patients experience an improvement in their visual acuity.

P1.52   C: Surgery is indicated in patients who do not wish to take long-term medication

Indications for surgery include severe oesophagitis, long-term complications, and inability or unwillingness to take long-term medication. Surgical options include laparoscopic fundoplication, laparoscopic placement of a Silastic prosthesis or use of the falciform ligament to reduce the hernia and maintain it, and open fundoplication. Long-term follow-up studies suggest that about a third of patients need proton pump inhibitors after surgery, compared with two-thirds of patients managed medically. Surgery is useful in sliding and rolling hernias; rolling hernias are more likely to obstruct. Patients should be able to eat normally after surgery.

P1.53   A: Ankylosing spondylitis

The presence of morning stiffness, age of onset <40 years, limited spinal flexion and improvement with exercise rather than rest is suggestive of ankylosing spondylitis. This can be confirmed with an X-ray of the lumbosacral spine showing sacroiliitis and HLA-B27 testing. Patients should be referred early for consideration of anti-TNF therapy. Fifty per cent of patients have associated non-spinal pathology such as iritis.

P1.54   D: Methotrexate frequently causes menstrual disturbances

Full blood count and LFTs should be done pre-treatment, after the initial dose and dose changes. Once stable, they can be done every 2–3 months. Falls in WCC and platelets, or increase in LFTs by a threefold factor or more, should prompt cessation. A mild increase in LFTs is common but a fall in albumin of >5 g/l is an early sign of liver toxicity. Folic acid is given on the 6 days a week when methotrexate is not taken. Methotrexate is teratogenic.

P1.55 A: Asperger syndrome

This child has typical features of Asperger syndrome. Children with this condition have a specific impairment in social functioning but have a normal IQ and often excel in certain areas. Patients can have a normal vocabulary but struggle with abstract language and metaphors, and have significant difficulties interpreting and using non-verbal communication.

Sleep disturbance

P1.56 A: Bed-time restriction

P1.57 E: Melatonin

P1.58 C: Intermittent short-term hypnotics

P1.59 D: Light therapy

Once other causes of sleep disturbance have been excluded, such as restless legs syndrome or chronic pain, insomnia should be classified as primary insomnia or delayed sleep phase syndrome (cannot get to sleep at night, cannot get up in morning). Delayed sleep phase syndrome is thought to be a disturbance of circadian rhythm and may respond to melatonin. Failing this, use of light boxes or exposure to natural light may help. Primary insomnia responds to a trial of at least 2 weeks of sleep restriction. Failing this, short-term intermittent use of hypnotics may be justified, with appropriate counselling.

P1.60 E: Ulipristal acetate

In this patient who has already tried anti-inflammatories and contraceptive pills and is awaiting surgery, the next step would be to try ulipristal acetate orally for 3 months. This is a progesterone receptor modulator and has been shown to be superior to placebo and GnRH analogues in both side effects and efficacy, reducing bleeding by 80%. It is licensed for use for up to 3 months before surgery. Danazol is not recommended for routine use by NICE due to side effects, whereas GnRH analogues are licensed to be used before planned surgery, but are associated with significant side effects. Mefenamic acid is unlikely to help if other NSAIDs have failed and HRT is unlikely to be effective in a premenopausal women.

P1.61 A: Cinnarazine is an effective treatment

Hyoscine is the most effective treatment, especially when used as a patch. Cinnarazine and promethazine are helpful but promethazine causes sedation and for most patients this limits its use, although it may be useful in children. Patients should be advised to stay on deck where possible, with a view of the horizon, and to try to stay in the middle of the boat where motion is minimal. Alcohol, heavy meals and pungent odours can exacerbate symptoms. Homeopathic treatments might be effective but trials have not shown any benefit from acupressure bands.

P1.62   D: Quantiferon testing is the investigation of choice in screening contacts

Quantiferon is a highly sensitive and specific test for TB-sensitised T cells, and patients with a positive test should be given chemoprophylaxis. Heaf testing is suitable for mass screening of populations whereas Mantoux testing is more specific and is a better choice for screening healthcare workers where Quantiferon is not available, although false positives can occur. Chest X-rays will pick up only pulmonary TB. Heaf testing might be positive in patients who have had avian TB or previous BCG vaccination.

P1.63   B: Oral doxycycline 100 mg once daily for 6 weeks

Blepharitis is a chronic condition and is managed in most cases with regular lid cleaning and compresses, with short courses of topical antibiotics for flare-ups. Where this is not helping and the diagnosis is not in question a 6-week course of a tetracycline is often helpful. Prednisolone drops should not be used in a red eye without ophthalmological review in case of underlying herpes simplex keratitis. Prolonged use of topical antibiotics is unlikely to help and will promote resistance.

P1.64   E: Refer immediately to the emergency department for an X-ray

This patient has symptoms of a fractured fibula, commonly seen after a fall wearing ski boots or inline skates. The common peroneal nerve might be damaged, causing numbness over the lateral border of the foot and weak dorsiflexion. Surgery might be necessary to keep the fibula reduced. Undisplaced fractures of the mid-shaft might not need a cast, but where there are signs of damage to the common peroneal nerve this should be treated actively to avoid lasting disability.

Abdominal pain

P1.65   G: Diverticulitis

This pattern of recurring attacks of left iliac fossa pain is usually due to diverticulitis. Colonic cancer would be the main differential in this age group and can be differentiated on barium enema or colonoscopy. In younger patients, irritable bowel syndrome can cause similar symptoms.

P1.66   K: Renal colic

Renal colic tends to radiate to the scrotum or labia and typically comes in waves. Dipstick testing usually shows haematuria.

P1.67   E: Crohn's disease

Crohn's disease usually starts in the terminal ileum or proximal colon and a mass can form in this part of the bowel. Diarrhoea, weight loss and fever are common. Diagnosis is usually made on endoscopy.

P1.68   C: Acute cholecystitis

Referred pain to the shoulder is usually a sign of diaphragmatic irritation, in this case due to inflammation of the gallbladder. Ectopic pregnancy or chlamydial perihepatitis should also be considered as possible causes in women. In cholecystitis there is right upper quadrant tenderness that is worse on inspiration.

P1.69   H: Gastric carcinoma

Progressive dysphagia with weight loss suggests a diagnosis of gastric or oesophageal cancer. An epigastric mass might be palpable and hepatomegaly is common.

P1.70   A: Ezetimibe has been reported to be associated with an increased risk of cancer

The SEAS (Simvastatin and Ezetimibe in Aortic Stenosis) trial looked at use of ezetimibe in combination with simvastatin in patients with mild aortic stenosis. It found no significant reduction in cardiovascular endpoints but did find increased incidence of all cancers. Ezetimibe is a cholesterol absorption inhibitor that has been shown in trial data to reduce low-density lipoproteins (LDLs), but it did not reduce clinical endpoints. Patients with a mixed hyperlipidaemia should be treated with a statin initially. Macrolides, amlodipine and antifungals interact with simvastatin and atorvastatin and should be used with caution in all patients on statins. Sleep problems are common, and there are increasing reports of impotence with statins. Patients with familial hyperlipidaemias should be treated to target.

P1.71   E: No treatment needed

Dead eggs (nits) often persist for many months after an episode of hair lice infestation and are not themselves an indication for treatment. If live lice are seen, wet combing with conditioner or simeticone is efficacious and not associated with resistance. Nits close to the scalp suggest recent infection, whereas those some distance from the scalp are likely to be old.

P1.72   C: Clinically asymptomatic cancers are being diagnosed earlier

The most likely explanation for the increase in cancer diagnoses over a short period is improved case finding. The time course is too short for a change in true prevalence and prostate cancer has a long lead time before symptoms appear. The lack of change in the death rate suggests that these cancers are not associated with reduced life expectancy, ie they are being diagnosed earlier but treatment and individual life expectancy are the same. Changes in life expectancy with new treatments can be compared only on a case–control basis. Advances in treatment might have led to improved life expectancy for individual patients, but many patients are treated with watchful waiting and die of other causes.

P1.73

Action group	Drug
μ-Opioid receptor antagonist	Methylnaltrexone
Stimulants	Bisacodyl
Osmotics	Macrogols
Softeners	Docusate sodium
Combined preparation	Co-danthramer

Macrogols can be used to treat faecal impaction as well as prevent constipation. They cause less wind than lactulose and are generally better tolerated. Methylnaltrexone is given as a single injection for severe opioid-induced constipation. Where there is rectal stool, glycerol or bisacodyl suppositories are useful, while an empty stool with a loaded colon can be effectively treated with arachis oil retention enema overnight.

P1.74   A: Glossopharyngeal neuralgia

Glossopharyngeal neuralgia is less common than trigeminal neuralgia but causes similar symptoms in the distribution of the glossopharyngeal nerve. Initial assessment should aim to exclude facial nerve involvement, tonsillar tumour and herpes zoster. Treatment usually aims to provide reassurance and avoidance of trigger factors where possible. Anticonvulsants can be helpful in some cases.

P1.75   Alcohol

These blood results show a macrocytosis with normal vitamin B_{12} and folate. The most likely cause of this is alcohol consumption. If the vitamin B_{12} or folate levels were low, primary vitamin deficiency should be considered. People with alcohol problems may also have low vitamin B_{12} and folate due to poor diet. The liver function tests show raised GGT, which is a sensitive but relatively non-specific marker of liver disease. It can be raised in pancreatic disease, MI, COPD, renal failure, diabetes, obesity and alcoholism. It may also be elevated in patients taking phenytoin and barbiturates. In this case normal HbA1c, renal function, vitamin B_{12} and folate in a patient on no regular medication strongly suggests alcohol abuse.

P1.76   C: Retrospective studies are quicker to conduct than prospective studies

Retrospective studies are more prone to bias but are cheaper and quicker to conduct. They have the advantage that the two groups are known to have different rates of a disease, whereas prospective studies do not have this advantage. It is not uncommon for an intervention group and a control group to have a statistically insignificant difference in event rates at the end of a long and expensive trial.

End-of-life care in patients with renal failure

P1.77   H: Ondansetron

Ondansetron, mirtazapine, aluminium hydroxide and gabapentin are all treatment options for itch in end-stage renal disease. If gabapentin is used, the dose should be reduced.

P1.78   E: Metoclopramide

Hiccups are common in end-stage renal failure. Metoclopramide is the first-line treatment of choice.

P1.79   A: Clonazepam

Clonazepam, pramipexole and gabapentin can all be used for restless legs, but again dose reduction is needed for gabapentin.

P1.80   I: Oxycodone

NSAIDs and codeine, morphine and diamorphine should not be used for pain. If oxycodone is not tolerated, fentanyl is an alternative.

P1.81   A: Basal cell carcinoma

Basal cell carcinomas are often seen in sun-exposed parts of the face and start with a small pearly white nodule, with telangiectatic blood vessels. Initially they may bleed and ulcerate, then heal again. In time the lesion expands to leave a rolled edge with central ulceration. These lesions are locally invasive and metastasis is rare. Treatment is with excision. Dermatofibromas usually grow rapidly on the legs of young to middle-aged women, forming a firm papule with brown pigmentation. Keratoacanthomas start as a nodule and rapidly grow over 3–4 weeks to form a nodule with a central plug of keratin. They naturally involute over 2–3 months. The main differential is squamous cell carcinoma. Seborrhoeic keratoses are well-demarcated brown macules with a stuck-on appearance, often multiple and oriented in line with skinfolds. Squamous cell carcinomas usually present as rapidly growing painless ulcerated nodules, which may have a cauliflower-like appearance

P1.82   E: Refer directly to the antenatal unit for biophysical profile

Reduced fetal movements are a common concern in the third trimester. Mothers should be asked to choose a set time every day and record how long it takes to feel 10 movements. If these are not felt by that time she should be referred to the antenatal unit for a biophysical profile, comprising cardiotocography (CTG), ultrasound examination of liquor volume, fetal tone, movements and breathing movements, giving a numerical score with 10 the maximum. If the score is between 0 and 2, immediate delivery is indicated, whereas a score of 8 or more is normal.

P1.83   E: Systematic desensitisation therapy

Antidepressants may help if there is associated depression or anxiety but anxiety is often secondary to the agoraphobia. Benzodiazepines should be avoided due to a risk of addiction. Systematic desensitisation consists of graded exposure and agreement of goals and homework where the patient continues to practice in real life. Up to 70% of patients report improvement although complete recovery of all symptoms is less common. The aim should be for a patient to be able to function normally. Hypnosis is sometimes used as part of this process but the graded exposure to the stimulus is key.

P1.84   B: Avoidance of nail rubbing

This condition is seen in people under stress who rub their thumbnails, causing typical central nail damage. Where this condition is unilateral, trauma to the nail bed should be considered. In fungal nail infections the infection normally starts distally, with discoloration of the nail, whereas a low calcium level causes brittle nails. Reassurance alone will not improve the condition and sometimes CBT might be appropriate to break up the stress response.

P1.85   D: Lymphoedema

Lymphoedema is a common incurable complication of breast cancer surgery, particularly where this involves axillary clearance. The arm is typically oedematous with no erythema and with non-pitting oedema. Infection can develop and fibrosis is common. Management involves elevation and massage, and four-layer bandaging, followed by compression hosiery, can be effective. Lymphoma would not normally affect a whole arm, and cellulitis and DVT are usually associated with erythema and tenderness.

P1.86   D: Start a smoking cessation programme and repeat the blood tests in 4 weeks

This pattern of blood results usually reflects secondary polycythaemia due to chronic hypoxia from COPD and smoking. Smoking cessation might be sufficient to bring his haemoglobin back to normal limits. If this fails to occur he should be investigated to confirm whether this is primary or secondary polycythaemia. Primary polycythaemia is associated with the JAK2 mutation and can be tested in most laboratories. The mainstay of management is venesection once secondary causes have been addressed.

P1.87   C: Suggest that she sees another doctor at the practice

GMC guidelines state that you should avoid treating people to whom you are close. Obviously, in life-or-death situations this can be waived, but convenience is not a reason to enter into a clinical situation where one's judgement might be impaired. If one has serious concerns about patient safety, it would be appropriate to raise these but clash of personalities is not an appropriate reason to instigate a complaint. GMC guidance further recommends that you should provide treatment only where you have adequate knowledge of the patient's health, and in the scenario described here there could be issues in your mother's medical history of which you are unaware.

Upper gastrointestinal disorders

P1.88   E: MALToma

Non-Hodgkin's lymphoma affecting the mucosa-associated lymphoid tissue (MALT) of the stomach is the most common non-epithelial malignancy of the stomach and accounts for 3% of stomach tumours. These tumours are associated with *Helicobacter pylori* infection and in low-grade tumours regression can occur after eradication of the infection.

P1.89   A: Achalasia

Achalasia is due to failure of relaxation of the gastro-oesophageal junction, resulting in progressive dilatation of the oesophagus. Regurgitation is common and many patients develop aspiration pneumonia. The symptoms progress more slowly than oesophageal cancer but often cause chronic malnourishment. In South America this condition is often seen in association with cardiomegaly in Chagas' disease, a trypanosomal infection.

P1.90   B: Barrett's oesophagus

Barrett's oesophagus is associated with a small risk of developing cancer and many authorities advocate routine endoscopic surveillance. The presence of dysplasia in biopsies is suspicious but at repeat endoscopy 75% of these will have resolved on treatment with a proton pump inhibitor (PPI). Where this has not occurred surgery should be considered.

P1.91   H: Oesophageal stricture

Oesophageal stricture is usually caused by acid reflux and often presents as bolus obstruction, but upper gastrointestinal endoscopy and biopsy are mandatory to exclude an underlying malignancy. Dilatation can be carried out at the time of endoscopy.

P1.92   I: Plummer–Vinson syndrome

Plummer–Vinson syndrome (also know as Patterson–Brown–Kelly syndrome) causes an oesophageal web and therefore dysphagia, together with iron-deficiency anaemia. It is associated with a significant increase in risk of oesophageal cancer.

P1.93   A: PSA screening has been shown to increase diagnosis of early prostate cancer

Large-scale studies of prostate cancer screening using PSA blood tests show that it increases the diagnosis of early prostate cancer but this does not translate into improved overall mortality or improved quality of life. Radical surgery for early screen-detected prostate cancer was shown in the PIVOT trial to have significant adverse effects, with no improvement in total or prostate cancer-related mortality.

P1.94   C: Each child has a 0% chance of being affected

Huntington's disease is an autosomal dominant trait that presents in middle age. Children of affected parents therefore have a 50% risk of inheriting the gene (assuming that the named parent is indeed the biological parent) and, in time, of becoming affected. If they are affected they will therefore have a 50% chance of passing the disease to each of their children, but if they are unaffected they will not have any risk of being a carrier or of developing the disease.

P1.95   E: Ultraviolet light used at the onset of symptoms may abort the attack

Cold sores are caused by reactivation of latent herpes simplex in the trigeminal ganglion, rather than primary infection. There is no evidence that topical aciclovir is effective but there is some evidence of efficacy for oral aciclovir. However, oral aciclovir is expensive and is not considered cost-effective. Where attacks are triggered by UV light, sunscreens might be effective. Small handheld UV light emitters are available on FP10, to be used at the onset of tingling, and have been shown to abort or shorten the duration of an attack.

P1.96   B: De Quervain's tenosynovitis

De Quervain's tenosynovitis is inflammation of the extensor pollicis brevis and abductor pollicis longus tendons. Finkelstein's test is positive if resisted abduction is painful. Treatment is usually steroid injection and a splint, but surgical decompression might be required in chronic cases. Carpal tunnel syndrome causes pain on pressure over the carpal tunnel (Tinel's test) or through forced flexion of the wrist (Phalen's test). Medial and lateral epicondylitis cause tenderness over the medial and lateral epicondyles respectively.

P1.97   B: Pelviureteric junction obstruction is more common in patients with duplex ureters

A Duplex ureter is seen in 0.2% of live births, and is more common in patients with a positive family history. It is usually picked up on antenatal ultrasound but in older patients might be discovered on routine ultrasound scanning. PUJ obstruction and urinary tract infection are more common in patients with this condition and this might require active management. Surgery is seldom necessary.

P1.98   E: Refer under the 2-week rule

This child has symptoms of retinoblastoma and should be referred under the 2-week rule. Early treatment carries a good prognosis because these tumours tend to metastasise late. Any child with new-onset squint, leukocoria or uveitis needs urgent assessment. The condition is familial and often there will be an affected first-degree relative.

P1.99   A: Bimanual examination

This woman has symptoms of an ovarian tumour and abdominal examination alone will miss pelvic tumours. Vaginal examination is mandatory in these cases, and where a mass is found referral under the 2-week rule is indicated. Ovarian tumours are often clinically silent in their early stages, becoming apparent only when they reach sufficient size to cause pressure effects or ascites, and a high index of suspicion should be maintained in patients with new symptoms, particularly those affecting the bladder or bowel, or those who have clinical evidence of ascites.

P1.100   B: IgA nephropathy

IgA nephropathy is the underlying pathology in 50% of cases of recurrent frank haematuria. It is usually seen in children and young adults and is more common in boys. Episodes are usually triggered by viral infections and usually resolve over days or weeks. Oral steroids are often used. Most patients have a good prognosis, but 15–20% of patients go on to develop chronic renal failure. Poor prognosis is associated with heavy proteinuria and hypertension. Bladder cancer would be very unusual in this age group. Wilms' tumours usually present in infancy and are palpable on examination as a flank mass, with microscopic haematuria. Polycystic kidneys are usually evident from birth in children, or develop in adulthood in the case of adult polycystic kidney disease.

P1.101   15 ml

The maximum number of milligrams that she can have is 3 × 50 = 150 mg; 1% lidocaine contains 1 g in 100 ml, or 10 mg/ml. The maximum safe dose is therefore 150/10 = 15 ml of 1% lidocaine.

P1.102   E: Presence of cataracts

The Guthrie test is done shortly after birth and involves taking a heel-prick test for congenital hypothyroidism. Coordination and patch testing are done at a later date when these skills have started to develop, usually by health visitors at the 8- and 18-month checks, and by an orthoptist around the age of 3 years. Newborn babies all have otoacoustic emission testing shortly after birth. Congenital cataracts must be picked up early to avoid amblyopia.

P1.103   D: Optic neuritis

This patient is suffering from retrobulbar neuritis, usually caused by multiple sclerosis. Papilloedema typically causes a peripheral visual field loss with normal acuity. CRVO usually causes engorgement of the retinal veins and a sunset appearance of the retina. Acute glaucoma causes severe pain in the eye, whereas amaurosis fugax causes retinal pallor and loss of vision in the whole eye and lasts for seconds or minutes.

P1.104   C: Sepsis

This patient fits the diagnostic criteria for systemic inflammatory response syndrome (two or more of fever >38.3°C, pulse >90 beats/min, RR >20/min, PCO_2 <4.3 kPa, BM >6.66 mmol/l, altered mental status, WBC >12 × 10^9/l). Where a patient is seen who fits these criteria, and the source is likely to be infection, sepsis is present. Leukocytes alone on a dipstick are unreliable for the diagnosis of a UTI and, although there are some signs of possible LRTI, the patient is clinically unwell and should be admitted promptly to hospital.

Childhood vaccinations

P1.105   D: HPV vaccine

HPV vaccination is given in a two-dose schedule to girls aged 12–13. Where the first dose is not given until age 15 years, a three-dose schedule is used due to a less responsive immune system.

P1.106   A: BCG

This should be offered to infants born in areas where there is a prevalence of ≥40/100 000, or where parents or grandparents were born in a country with a prevalence >40/100 000.

P1.107   E: Influenza vaccine

Live attenuated nasal influenza vaccine is offered to children from age 2 as a single nasal dose in low-risk groups, with a second booster dose 4 weeks later for those in high-risk groups.

P1.108   I: Rotavirus vaccine

This is given at 8 weeks and a second dose at 12 weeks.

P1.109:   D: Contact the regional Responsible Officer to report your concerns

The GMC guidance is explicit in stating that 'All doctors have a duty to raise concerns where they believe that patient safety or care is being compromised by the practice of colleagues or the systems, policies and procedures in the organisations in which they work'. It would be good practice to contact your indemnity provider and to encourage him to seek treatment through his GP. The local Responsible Officer is responsible for clinical governance, fitness to practice and liaising with the GMC where appropriate.

P1.110   D: There is a 1% annual risk of developing malignancy in patients with Barrett's oesophagus

Barrett's oesophagus is metaplastic change in the distal oesophagus caused by longstanding acid reflux. There is a 1% annual risk of malignant transformation and many centres carry out routine surveillance. Treatment is of the underlying reflux, with proton pump inhibitors for life. Photodynamic therapy is available in some centres. There is no association between *H. pylori* and Barrett's oesophagus.

P1.111   E: Tiotropium should be considered at step 2 in COPD management

The POET-COPD trial (*N Engl J Med* 2011) compared long-acting β agonists and tiotropium in stage 2 of COPD management and found evidence of reduced exacerbations in the tiotropium group. There is mounting evidence that β blockers are safe and effective in patients with COPD, because these patients often have coexistent ischaemic heart disease, and there is some evidence that exacerbations of COPD are reduced with β blockers. Indacaterol is a new longacting β agonist that can be given once a day, and studies suggest a beneficial impact on FEV_1 compared with salmeterol. Patients with a resting SpO_2 of >95% can usually fly without oxygen, whereas those with a resting SpO_2 of <92% will need supplemental oxygen. A hypoxic challenge test can be carried out in these patients.

P1.112   A: Acute angle-closure glaucoma

This is a typical history of acute angle-closure glaucoma. On examination the pupil is often fixed in a semi-dilated position and is oval. The eye feels stony-hard and the pain is extreme. Cluster headache can cause pain localised around the eye, but is not usually associated with fixation of the pupil. Anyone with a temporal headache should be examined to exclude temporal arteritis. Migraine would not normally cause pupillary changes and subarachnoid haemorrhage causes a more generalised headache with no loss of vision, although cranial nerve lesions can be seen.

P1.113   B: Each patient has a 70% chance of improving after the intervention

Cates's plots are designed to assist patients in understanding the likely pros and cons of a treatment. They are usually expressed as a table of 100 people, with patients improving being represented as a smiling face and patients being worse off as a sad face. Patients harmed by treatment may also be shown, eg for antibiotics in otitis media, patients with resultant diarrhoea are represented by a face with a cross through, and patients who are prevented from having an adverse outcome (ie saved) by a different colour smiling face. If the number of sad and smiling faces is equal, there is a 50% chance of improving and 50% chance of deteriorating with a treatment, ie no net effect. If there are >50% of the faces smiling, the chance of an individual being better off is >50%. This relates to individual chance of improvement, not level of improvement in an individual. No conclusions regarding cost-effectiveness can be drawn without data on cost.

P1.114   B: Achilles tendinopathy

Quinolone antibiotics are associated with tendinopathy. This usually settles with cessation of the drug, rest and ice, together with non-steroidal anti-inflammatories. Rupture would usually be suggested by a palpable step in the tendon and reduced plantarflexion. Overuse injury may cause tendonitis but is usually seen when there has been a change in training or footwear. Polymyalgia rheumatica tends to cause a pelvic girdle rather than an ankle pain.

P1.115   D: Extrinsic allergic alveolitis

This patient has symptoms of farmers' lung, an acute extrinsic allergic alveolitis. Symptoms typically come on 4–8 hours after exposure to fungal spores and in time the condition can progress to pulmonary fibrosis. Similar symptoms are seen with bird fanciers, maltworkers and mushroom farmers. An occupational history is vital in diagnosing these patients. Management is with avoidance and steroids if severe. Bronchiectasis would tend to present with recurrent chest infections from childhood, whereas pulmonary fibrosis would usually be associated with chronic rather than relapsing and remitting symptoms, and clubbing.

P1.116 B: The combined oral contraceptive has a number needed to treat of 5 for management of primary dysmenorrhoea

A Bandolier review found that, in general, NSAIDs are the most effective treatment, with ibuprofen having the best risk:benefit ratio. Aspirin was the least effective. COX-2 inhibitors are effective, with good tolerability. There is no evidence to support the use of spinal manipulation and paracetamol has very weak efficacy in pain relief in this condition.

P1.117 E: Where a partnership agreement does not exist, the partnership can be terminated at any time by one of the partners

Where no formal partnership agreement exists, the partnership is considered a 'partnership at will' and can be terminated at any time without prior discussion. A partnership agreement should include all names and profit shares and therefore should be updated with all partnership changes. All decisions are by a majority, unless specified in the partnership agreement. Non-GP partners are legal, but might require complex calculations regarding remuneration.

Bowel symptoms

P1.118 A: Check CA-125

New-onset symptoms of IBS in a women aged >50 are rarely due to IBS. Examination and investigation should aim to exclude ovarian cancer, initially with a CA-125 and consideration for a pelvic ultrasound scan.

P1.119 D: Refer for colonoscopy

These are typical symptoms of inflammatory bowel disease and require urgent assessment to confirm the diagnosis and exclude colonic malignancy.

P1.120 C: Mebeverine

This patient has typical symptoms of IBS. Trial of antispasmodics or peppermint oil should be first line for cramps and bloating. Constipation should be treated with bulk-forming agents and diarrhoea with loperamide. Second-line prophylaxis is usually tricyclic antidepressants.

P1.121 E: Refer for gastroscopy

This man has symptoms of either a peptic ulcer or gastro-oesophageal cancer. In the absence of abnormal blood tests a trial of acid suppression may be helpful, but patients not responding should have upper GI endoscopy.

P1.122 Trephining

Subungal haematoma is caused by trauma to the nailbed. Untreated the nail will be lost, and the haematoma causes acute pain. This can be relieved with a red-hot paperclip or a bevelled needle used as a drill. The nail is often lost over the next few weeks and can take some months to re-grow. This appearance in the absence of trauma may be a sign of subungal melanoma.

P1.123   C: The earliest possible fertile ovulation is around 28 days postpartum

Ovulation precedes the onset of a period so patients should be advised not to have unprotected sex before their first period after childbirth. The pill should not be used in the early postpartum phase due to the risk of thromboembolism. In the absence of breastfeeding, the earliest the pill should be considered is 21 days, but patients who have suffered from HELLP syndrome or pregnancy-induced hypertension are at increased risk of thrombosis and should not start the COCP until biochemically normal and normotensive. The COCP interferes with breastfeeding, so the mini-pill is a better choice in lactating mothers. Mothers should be warned that breastfeeding has poor efficacy as a contraceptive.

Management of back pain

P1.124   E: Red flag symptoms

P1.125   B: GP management

P1.126   H: Review in 2 weeks

P1.127   D: Physiotherapy

P1.128   G: Refer to secondary care

P1.129   C: He should have an MMR booster immediately

A single dose of MMR confers immunity in 70–85% of patients. In the case of an outbreak, a booster dose is recommended which will boost coverage to 95%, and can be given from 4 weeks after the previous dose. Single measles vaccines are not licensed or available in the UK. Failure to vaccinate with the booster at this time makes him prone to infection and carriage of the vaccine. Where children have received a booster before the age of 18 months, the usual preschool booster should also be given because response below the age of 18 months can be suboptimal.

P1.130   D: It can be associated with palpitations

The typical patient with mitral valve prolapse is a young slim woman. It is frequently asymptomatic and is often picked up on routine examination as a diastolic murmur or systolic click. It is associated with atypical chest pain and palpitations, and rarely causes congestive cardiac failure or embolic phenomena. β Blockers or antiplatelet therapy might be indicated. Patients with no other abnormalities on echocardiography and no other cardiac risk factors have a long-term survival rate similar to that of the general population.

P1.131   D: Nasal polyps

Nasal polyps are by far the most common cause of reduced smell and taste. Tumours of the frontal lobe, meningiomas or ethmoid tumours are all very rare and usually associated with other symptoms. Overuse of decongestants causes rhinitis rather than loss of smell. Nasal polyps can cause reduced sense of smell without complete nasal obstruction and are often not visible without Thudichum's speculum. A trial of steroids, either nose drops or orally, will produce a dramatic improvement if nasal polyps are the cause. They can be removed surgically, but 50% recur within 2 years.

Causes of pneumonia

P1.132   G: *Mycoplasma pneumoniae*

Mycoplasma pneumoniae causes a flu-like respiratory illness that affects children. It can be associated with erythema multiforme, myalgia and diarrhoea. Treatment is with a macrolide or tetracycline for 10–14 days.

P1.133   F: Measles

Measles starts with a prodromal illness with respiratory symptoms and can go on to develop into pneumonia in around one in six patients, with bronchiectasis as a late complication.

P1.134   A: Aspergillosis

Aspergillosis tends to affect people with HIV or on immunosuppressants, or chronically ill individuals. It is usually diagnosed in patients who fail to respond to antibiotic therapy. It has been noted *post mortem* in 4% of patients dying in hospital.

P1.135   L: Varicella

Varicella frequently causes a primary viral pneumonia in adults but less commonly in children. X-rays show multiple small pulmonary lesions. Treatment is with aciclovir.

P1.136   E: Legionnaires' disease

Legionella sp. has an incubation period up to 10 days and is often associated with altered mental status. Respiratory symptoms and signs are often mild initially, and renal failure can develop. Treatment is with a macrolide and supportive care.

P1.137   C: This condition often has an infectious cause

There are many causes of erythema multiforme. Mycoplasma and herpesvirus infections are common causes and should be excluded, particularly if oral steroids are contemplated. Itch often responds to antihistamine or topical steroids. This condition can be associated with mouth and genital ulcers in Stevens–Johnson syndrome or with toxic epidermal necrolysis. Erythema nodosum causes tender nodules on the legs that fade to look like bruises.

P1.138   E: Report the incident to the police

Since 2015 it has been a mandatory requirement for healthcare and social care workers to report cases where they suspect female genital mutilation has occurred in a child aged <18 years. Complying with the duty does not breach confidentiality and the individual who became aware must make the report; this responsibility cannot be transferred. It applies only to cases where the age of disclosure (not the age at which FGM took place) is <18. It does not apply when someone other than the patient makes a disclosure, but consideration should be given to safeguarding issues.

P1.139   C: Ventricular bigeminy

This ECG shows ventricular bigeminy, where a normal sinus beat is followed by a premature ventricular contraction. There is often a compensatory pause after the ectopic beat. In the absence of other cardiovascular disease it is seldom of consequence. A history should be taken, aimed at identifying any factors that might increase ectopic activity, such as thyroid disease, caffeine or alcohol, but usually no treatment is needed. Paroxysmal atrial fibrillation consists of runs of atrial fibrillation interspersed with normal sinus rhythm whereas Wenckebach's phenomenon is characterised by an increasing PR interval until a ventricular beat is missed. AV dissociation shows atrial activity and ventricular activity that are not coordinated, whereas 2:1 heart block shows two P waves for each QRS complex.

P1.140   C: Sildenafil

NHS treatment for erectile dysfunction is restricted to patients who have erectile dysfunction due to medical or surgical reasons, eg diabetes, Parkinson's disease, multiple sclerosis or spinal cord injury, or after surgery. Patients falling into this category should have their prescriptions annotated 'SLS' to obtain the drug as an NHS prescription. Generic sildenafil and apomorphine hydrochloride, moxisylyte and thymoxamine are no longer covered by these rules, although Viagra is.

Difficult patients

P1.141   B: Entitled demanders

Entitled demanders seek medical attention and try to control the direction through intimidation and induction of guilt. They might also attempt to use litigation or the threat of this to get their own way.

P1.142   D: Heartsink patient

'Heartsinks' are a function of the doctor–patient relationship rather than purely a character trait of the patient. Female GPs identify fewer heartsinks than their male colleagues, and doctors who are stressed and showing signs of burnout typically report higher numbers of heartsinks.

P1.143   F: Self-destructive denier

The possibility of underlying depression should be considered in these patients, but often these patients seem to derive satisfaction from their plight, in an extension of the sick role. An example would be the patient with poorly controlled diabetes who is rapidly going blind but continues to ignore advice on diet and medication.

P1.144   E: Manipulative help rejector

Manipulative help rejectors are usually pleasant in a consultation but believe that they are beyond help and seem to enjoy the physician's inability to cure them of their symptoms, which are usually mild and not life threatening. Where a symptom is cured they will often present with a new, equally difficult symptom.

P1.145   C: Frequent attenders

One should always avoid subjective terms that imply a character judgement such as 'dependent clinger' or 'heartsink' when writing in medical notes.

P1.146   A: Check thyroid autoantibodies

The most likely cause in this patient is thyroid eye disease, usually seen in Graves' disease, but it can precede the development of hyperthyroidism. Myasthenia gravis causes ptosis rather than proptosis and can be tested for with anti-acetylcholine receptor antibodies. A brain tumour would not usually cause proptosis and tumours in the orbit would usually cause visual signs and pain. Orbital cellulitis can cause proptosis but is usually clinically obvious, with erythema, pain and fever, together with ophthalmoplegia and, later, loss of colour vision. Following blood tests for Graves' disease, she should be referred to ophthalmology.

P1.147   B: Cryptosporidia can be resistant to chlorination of water

Some strains are resistant to chlorination, although all strains of these organisms should be killed by chlorine dioxide ozone if used correctly. Transmission is faeco-oral, with humans or animals passing spores in the faeces. Affected children should remain off school until 48 hours after symptoms have settled. Most cases are mild but children and immunocompromised individuals can develop a chronic illness. Transmission is usually through drinking, but can also be through swimming in lakes and rivers, drinking from streams (eg when hiking) or sexual intercourse.

Driving and neurological disorders

P1.148   C: Must not drive for 1 month and must inform DVLA

Group 2 holders must not drive for 3 months. There are no restrictions where typical vasovagal syncope with prodrome occurs when standing.

P1.149   F: Must notify DVLA but may continue to drive as long as safe control maintained at all times

Both Group 1 and 2 licence holders may continue to drive as long as there is no impairment or variability in function.

P1.150   B: Must not drive and must notify DVLA

Group 1 drivers suffering a single TIA must not drive for 4 weeks but need not inform the DVLA. Group 2 licence holders must notify the DVLA and cannot drive for 12 months after a stroke or TIA.

P1.151   B: Must not drive and must notify DVLA

Driving is prohibited for 6 months from the date of the first seizure. For Group 2 licence holders driving is prohibited for 5 years from the date of the seizure.

P1.152   E: Must not drive for 1 month but need not inform the DVLA

This is the case if there is no residual neurological deficit 4 weeks after a single stroke. Minor limb weakness does not need notification as long as no vehicle adaptations are required.

P1.153   B: It is a cause of sudden death in young athletes

HOCM is the most common genetic cardiac disease and is inherited as an autosomal dominant trait, although many cases are the result of spontaneous mutation. It frequently presents with sudden death in young athletes, and in some countries high-school athletes are required to have echocardiography as a screening test. Less frequently it can present with chronic heart failure or arrhythmia, but treatment usually controls symptoms only without affecting outcome. It can also be detected as an asymptomatic finding in older patients.

P1.154   Dupuytren's contracture

This is caused by thickening of the palmar fascia resulting in permanent flexion of the MCP joints. It is usually bilateral, starts on the fourth and fifth fingers and may also involve the feet. There is often a strong family history and it is often seen in men of northern European descent; it is thought to be an autosomal dominant trait with variable penetrance. No treatment is needed where there is no functional limitation. Where there is limitation, surgical release is an option but there is a complication rate of 46% with persistence or recurrence of contractures in 15%.

P1.155   B: Change to a triphasic pill

Breakthrough bleeding is common in the first 6 months on the combined pill. If it persists and no other cause can be found, the patient should be changed to a higher oestrogen dose pill or a triphasic pill. There is little justification for taking two combined pills a day because the dose of oestrogen would pose a significant risk of side effects. The mini-pill is a common cause of spotting and would not be an appropriate alternative in this instance. A Mirena IUS would be technically difficult to fit in a nulliparous woman, but might be appropriate if symptoms could not be controlled with medication or if estrogen was contraindicated.

P1.156   A: Carbon monoxide poisoning

Exposure to low levels of carbon monoxide may cause symptoms suggestive of food poisoning or influenza, but, where altered consciousness and headache are present, carbon monoxide poisoning should be excluded. Other common symptoms include vertigo, focal neurological defects and tachycardia. The characteristic cherry-red skin colour is usually seen only in fatal poisoning. Meningitis is usually a more acute presentation. Haemolytic–uraemic syndrome is usually seen in children after a diarrhoeal illness and is usually associated with symptoms of renal failure.

Treatment of prostate cancer

P1.157   E: External-beam radiotherapy

Approximately 12% of patients receiving external-beam radiotherapy suffer proctitis and haemorrhage. This is significantly less common with brachytherapy.

P1.158   I: Watchful waiting

Radical prostatectomy was shown to reduce deaths from prostate cancer but not overall mortality when compared with watchful waiting.

P1.159   D: Docetaxel

Docetaxel chemotherapy can be effective in non-hormone-responsive recurrences. Bisphosphonates might be useful in managing bone pain as an adjunct to radiotherapy or NSAIDs.

P1.160   G: Orchidectomy

NICE recommend offering bilateral orchidectomy to all patients with hormone-sensitive tumours as an alternative to LHRH agonists.

P1.161   F: LHRH analogue

LHRH analogues cause an initial flare in testosterone production followed by suppression to the equivalent of castration. Initial treatment should be covered with an anti-androgen to prevent tumour flare, especially where there are spinal metastases. Cord compression has been reported in some patients in whom LHRH analogues are used alone.

P1.162   E: Patients who are intolerant of colchicine or NSAIDs should be treated with prednisolone

Most cases of gout are due to an inherited metabolic defect or are iatrogenic, common triggers including thiazides, furosemide and low-dose salicylates. The traditional purine-rich duet is rarely seen as a cause. Uric acid often drops during an acute attack. Joint aspiration reveals clear fluid, with crystals seen on microscopy. Colchicine should be given as 500 mcg three times a day. Prophylaxis should be considered if patients are having more than two attacks a year, but should not be started during an acute attack, and patients should be warned that prophylaxis can trigger an acute attack.

P1.163   D: Seborrhoeic keratosis

Seborrhoeic keratoses are common lesions usually seen on the torso from the age of 40 onwards. No evidence of viral infection has been found, and although unsightly no treatment is needed, other than on cosmetic grounds.

P1.164   C: Candidal infection is more common in pregnancy

A fishy smell suggests bacterial vaginosis or infection with *Trichomonas* sp. These are both treated with metronidazole orally or clindamycin pessaries. There is no need for condoms or partner treatment with bacterial vaginosis. Bacterial vaginosis is often discovered incidentally on swabs or smears. Thrush is more common in sexually active people, pregnant women and immunocompromised individuals. Trichomoniasis is a sexually transmitted infection that causes a urethritis in men and a foul-smelling mucopurulent discharge in women. Diagnosis is on microscopy.

P1.165   B: The data show a statistically significant weight loss at 3 months

The data show an 80% drop-out rate by 12 months. The data are not presented on an intention-to-treat basis. Assuming that the patients who drop out regain their weight loss, the average weight loss is likely to be <1 kg. The high dropout rates imply poor concordance with treatment. Weight loss is maintained in the 20% of patients who are still in the programme at 12 months.

Viral infections

P1.166   E: Human papillomavirus

P1.167   H: Norovirus

P1.168   I: Parvovirus B19

P1.169   B: Coxsackievirus

P1.170   C: Epstein–Barr virus

HPV is responsible for increasing numbers of cases of oral cancer, often in patients without the traditional risk factors of alcohol and smoking. Norovirus is the leading cause of infectious gastroenteritis in developed countries and is highly infectious, causing particular problems in hospitals, hotels and cruise ships. Slapped cheek is a common viral condition affecting preschool children. It is rarely dangerous in children but unexposed pregnant women have a small risk of fetal hydrops. Hand, foot and mouth disease affects toddlers and causes characteristic vesicles on the buccal mucosa, hands and feet. It is self-limiting and usually caused by Coxsackie A virus or enteroviruses. Both the sporadic and the endemic (usually equatorial Africa) forms of Burkitt's lymphoma are associated with EBV infection.

P1.171   C: Perthes' disease

Perthes' disease, avascular necrosis of the femoral head, is usually seen in children between the ages of 5 and 10 years, and 80% of cases are seen in boys. Initially it presents as an irritable hip but later the joint becomes fixed and movements improve, albeit with a positive Trendelenburg gait. Congenital dislocation of the hip usually presents earlier as asymmetrical creases, or is picked up at child health surveillance. Slipped upper femoral epiphysis is typically seen in boys between the ages of 10 and 15 years, and presents with a shortened and rotated leg. Septic arthritis is usually associated with a raised CRP and WCC. The main differential is irritable hip but this does not usually persist as long and can be excluded on X-ray.

P1.172   C: Patients diagnosed with osteoporosis should be investigated for coeliac disease

Bisphosphonates are available in oral and intravenous formulations. They have been shown to increase bone density and reduce fractures. In patients who are intolerant, strontium can be used as a second-line treatment. A T score <2.5 is diagnostic, and all patients should be assessed to exclude secondary osteoporosis, eg due to coeliac disease or hypogonadism. Bisphosphonates should usually be prescribed for 5 years. Where patients have refractory osteoporosis, PTH or teriparatide can be used under specialist supervision.

P1.173   A: All patients should be advised to exercise regularly

All patients with clinical symptoms and signs of osteoarthritis should be advised to exercise regularly, although they should be advised to avoid high impact or twisting/loading movements (eg basketball). X-rays seldom add to clinical findings and correlate poorly with symptoms. Patients should be screened for associated depression or anxiety, which may impede progress. All patients who are overweight or obese should try to lose weight, aiming for >5% of initial body weight. Patients who fail to respond to oral or topical analgesia, lifestyle changes and physiotherapy, or who have severe symptoms should be referred for consideration of joint replacement. Arthroscopy is indicated only for mechanical symptoms such as locking.

P1.174   B: Benign intracranial hypertension

Benign intracranial pressure causes headache in the mornings and evenings, relieved by standing. It is associated with papilloedema and in time visual fields may be lost and a VIth nerve palsy may develop. It usually affects young obese women and is due to impaired absorption of cerebrospinal fluid. It is usually idiopathic or may be seen in endocrine abnormalities, pregnancy or as a reaction to medication such some drugs. Treatment with lumbar puncture provides rapid relief at presentation, and recurrence may be prevented with acetazolamide or shunt insertion in refractory cases. Acute glaucoma affects the pupils early and is constant, whereas pre-eclampsia would not normally be seen at this stage of pregnancy, and would be associated with hypertension and proteinuria. The main differential diagnosis is a space-occupying lesion.

Management of abnormal smears

P1.175   A: Refer for colposcopy

Patients with 'borderline change with endocervical changes' should be referred for colposcopy after one abnormal smear. Patients with 'borderline smear with squamous changes' should be referred after three abnormal smears.

P1.176   D: Repeat in 6 months

Three inadequate smears should prompt referral for colposcopy.

P1.177   H: Smear no longer necessary

Local protocols vary but most areas invite women for their first smear at 25, then 3-yearly to 49 and 5-yearly to 64. Patients aged over 65 need have a smear only if they have had a previous abnormal result.

P1.178   D: Repeat in 6 months

Again, local protocols vary but it is considered acceptable after one smear showing mild dyskariosis to repeat this and refer for colposcopy if the follow-up smear is abnormal.

P1.179   B: Refer under 2-week rule

Smears that are suspicious of cancer should be referred under the 2-week rule. Note that cervical smears are a screening test rather than a diagnostic test and cannot rule out cancer. Where a cervix looks abnormal or there is a suspicious history, a clinical diagnosis should prompt a 2-week referral.

P1.180   C: Prescribe vitamin D analogues

This patient has psoriasis. The use of emollients will often improve the dry scaly appearance, leaving red papules. The improvement in symptoms with ultraviolet light is characteristic. Steroids will often produce a dramatic improvement, which relapses, however, on cessation of the steroid. Vitamin D analogues are the first-line treatment for most patients. Patients with new-onset psoriasis should have a thorough drug history to exclude causative agents such as β blockers.

P1.181   A: She should be offered incision and curettage

Chalazions are cysts that develop in the meibomian glands. They often enlarge slowly but a third resolve within 3 months and almost all resolve within 2 years. If they become infected they should be treated with a short course of antibiotic ointment. Definitive treatment is incision and curettage, which can be done in general practice if the right equipment is available. If large they can compress the eyeball, causing astigmatism. Lesions around the eye should always be examined for evidence of malignancy (eg basal cell carcinoma, squamous cell carcinoma), although this would be unusual in this age group. Cryotherapy is not appropriate in this area due to the risk of cicatrising scars.

P1.182   A: All pregnant women should take vitamin D supplements

Patients with pre-existing hypertension are at increased risk of pre-eclampsia and should be monitored for this. Consideration should be given to using aspirin and changing antihypertensives to nifedipine, labetalol or methyldopa. ACE inhibitors and angiotensin receptor blockers are teratogenic. All patients should take folic acid 400 mcg and vitamin D. Doses of these should be higher in high-risk patients, eg patients with diabetes, those with a personal or family history of neural tube defects and those on anticonvulsants should take 5 mg folic acid a day. Alcohol should be limited to 1–2 units once or twice a week and every effort should be made to stop smoking. Nicotine replacement therapy is safe in pregnancy. Overweight patients should be advised and supported to lose weight pre-conception, because obesity increases risk of diabetes and hypertension. Attention should also be paid to patients with a history of substance abuse.

P1.183   C: *Salmonella* sp.

Salmonellosis has an incubation period of 12–48 hours and typically causes vomiting followed by diarrhoea, which usually settles over 72 hours. In some cases it can cause a reactive arthritis and approximately 1% of patients go on to become carriers. Treatment is supportive, and antibiotics are not recommended for most patients. *Campylobacter* sp. causes diarrhoea and malaise but vomiting is rare; prolonged excretion can occur and this might be relevant for care-home or nursing staff. *Shigella* sp. is unusual in the UK but should be suspected in travellers who return with bloody diarrhoea. *Cryptosporidium* sp. usually affects children, whereas typhoid has a much longer incubation period and a more protracted clinical course.

P1.184   B: Cupping of the disc indicates damage to the eye despite normal intraocular pressure

Normal pressure glaucoma is a condition where there are signs of damage to the optic nerve with normal pressure. These patients should be started on treatment and have regular visual field monitoring. Laser iridotomy is useful for acute angle-closure glaucoma. Relying on patient symptoms is a poor indicator of disease progression because most patients are unaware of their peripheral visual field loss.

P1.185   C: Multiple myeloma

This pattern of symptoms and blood results is suggestive of myeloma. Urine should be sent for Bence Jones protein and he should be referred under the 2-week rule. CLL would usually cause a raised white cell count and symptoms are unusual, whereas lung cancer would usually cause respiratory symptoms. Metastatic prostate cancer can cause bony pain but would be unusual in patients without urinary symptoms. Persistent backache in young patients with systemic signs should prompt investigation to exclude sarcoma or infection.

P1.186   C: Patients should be monitored with regular bhCG levels for 2 years

Around 10% of molar pregnancies go on to develop neoplastic disease, but if treated early there is a very good prognosis. Recurrence risk for molar pregnancy is approximately 1 in 80 and most women go on to have a normal pregnancy afterwards. The COCP should not be used until bhCG levels are undetectable because it can delay tumour regression. All patients should be referred to specialist centres for follow-up.

The Mental Health Act

P1.187   **I:**   None of the above

Detention is specifically excluded in patients without mental illness who are sexually deviant, suffer from drug and alcohol addiction, or commit disorderly acts, or on the grounds of religious or cultural beliefs.

P1.188   **H:**   Section 136

Section 136 allows the police to take a patient to a place of safety for up to 72 hours. They cannot enter a private residence without consent to do so, however.

P1.189   **C:**   Section 4

Section 4 of the Mental Health Act allows admission for 72 hours for assessment and allows for emergency detention and assessment. It requires one doctor and the application can be made by the nearest relative or an Approved Mental Health Professional. It should be used only where delay would pose a significant risk of harm to the patient or others.

P1.190   **I:**   None of the above

Severe learning disabilities in the absence of other mental health problems are specifically excluded under the 2007 amendments to the Mental Health Act. This situation would best be resolved through the Court of Protection.

P1.191   **F:**   Section 17

Section 17 is an amendment introduced in 2007 to allow supervised community treatment orders and includes provision for failure to comply and the conditions under which re-admission would be needed.

Management of heavy menstrual bleeding

P1.192   **C:**   Fibroids present on ultrasound

P1.193   **H:**   Refer under 2-week rule

P1.194   **A:**   Contraceptive pill

P1.195   **I:**   Tranexamic acid

P1.196   **E:**   Mirena

P1.197   **B:**   Cessation of alcohol for at least 4 weeks

Simple snoring can have a significant impact on quality of life of spouses and many snorers present only because of spousal pressure. Sleep apnoea should be excluded on the history and significant causes of obstruction such as large tonsils, a large tongue base or nasal obstruction identified. Simple measures that can help include weight loss, avoidance of sedatives and alcohol, and positional measures if the snoring is postural. Thyroid function should always be checked. Where simple measures fail, UVPP might be considered but it is very painful and is associated with a significant risk of nasal escape.

P1.198   B: A 23-year-old man who has recently returned from a year travelling in south-east Asia with a new tattoo

At-risk groups include those who have had blood transfusions before 1987, those who have had dental treatment, invasive medical procedures or body piercing in the developing world, those with a history of intravenous drug use, people with a raised ALT level and people who have had contact with these groups. Singapore is a developed country and not high risk; patients who live abroad as expats, but who do not use local facilities for health care, are not at high risk.

P1.199   C: Exostoses

Exostoses and osteomas are benign bony growths of the external auditory meatus, seen particularly in people habitually exposed to cold water. They are usually asymptomatic but when large may cause wax and water trapping, and predispose to otitis externa. Cholesteatoma is a collection of squamous debris close to the tympanic membrane. Inflammatory polyps usually have a more erythematous appearance. The swelling here is subepithelial, as indicated by capillaries running over the lump. Chronic otitis externa usually has a more atrophic appearance to the skin of the external auditory meatus and there is usually considerable squamous debris.

P1.200   C: Moderate depression

PHQ-9 is an assessment tool for classifying the severity of depression based on the nine criteria listed in DSM-IV, looking at symptoms in the 2 weeks before the test. It is not a diagnostic test. The classification of depression severity according to PHQ-9 score is as follows:

0–4:	Normal
5–9:	Mild
10–14:	Moderate
15–19:	Moderately severe
20–27:	Severe

Paper 2
Questions

Total time allowed is three hours and ten minutes.

P2.1   Minor injuries
While working in the local minor injury unit a young man comes in with the injury shown below.

Which ONE of the following would be the SINGLE MOST appropriate strategy to remove the hook?

O   A   Cut the hook where it enters the skin and push the distal end through the skin

O   B   Making an incision along the skin overlying the barb and removing the hook

O   C   Pull the hook back out through the entry wound

O   D   Push the hook through and out of the skin before cutting off the barb

O   E   Refer to on-call plastic surgery team to remove under general anaesthetic

P2.2 Joint pain

A 7-year-old boy is seen with his mother complaining of a 6-week history of joint pain, lethargy and headache. He has been getting recurrent episodes of sore throat and has persistently enlarged lymph nodes. On examination he is pale and has some petechiae on his back. Which ONE of the following is the SINGLE MOST appropriate next step in this patient? Select ONE option only.

O   A   Prescribe a 10-day course of phenoxymethylpenicillin (penicillin V)

O   B   Reassure the mother that he probably has post-viral fatigue and review in 6 weeks if no better

O   C   Check his full blood count (FBC)

O   D   Prescribe a non-steroidal drug for his arthralgia

O   E   Reassure the mother that the probable diagnosis is Henoch–Schönlein purpura, which should resolve without any complications

Lower urinary tract symptoms in men

P2.3–P2.7

Options

A   5α-Reductase inhibitor
B   α Blocker
C   α Blocker plus 5α-reductase inhibitor
D   Anticholinergic
E   Bladder training
F   Desmopressin
G   GnRH analogue
H   None of the above

Complete the table below describing the management of lower urinary tract symptoms. Each option may be used once, more than once or not at all.

Symptoms	Moderate-to-severe LUTS	Detrusor instability	LUTS with enlarged prostate	LUTS with enlarged prostate despite treatment with 3	Nocturnal polyuria
Treatment	[P2.3]	[P2.4]	[P2.5]	[P2.6]	[P2.7]

P2.8   Psoriasis
A 14-year-old girl with psoriasis comes to see you begging for something to be done for the lesions on her face. These respond to short courses of potent topical steroids but quickly return on stopping. Which one of the following would be the single most appropriate management option for her?

○   A   Betamethasone cream for 8 weeks

○   B   Coal tar

○   C   Emollients

○   D   Topical tacrolimus

○   E   Vitamin D

P2.9   Hip problems in infancy
Which of the following statements about screening for congenital dislocation of the hip is true? Select ONE option only.

○   A   The Ortolani test is used to detect a dislocatable hip

○   B   The Barlow test is used to detect a dislocated hip

○   C   Ultrasonography is much more sensitive and specific than clinical testing

○   D   Most children who are discovered to have the condition will require surgery

○   E   Breech presentation is a risk factor

P2.10   Rectal bleeding
A 37-year-old man complains of severe pain every time that he passes a stool, with fresh blood on the toilet paper. This has not improved with Anusol. Examination reveals a small skin tag and exquisite tenderness just inside the anal margin, but no mass. Which of the following is the SINGLE MOST appropriate management in this case? Select ONE option only.

○   A   Anal stretch

○   B   Instillagel

○   C   Ciprofloxacin

○   D   Haemorrhoidectomy

○   E   Topical glyceryl trinitrate

P2.11   Drug doses in end-of-life care
Breakthrough pain in patients taking regular opioids should be treated with bolus doses equivalent to one-sixth of the patients' daily background opioid dose.

A patient being treated for prostate cancer has normal renal and liver function and weighs 75 kg. He is taking sustained-release morphine 60 mg twice daily.

What would be an appropriate bolus dose of oral morphine for this patient? Write your answer in MILLIGRAMS in the box below.

P2.12   Shortness of breath
A 74-year-old former boilermaker complains of progressive dyspnoea and weight loss over the last 18 months. He is an ex-smoker but has no other previous medical history of note. On examination he has bilateral inspiratory crackles and is clubbed. You arrange a chest X-ray, which shows diffuse shadowing and pleural plaques. What is the SINGLE MOST likely diagnosis? Select ONE option only.

○ A   Asbestosis

○ B   Bronchogenic carcinoma

○ C   Chronic obstructive pulmonary disease

○ D   Extrinsic allergic alveolitis

○ E   Left ventricular failure

P2.13   Hypoglycaemia
You visit a 24-year-old man with type 1 diabetes who is drowsy, slurred and confused. He has had gastroenteritis and his mother thinks that he has not been eating. You measure his blood sugar level at 1.6 mmol/l. You decide to give him intramuscular glucagon. Write the appropriate dose in milligrams in the box below.

Common infections

P2.14–P2.17

Options

A	1 day
B	4 days
C	1 week
D	2½ weeks
E	3 weeks
F	6 weeks
G	3 months

For each of the common self-limiting infections seen in primary care, select the usual duration of symptoms from the list of options above. Each option may be used once, more than once or not at all.

P2.14	Acute tonsillitis
P2.15	Acute bronchitis
P2.16	Acute sinusitis
P2.17	Acute otitis media

P2.18 Heel pain

A 37-year-old recreational marathon runner complains of recurrent pain in his right heel. He has tried anti-inflammatories and several different insoles and different shoes with no benefit. He has seen a sports therapist who has taped his foot to no avail. Examining him he has marked local tenderness. You give him a steroid injection into the point of maximal tenderness but when he fails to improve arrange an X-ray, which shows a heel spur. Which one of the following would be appropriate in his management at this stage?

- O A Bed rest
- O B Botox injections
- O C Refer for excision of his heel spur
- O D Refer for lithotripsy
- O E Repeat cortisone injection

P2.19   Fatigue
A 67-year-old woman presents with dizziness and fatigue. Her
electrocardiogram (ECG) is shown below.

Heart rate: 32 beats/min
QT interval: 604 ms

**Which ONE of the following statements is true with regard to this case?
Select ONE option only.**

○   A   The diagnosis is Möbitz type 2 heart block

○   B   She should be treated with a cardioselective β blocker

○   C   This condition is usually iatrogenic

○   D   If the patient is well in herself she can be referred to the outpatient
department

○   E   She should be treated with a permanent pacemaker

P2.20   Vasectomy
One of your patients comes to see you to request a vasectomy. He has four
children already and feels that he cannot afford to have any more. You
counsel him about the pros and cons of vasectomy. Which of the following
statements about vasectomy is true? Select ONE option only.

○   A   It is usually carried out under general anaesthetic

○   B   Sterility is immediate after the procedure

○   C   Bruising is uncommon and should be investigated

○   D   The lifetime failure rate is approximately 1%

○   E   Vasectomy is reversible in only 50% of cases

P2.21   Nosebleeds
With regard to the management of epistaxis in a 76-year-old man, which of the following statements is correct? Select ONE option only.

O   A   Most bleeds are posterior

O   B   Bleeding comes from branches of the internal jugular vein

O   C   The majority of cases are caused by high blood pressure

O   D   Anterior bleeds are never fatal

O   E   Silver nitrate cautery may cause septal perforation

P2.22   Eye symptoms
A 56-year-old office worker with no previous history of note presents with a painful red eye of 3 days' duration. There is no history of trauma or foreign body, and he does not wear contact lenses. He has tried over the counter chloramphenicol with no benefit. Examination reveals reduced corneal sensation and fluorescein staining reveals the appearance below.

Which of the following is the SINGLE MOST likely diagnosis? Select ONE potion only.

O   A   Dendritic ulcer

O   B   Iritis

O   C   Acute conjunctivitis

O   D   Corneal foreign body

O   E   Recurrent corneal erosion

P2.23 Cardiovascular side effects of drugs

A 63-year-old woman registers at your practice and is found to have persistently raised blood pressure. As part of her baseline investigations an ECG is recorded. Part of this is shown below, together with the automatic measurements.

Which ONE of the following drugs is associated with this condition? Select ONE option only.

O   A   Amoxicillin

O   B   Clarithromycin

O   C   Doxycyline

O   D   Terbinafine

O   E   Trimethoprim

P2.24 Memory problems

A 76-year-old man is brought into the surgery by his wife. He claims not to know why he is there but she tells you that she is worried that he may be starting to develop dementia. Which ONE of the following statements is NOT true about dementia? Select ONE option only.

O   A   Dementia is usually associated with altered cognition and consciousness

O   B   It is usually seen in many spheres of intellectual function

O   C   All patients should have baseline biochemical and haematological investigations before referral

O   D   *Gingko biloba* is of some benefit in slowing memory impairment

O   E   HIV testing is appropriate in young patients

Liver function tests

P2.25–P2.29

Options

A   Gallstones
B   Gilbert syndrome
C   Haemochromatosis
D   Haemolysis
E   Hepatitis
F   Iatrogenic
G   Malnutrition
H   Physiological

For each of the descriptions below, select the SINGLE MOST appropriate diagnosis from the list of options. Each option may be used once, more than once or not at all.

P2.25   A 34-year-old man has recently suffered flu-like symptoms. His bloods show a raised bilirubin only and a normal FBC.

P2.26   A 56-year-old man with epilepsy attends for liver function tests (LFTs) as part of an insurance medical. He has a raised γ-glutamyltransferase (GGT), normal bilirubin, ALT (alanine transaminase) and alkaline phosphatase (ALP).

P2.27   A 12-year-old girl has blood tests as part of investigations for recurrent urinary tract infections. Her ALP level is raised, although bilirubin and ALT are normal.

P2.28   A 34-year-old man has recently returned from a holiday where he had a brief romance. He has now developed jaundice. His blood tests show an ALT five times normal levels, bilirubin elevated and a normal ALP.

P2.29   A 47-year-old woman presents with acute abdominal pain. Her urine has darkened and her stools are pale. Bloods show raised ALT, raised bilirubin and raised ALP. GGT is normal.

P2.30   Tremor
A 78-year-old man comes to see you with his wife and daughter. They have noticed a tremor recently and are concerned that he may have Parkinson's disease. Which ONE of the following statements is true about the clinical diagnosis of Parkinson's disease? Select ONE option only.

O   A   Nystagmus is a common finding in Parkinson's disease

O   B   Parkinson's disease tends to cause reduced tone in the affected limb

O   C   Postural instability is a key symptom of Parkinson's disease

O   D   Symptoms in Parkinson's disease are always bilateral

O   E   Tremor in Parkinson's disease is not usually present at rest

P2.31   Abdominal pain

A 45-year-old man presents with acute onset of severe pain in his loin that is radiating to the flank and groin. On examination he is slightly tender in the renal angle but has no fever. His urine is positive to blood on dipstick testing. Which ONE of the following statements about this situation is true? Select ONE option only.

-   A   He should be given fluids and a broad-spectrum antibiotic
-   B   This condition is usually the result of raised urate levels
-   C   A non-steroidal anti-inflammatory drug (NSAID) is contraindicated due to the risk of renal failure
-   D   Plain radiographs will usually show a stone if one is present
-   E   This could be a presentation of a renal tumour

Erectile dysfunction

P2.32–P.36

Options

A   All of them
B   Caverject
C   MUSE (medicated urethral system for erection)
D   None of them
E   Sildenafil
F   Tadalafil
G   Vacuum pump

For each statement relating to treatments for erectile dysfunction, select the SINGLE MOST appropriate treatment from the list of options. Each option may be used once, more than once or not at all.

P2.32   The treatment may cause disturbance of colour vision.
P2.33   It is contraindicated in sickle cell disease.
P2.34   It is contraindicated in urethral stricture.
P2.35   Its efficacy may persist for 36 hours after use.
P2.36   It may be prescribed on the NHS to men with Parkinson's disease.

P2.37 Data interpretation

A local reflexologist writes to your practice asking if you would like to set up a reflexology service under practice-based commissioning. She cites a recent paper that showed significant benefits for patients with depression. You look the paper up on the internet and find the following abstract:

Qualitative study of the efficacy of reflexology in patients with mild depression

A retrospective postal survey was sent to 18 patients who had received reflexology for mild depression in the 6 months before the survey. The survey dealt with efficacy and satisfaction measures using a 10-point scale. The results showed that 16/18 (89%) of patients reported improvement in their depression after treatment, while no patients reported adverse effects; 13/18 described themselves as very satisfied with the service and 5/18 were quite satisfied. The mean number of sessions was 11, with each session lasting 45 minutes. These data suggest that reflexology is a cost-effective and efficacious alternative to drugs in the management of depression.

Which ONE of the following statements is true with regard to this research? Select ONE option only.

O A   The data support the suggestion that reflexology is a cost-effective alternative to drug therapy

O B   The study follows a valid protocol

O C   Qualitative studies are less prone to bias than quantitative studies

O D   The results should be treated with caution because of inclusion bias

O E   The improvement rates are significantly better than those seen with antidepressants

P2.38 Abdominal pain

A 53-year-old woman presents with mild right iliac fossa pain of 2 months' duration. Examination shows no abnormality but blood tests show a mild iron-deficiency anaemia. Which of the following statements about investigation is correct? Select ONE option only.

O A   Refer for colonoscopy

O B   Refer for sigmoidoscopy

O C   If a barium enema is normal she may be reassured

O D   Refer for ultrasonography

O E   A raised ESR suggests that infection is a probable cause

P2.39   Suicide
        **Which ONE of the following statements about suicide is true? Select ONE
        option only.**

   O   A   Approximately 4000 people a year commit suicide in England and
           Wales

   O   B   Young women are a high-risk group

   O   C   It is more likely in those living in rural communities

   O   D   Cutting the wrists is the most common mode of attempted suicide

   O   E   There is a 20% risk of a patient who has had an episode of deliberate
           self-harm committing suicide within the next 12 months

Child development

P2.40–P2.42

Options

A   6 weeks
B   6 months
C   9 months
D   12 months
E   15 months
F   18 months
G   24 months
H   36 months

For each developmental milestone below, select the SINGLE most appropriate age
at which it would be expected to be seen in a child.

P2.40   Smile back at parent
P2.41   Use a knife and fork
P2.42   Respond to its name

P2.43 and P2.44   Malaise

A 14-year-old boy complains of a 1-week history of flu-like symptoms and sore throat. On examination there is evidence of tonsillitis and lymphadenopathy. You arrange blood tests, the results of which are shown below:

Hb	13.4 g/dl
WBC	$17.3 \times 10^9/l$
Platelets	276
Atypical lymphocytes	15%
Bilirubin	36 (<21) µmol/l
AST	96 (8–48) U/l

Part A

What is the most likely diagnosis? Write the answer in the box below.

Part B

Which ONE of the following is the most appropriate management at this stage? Select ONE option only.

○ A   Amoxicillin

○ B   Ampicillin

○ C   Co-amoxiclav

○ D   Phenoxymethylpenicillin

○ E   None of the above

P2.45 Private fees

Your practice manager has been reviewing the private fees charged in your practice and has suggested that these be increased. Which ONE of the following statements is true with regard to private services? Select ONE option only.

○ A   Private fees can be set at whatever level the practice wishes

○ B   The British Medical Association publishes recommended levels for each service annually

○ C   Private fees cannot increase by more than the level of inflation

○ D   Private fees are covered by the GMS Contract

○ E   Private fees can be charged only if the practice is registered for VAT

P2.46 Hip surgery

A 61-year-old woman comes to see you for advice about whether she should have her hip replaced (as recommended by her orthopaedic surgeon). Which ONE of the following statements about hip replacements is true? Select ONE option only.

○ A   Ninety per cent of hip replacements last for more than 10 years

○ B   There is a 10% infection risk for hip replacement surgery

○ C   Once pain free, there are no restrictions on movement

○ D   The incidence of DVT is 10% after total hip replacement

○ E   Hip resurfacing is superior to conventional arthroplasty in advanced osteoarthritis

Headache

P2.47–2.51

Options

A   Cluster headache
B   Cervicogenic headache
C   Medication overuse headache
D   Migraine
E   Tension headache
F   None of the above

Complete the diagnosis row in the table below designed to aid in the classification of headache, using the list of options above. Each option may be used once, more than once or not at all.

Frequency	1 to several per month	Variable	Alternate days to 8/day	Daily for weeks	>15 days a month
Severity	Moderate–severe	Mild–moderate	Severe	Moderate–severe	Mild–severe
Site of headache	Unilateral or bilateral	Bilateral	Unilateral	Posterior unilateral	Bilateral
Pain type	Throbbing/pulsing	Pressure/tightening	Severe unilateral pain	Ache from occipital region	Diffuse ache/pressure
Aura?	In 33%	None	In some patients	None	None
Duration	4–72 h	Variable	15–180 min	Hours/constant	Hours/constant
Photophobia	Severe	Mild	Mild, may be ipsilateral	None	None
Nausea/vomiting	Moderate–severe	Mild	Mild–moderate	Mild	None
Patient activity	Lie still	Normal	Agitated	Worse with head movement	Normal
Examination findings	Normal	Trigger points in scalp	Epiphora	Pain on neck movement	Normal
Diagnosis	[P2.47]	[P2.48]	[P2.49]	[P2.50]	[P2.51]

P2.52   Febrile illness in childhood

A 3-year-old boy is brought in by his mother with a 6-day history of fever, conjunctivitis, cracked lips and a red tongue, with red swollen hands and feet. She reports that in the first few days of the illness he had a rash on his abdomen, but this has now faded. On examination of his heart sounds he has a gallop rhythm and the heart sounds appear muffled. Which ONE of the following is the MOST likely diagnosis? Select ONE option only.

- ○   A   Kawasaki's disease
- ○   B   Measles
- ○   C   Rubella
- ○   D   Scarlet fever
- ○   E   Takayasu's disease

P2.53   Oedema

A 73-year-old man with a history of hypertension and diabetes presents with 4 weeks of increasing breathlessness on exertion. Over the last 10 days he has had trouble sleeping and cannot get his shoes on as a result of swollen legs. On examination he is afebrile with bilateral basal crepitations and a regular pulse, which you measure as 100 at rest. Which ONE of the following diagnoses is probable in this case? Select ONE option only.

- ○   A   New-onset atrial fibrillation (AF)
- ○   B   Pulmonary fibrosis
- ○   C   Right ventricular failure
- ○   D   Cor pulmonale
- ○   E   Biventricular failure

P2.54   Sore penis

A 5-year-old boy is brought in by his father because he says that it hurts to pass urine. On examination he has balanitis. Which ONE of the following statements is true with regard to management of this condition? Select ONE option only.

- ○   A   *Staphylococcus aureus* is the most common organism
- ○   B   Topical treatment is rarely helpful
- ○   C   All patients should be referred for circumcision
- ○   D   It may cause phimosis
- ○   E   Ninety per cent of 6-year-olds should be able to retract the foreskin

P2.55 Contraception
You see a 19-year-old woman who requests the morning-after pill, and asks if she can go on the pill afterwards. You prescribe ulipristal acetate. Which ONE of the following statements is true about starting the combined oral contraceptive pill in this situation? Select ONE option only.

○ A   She can start taking the combined oral contraceptive pill immediately and need use no other precautions

○ B   She can start taking the combined oral contraceptive pill immediately but should use condoms or avoid sex for 2 days

○ C   She can start taking the combined oral contraceptive pill immediately but should use condoms or avoid sex for 7 days

○ D   She can start taking the combined oral contraceptive pill immediately but should use condoms or avoid sex for 9 days

○ E   She can start taking the combined oral contraceptive pill immediately but should use condoms or avoid sex for 14 days

P2.56 Visual problems
A 24-year-old man comes to see you for advice. He has been told by his optician that he has keratoconus and has been referred to see an ophthalmologist. He is understandably concerned and would like to know more about the condition. Which ONE of the following is correct regarding this condition? Select ONE option only.

○ A   The condition is always bilateral

○ B   The condition is caused by nutritional deficiency

○ C   The condition is non-progressive

○ D   The condition may be associated with corneal thinning

○ E   The only treatment for this condition is corneal grafting

P2.57 Back problems
A 13-year-old girl attends with her mother. She is becoming increasingly concerned about the appearance of her back and has stopped going swimming because of this. On examination she has a prominent scoliosis. Which ONE of the following statements about scoliosis is true? Select ONE option only.

○ A   Spontaneous resolution never occurs

○ B   Scoliosis is always evident from infancy

○ C   Scoliosis in adolescence is more common in boys

○ D   Scoliosis usually affects the lumbar spine

○ E   Scoliosis may be associated with deformity of the skull and ribcage

Bleeding in early pregnancy

P2.58–P2.62

Options

A   Blighted ovum
B   Cervical incompetence
C   Complete abortion
D   Ectopic pregnancy
E   Missed abortion
F   Septic abortion
G   Threatened abortion

For each of the descriptions below, select the SINGLE MOST appropriate diagnosis from the list of options. Each option may be used once, more than once or not at all.

P2.58   A woman with heavy bleeding in week 7 of pregnancy, which initially settled. She now feels unwell and has an offensive vaginal discharge.

P2.59   A woman with a positive pregnancy test has bleeding and abdominal pain in the sixth week of her pregnancy. Ultrasonography shows an empty uterus. Her quantitative bhCG (β-human chorionic gonadotrophin) level is maintained over 72 hours.

P2.60   A woman with a previous history of dilatation and curettage presents with bleeding and mild cramps in week 14 of pregnancy.

P2.61   A woman with painless bleeding in week 7 of pregnancy. On examination her external os is closed.

P2.62   May be accompanied by light bleeding only with severe abdominal pain.

P2.63   Respiratory problems in babies
A 3-month-old baby is brought to the out-of-hours treatment centre by his parents with a cough and failure to feed. He had previously been well and was born after an uneventful pregnancy. He has had coryzal symptoms for the last 3 days. On examination he is tachypnoeic, cyanosed and has a temperature of 40°C. Examination of his chest reveals widespread wheeze and crepitations. What is the SINGLE MOST likely diagnosis? Select ONE option only.

O   A   Asthma

O   B   Bronchiolitis

O   C   Inhaled foreign body

O   D   Pertussis

O   E   Pneumonia

P2.64 **Discrimination**
One of your receptionists decides to retire and you advertise for a replacement. Several of the applicants are aged over 60 years. The practice retirement age is set at 60. Which ONE of the following statements is true about this situation? Select ONE option only.

○ A Age discrimination laws are designed specifically to protect elderly people

○ B Mandatory retirement is 60 years for women and 65 years for men

○ C Employers must write to employees in advance of their retirement date and advise them of their rights to apply to work beyond this date

○ D Employment benefits with length of service are legal as long as the length of service to qualify is no more than 10 years

○ E Dismissal on the basis of age is unlawful regardless of age

P2.65 **Sore throat**
You see a 5-year-old boy with a sore throat, headache and fever. On examination you note tonsillitis with a white furry tongue and enlarged papillae, and a fine red blanching rash on the abdomen and chest. You prescribe antibiotics and advise the mother to keep the boy off school.

How long after commencing the antibiotics can the child return to school? Write the number of hours in the box below, in numbers.

P2.66 **Treatment of chest infections**
A 76-year-old man with controlled hypertension is diagnosed with pneumonia. Which ONE of the following statements about management is correct? Select ONE option only.

○ A He should receive a broad-spectrum cephalosporin

○ B He should be treated with a macrolide

○ C First-line treatment should be amoxicillin 250 mg three times daily

○ D If he fails to respond to a first-line antibiotic the dose should be increased

○ E If *Staphylococcus* sp. is suspected flucloxacillin should be added

P2.67 Premature ejaculation
You see a 28-year-old man and his partner, who complain that since the start of their relationship he has been plagued by premature ejaculation. This is starting to cause problems in their relationship. Which ONE of the following statements about management of this condition is true? Select ONE option only.

O   A   The problem affects 5% of men questioned in surveys

O   B   Clomipramine taken before intercourse is no more effective than placebo

O   C   Paroxetine can increase the period before ejaculation up to eight times longer than placebo

O   D   Fluoxetine is very effective when taken once a day

O   E   Chlorpromazine is the treatment of choice for resistant patients

Management of epididymitis

P2.68–P2.70

Options

A   Amoxicillin
B   Benzylpenicillin
C   Ciprofloxacin
D   Contact tracing
E   Doxycyline
F   Screen for *Chlamydia* sp.
G   Trimethoprim

Complete the algorithm below for the management of acute epididymo-orchitis, from the list above. Each option may be used once, more than once or not at all.

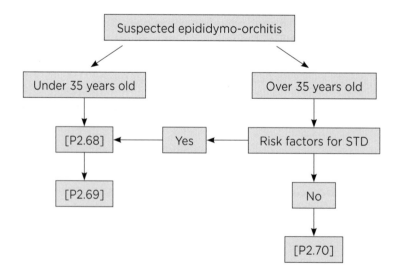

P2.71   Lithium
Your practice decides to do an audit of lithium prescribing as a result of a significant event. Which ONE of the following statements is correct regarding the use of lithium in general practice? Select ONE option only.

O   A   Lithium has a wide therapeutic range

O   B   Lithium has few side effects

O   C   Lithium is associated with an increase in risk of hypothyroidism

O   D   Lithium is safe to use in renal impairment

O   E   Lithium toxicity is rare

P2.72 and P2.73   Speech problems
Which TWO of the following statements are CORRECT with regard to speech delay? Select TWO options only.

O   A   Language delay has a worse prognosis than speech delay

O   B   Speech and language delay are more common in girls

O   C   Speech and language delay is always a primary neurological condition

O   D   Speech and language delay is rare in children entering primary school

O   E   There is often a family history of speech and language delay

P2.74   Use of ACE inhibitors
A 67-year-old hypertensive woman is started on aspirin and ramipril after suffering a transient ischaemic attack. One week after starting the ramipril she attends for renal function testing and her creatinine has increased from 83 mmol/l to 133 mmol/l. Which ONE of the following statements about her management is true? Select ONE option only.

O   A   The dose of ramipril should not be increased further and she should have a repeat blood test in 1 week

O   B   As long as she is not hypotensive and her creatinine <150 mmol/l she can be reassured

O   C   The ramipril should be stopped and specialist advice sought

O   D   The ramipril should be changed to an angiotensin II receptor blocker

O   E   She should have her aspirin stopped

P2.75 Prescribing controlled drugs
Which ONE of the following statements is correct with regard to the prescribing of controlled drugs in primary care? Select ONE option only.

○ A   All prescriptions for controlled drugs must be hand written

○ B   All prescriptions for controlled drugs must specify the quantity in words and numbers

○ C   Prescriptions for controlled drugs may be sent to the pharmacy electronically

○ D   The date on the prescription must be handwritten

○ E   The patient's age and date of birth must be specified on the prescription

P2.76 Vertigo
A 54-year-old woman presents with vertigo. Which ONE of the following symptoms would be consistent with a diagnosis of benign paroxysmal positional vertigo? Select ONE option only.

○ A   Hallpike testing provokes instantaneous onset of symptoms

○ B   It worsens with repeat Hallpike testing

○ C   It is typically triggered by particular head movements

○ D   It is associated with unilateral tinnitus

○ E   It may be treated with Stemetil

P2.77　Moles

A 32-year-old woman attends for a mole check after reading a newspaper article about skin cancer. The lesion shown below is particularly worrying her, because it has recently grown significantly.

What is the SINGLE MOST likely diagnosis? Select ONE option only.

○　A　Seborrhoeic keratosis

○　B　Intradermal naevus

○　C　Histiocytoma

○　D　Malignant melanoma

○　E　Squamous cell carcinoma (SCC)

P2.78　Eating disorders

Which ONE of the following statements is true with regard to anorexia nervosa? Select ONE option only.

○　A　Patients can be screened for this condition using the SCOFF questionnaire

○　B　The prevalence in the UK is estimated to be 10%

○　C　It is seen exclusively in females

○　D　It is characterised by obsession with exercise

○　E　It can be diagnosed in those with a BMI <20 kg/m² and food avoidance

Cardiovascular drugs

P2.79–P2.86

Options

A   Amiodarone
B   Atorvastatin
C   Clopidogrel
D   Dipyridamole
E   Flecainide
F   Furosemide
G   Indapamide
H   Isosorbide mononitrate
I   Metoprolol
J   Ramipril
K   Sacubitril
L   Sotalol
M   Spironolactone
N   Valsartan
O   Verapamil
P   Warfarin

For each clinical scenario above, select the most appropriate therapy from the list of options. Each option may be used once, more than once or not at all.

P2.79   It reduces triglycerides as well as total cholesterol.
P2.80   It is used for prophylaxis of atrial fibrillation.
P2.81   It may be used in left ventricular dysfunction where ACE (angiotensin-converting enzyme) inhibitors are not tolerated.
P2.82   It is contraindicated in patients on β blockers.
P2.83   It often causes headache, flushing and postural hypotension.
P2.84   It should be considered in patients with heart failure already on an ACE inhibitor and thiazide.
P2.85   It may cause corneal microdeposits and phototoxicity.
P2.86   It may be safely used in young patients with hypertension and renal artery stenosis.

P2.87 Aspirin
A 52-year-old businessman comes to see you for a well man check. He is normotensive and his cholesterol and glucose levels are normal. He asks you about the merits of taking daily aspirin. Which ONE of the following statements is correct regarding the pros and cons of aspirin in primary prevention? Select ONE option only.

O   A   Aspirin may increase the risk of cancer

O   B   Aspirin use in primary prevention reduces risk of non-fatal myocardial infarction

O   C   Clopidogrel should be used for primary prevention due to an improved safety profile

O   D   The risk of gastrointestinal bleeding remains constant regardless of duration of aspirin use

O   E   There are no significant side effects from taking aspirin

P2.88 Treatment of skin lesions
A 12-year-old girl has had the skin lesion below for 18 months. She has tried topical salicylic acid and topical glutaraldehyde without benefit.

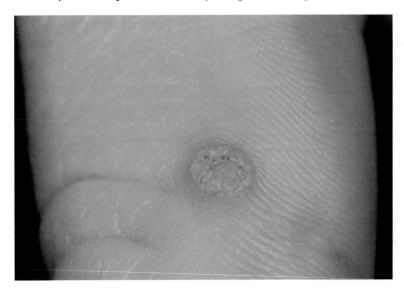

Which ONE of the following would be the SINGLE MOST appropriate next step in her treatment? Select ONE option only.

O   A   Bleomycin

O   B   Cryotherapy

O   C   Excision

O   D   Podophyllin

O   E   No treatment

P2.89 Palpitations
A 33-year-old marketing executive complains of palpitations at night. These come and go and, although he does not feel unwell with them, he gets a fluttering sensation in his chest for 30–60 seconds. He is otherwise well and takes no regular medication. His bloods and ECG are normal; however, a 24-hour ECG reveals short runs of atrial fibrillation. Which ONE of the following statements about paroxysmal atrial fibrillation is true? Select ONE option only.

- A It affects approximately 10% of the population at some time in their lives
- B All patients should be anticoagulated because of the risk of stroke
- C Digoxin is effective in this patient group
- D Lifestyle has little effect on symptoms
- E Patients with recurrent symptoms can use flecainide as a 'pill-in-the-pocket' treatment

P2.90 Abdominal pain
A 37-year-old woman complains of recurrent severe pain in the right upper quadrant after meals. On examination she is tender in the right upper quadrant on deep inspiration. Which ONE of the following statements is true? Select ONE option only.

- A If caused by gallstones the pain usually settles within a few minutes
- B When associated with jaundice the cause is usually malignant
- C Symptoms usually settle spontaneously with a change in diet
- D She should be referred for endoscopic retrograde cholecystopancreatography
- E Raised alkaline phosphatase (ALP) suggests that the diagnosis is gallstones

P2.91 Sore throat
A 21-year-old who was started on antibiotics for tonsillitis 2 days ago presents with signs of a quinsy. Which ONE of the following statements about this condition is true? Select ONE option only.

- A It is usually caused by infection with *Haemophilus influenzae* type B
- B It is an abscess within the tonsillar crypts
- C Earache, trismus and dysphagia are typical symptoms
- D It should be treated by adding in metronidazole tablets
- E It does not recur

P2.92   Skin lump
A 79 year old has noticed a lump on his leg over the last 4 weeks. This has grown rapidly and he thinks started after he scratched himself gardening. The lump is shown below.

Which ONE of the following would be the MOST APPROPRIATE treatment for this lesion? Select ONE option only.

○   A   Cryotherapy

○   B   Excision biopsy

○   C   Topical 5-fluorouracil (Efudix)

○   D   Topical ingenol mebutate (Picato)

○   E   Watchful waiting

Travellers' diarrhoea

P2.93–P2.95

Options

A   *Cambylobacter jejuni*
B   *Cryptosporidium* spp.
C   *Entamoeba histolytica*
D   Enterotoxigenic *Escherichia coli* (ETEC)
E   *Giardia lamblia*
F   *Shigella* spp.
G   *Vibrio cholerae*

For the patient described, select the SINGLE MOST likely diagnosis from the list of options. Each option may be used once, more than once, or not at all.

P2.93   A 23-year-old woman has been backpacking in Cambodia for 3 months. She develops bloating and belching followed by diarrhoea and steatorrhoea with excessive flatus. These symptoms last for several weeks.

P2.94   A 19-year-old gap-year student has been in Peru for 2 weeks. He develops abdominal cramps and nausea followed by 36 hours of profuse watery diarrhoea. The symptoms settle spontaneously within 48 hours.

P2.95   A 34-year-old volunteer working in Haiti develops nausea and then profuse watery diarrhoea, causing him to feel faint on standing.

P2.96 and P2.97   Chest infection

You see a 68-year-old patient who has been suffering from a cough for the last 72 hours, and has now developed mild pleuritic pain. He is normally fit and well and takes no regular medication. On examination he has left basal crepitations, is not confused and has the following observations:

Pulse	83 beats/min
Respiratory rate	32/min
Blood pressure	112/74 mmHg
Temperature	38.1°C
Oxygen saturation	94%

Part A

What is his CRB-65 score? Write the answer in numbers in the box below

Part B

Which of the following is the SINGLE MOST appropriate action in this situation? Select ONE option only.

- O A Admit to hospital
- O B Prescribe antibiotics and arrange review in 48 hours
- O C Prescribe antibiotics and give safety-netting instructions
- O D Prescribe deferred antibiotics with instructions on when to use
- O E Prescribe non-steroidal anti-inflammatories

P2.98 Deafness

A 35-year-old woman presents with steadily increasing deafness that is causing her to struggle to hear on the telephone. Which ONE of the following statements about otosclerosis is true? Select ONE option only.

- O A It causes a sensorineural deafness, worse in low frequencies
- O B It typically presents in the fifth decade
- O C Its incidence is rising
- O D It often gets worse during pregnancy
- O E Hearing aids are the only treatment

P2.99 Boils

A 25-year-old woman presents complaining of recurrent boils in her axillae. These come on for no obvious reason and she has had numerous courses of antibiotics over the last 5 years. She says that she is fed up and has had to stop shaving her armpits, which she finds very distressing. Which ONE of the following statements about treatment of this condition is true? Select ONE option only.

- O A Botox injections may reduce the frequency of attacks
- O B Anhydrol Forte may be helpful in place of antiperspirant
- O C A low-dose combined oral contraceptive may be helpful
- O D Long-term oral tetracycline is effective in reducing frequency of attacks
- O E She should be referred at this point for surgical excision and skin grafting

P2.100 Arm pain

A 73-year-old woman noticed a sudden popping sensation in her left arm. On examination her arm has the following appearance.

What treatment is required? Select ONE option only.

○ A   Referral to physiotherapy for ultrasound therapy

○ B   Referral to orthopaedics for repair

○ C   Collar-and-cuff sling

○ D   Steroid injection into the rotator cuff

○ E   None

P2.101 Epiglottitis

Which ONE of the following is NOT a feature of epiglottitis? Select ONE option only.

○ A   The patient is unwell and looks septic

○ B   The voice is muffled

○ C   There is increasing dysphagia

○ D   There is drooling

○ E   It is exclusively seen in children

P2.102 Head lump

A 55-year-old man complains of a lump behind his left ear. This has been slowly growing for a number of years. It is 2.5 cm in diameter, non-tender, mobile with no punctum and there is no history of discharge. The lump is shown below.

Which ONE of the following statements is the SINGLE MOST APPROPRIATE primary care management of this condition? Select ONE option only.

○ A Excise for histology

○ B Needle aspiration

○ C Reassurance with safety-netting advice

○ D Refer for routine ultrasound scan

○ E Refer under the 2-week rule

P2.103 Constipation

A 63-year-old woman has been struggling with constipation for several years. She has tried bulk-forming laxatives, stimulating laxatives and high-fibre diet. None of these has been successful. She takes no other medication and has no other previous history of note and a recent colonoscopy was normal. Which ONE of the following treatments would be indicated at this point? Select ONE option only.

- O A Co-danthrusate
- O B Lactose-free diet
- O C Methylnaltrexone
- O D Prucalopride
- O E Sodium picosulfate

P2.104 Hand injuries

You see a 23-year-old man at the walk-in centre who has cut his knuckles on someone else's teeth during a pub fight the night before. On examination he has several puncture wounds over the knuckles and the hand is swollen. Which ONE of the following statements about his management is NOT true? Select ONE option only.

- O A He should be given co-amoxiclav 625 mg three times daily and advised to return for review the following day
- O B The wounds should be cleaned with saline, and closed
- O C An X-ray should be taken of the hand to exclude underlying fracture or broken teeth
- O D Consideration should be given to HIV testing
- O E He should receive a tetanus booster

P2.105 **Tennis elbow**

An audit of minor surgery carried out in your surgery reveals that a significant number of patients treated with cortisone injections for tennis elbow return for further treatment. You review the evidence with a view to creating a practice protocol. Which ONE of the following statements is correct about current evidence-based management of this condition? Select ONE option only.

○ A All patients not improving after 4 weeks of physiotherapy should be referred for consideration of Botox therapy

○ B Graduated loading with eccentric exercises should be used as firstline treatment

○ C Most cases are seen in racket sport players, and they should be advised to modify their technique

○ D Steroid injections provide long-term benefit, although they may cause side effects

○ E Topical non-steroidal anti-inflammatory drugs do not have any effect in this condition

Drug management of Parkinson's disease

P2.106-P2.109

Options

A Amitriptyline
B Chlorpromazine
C Citalopram
D Clozapine
E Domperidone
F Levodopa and dopa decarboxylase inhibitor
G Pramipexole
H Rivastigmine
I Selegiline
J None of the above

For each of the statements regarding drug management of Parkinson's disease below, select the SINGLE MOST appropriate option from the list above. Each option may be used once, more than once or not at all.

P2.106 Associated with impulse control symptoms, particularly in young men
P2.107 Useful for depressive symptoms in patients with Parkinson's disease
P2.108 Co-prescription with levodopa agents allows a lower dose of dopamine
P2.109 Indicated for psychotic symptoms

P2.110 Dizziness

You visit an 82-year-old man with a history of ischaemic heart disease who complains of dizziness. He reports that he has developed vertigo and double vision, and has dysarthria when you speak to him. Neurological examination also shows some loss of sensation and loss of power in both arms. He has no signs of middle-ear disease and his cardiovascular observations are normal. Which ONE of the following is the SINGLE MOST likely diagnosis? Select ONE option only.

- ○ A   Labyrinthitis
- ○ B   Ménière's disease
- ○ C   Migraine
- ○ D   Vestibular neuronitis
- ○ E   Vertebrobasilar stroke

P2.111 Rash

A 3-year-old girl presents with a vesicular rash on her face and body. She was previously well until she developed a flu-like illness 3 days ago. She has no eye or chest symptoms. Her face has the following appearance.

What is the diagnosis? Select ONE option only.

- ○ A   Measles
- ○ B   Rubella
- ○ C   Shingles
- ○ D   Parvovirus B19
- ○ E   Chickenpox

Prescription charges

P2.112–P2.116

Options

A   Apply under low-income scheme
B   Automatically entitled to free prescriptions
C   Entitled to free NHS dental treatment
D   Entitled to free NHS sight tests
E   Entitled to free prescriptions on applying for an exemption certificate
F   Not entitled to free dental treatment
G   Not entitled to free NHS sight test
H   Not entitled to free prescriptions
I   Prescription pre-payment certificate

For each of the patients described below, select the SINGLE MOST appropriate rule about health charges. Each option may be used once, more than once or not at all.

P2.112   A 56-year-old businessman with diet-controlled diabetes who needs antibiotics.

P2.113   A 33-year-old woman who gave birth 9 months ago needs a dental crown.

P2.114   A 57-year-old accountant who takes thyroxine needs an eye test.

P2.115   An 18-year-old student who needs antibiotics.

P2.116   A 35-year-old person with newly diagnosed epilepsy taking phenytoin.

P2.117 Skin problems

A 76-year-old man presents with a rash on both legs for 2 years. It is itchy and he has been using E45. He has no previous history of note and is otherwise well. The rash is shown below.

What is the diagnosis? Select ONE option only.

○ A   Asteatotic eczema

○ B   Varicose eczema

○ C   Pompholyx

○ D   Psoriasis

○ E   Contact dermatitis

Examination of the eye

P2.118–P2.122

Options

A   Acute angle-closure glaucoma
B   Cataract
C   Chronic glaucoma
D   Corneal abrasion
E   Keratoconus
F   Optic atrophy
G   Recurrent uveitis
H   Retinoblastoma

For each of the scenarios described below, select the SINGLE MOST appropriate diagnosis from the list of options. Each option may be used once, more than once or not at all.

P2.118   The red reflex appears white.
P2.119   On fundoscopy the disc appears pale compared with the other eye.
P2.120   The pupil is fixed but round.
P2.121   The pupil is fixed but irregular.
P2.122   The disc has a cupped appearance.

P2.123 Birthmarks
A 5-year-old girl is noted to have the lesion below by her grandmother, who is looking after her while her parents are on holiday. She is concerned as to the significance. The child has no previous history of note and there is no family history of note. Examination reveals a total of two such lesions on her body both <1 cm in diameter.

What is the SINGLE MOST likely diagnosis? Select ONE option only.

O   A   Albright syndrome

O   B   Bloom syndrome

O   C   Neurofibromatosis

O   D   Tuberous sclerosis

O   E   None of the above

P2.124 Eyelid problems

A 21-year-old man presents with a painless swelling in his left lower eyelid for 3 months. On examination there is no erythema or discharge. Which ONE of the following is the SINGLE MOST likely diagnosis? Select ONE option only.

- ○ A   Basal cell carcinoma
- ○ B   Stye
- ○ C   Xanthelasma
- ○ D   Chalazion
- ○ E   Conjunctivitis

Antibiotic prescribing

P2.125–P2.129

Options

A   Aciclovir
B   Amoxicillin
C   Co-amoxiclav
D   Benzylpenicillin
E   Cefradine
F   Ciprofloxacin
G   Chloramphenicol
H   Erythromycin
I   Flucloxacillin
J   Fusidic acid
K   Metronidazole
L   Nitrofurantoin
M   Phenoxymethylpenicillin
N   Trimethoprim

For each infection described below, select the SINGLE MOST appropriate antibiotic from the list of options. Each option may be used once, more than once or not at all.

P2.125   A 67-year-old woman who requires prophylaxis against recurrent urinary tract infections and has had a severe allergic reaction to Septrin (co-trimoxazole).

P2.126   A 21-year-old student who has been in close contact with a patient with meningococcal meningitis.

P2.127   A 4-year-old child with tonsillitis.

P2.128   A 35-year-old man with a chest infection who is allergic to penicillin.

P2.129   A 34-year-old veterinary nurse who has received a dog bite to the hand.

P2.130 Diabetic ketoacidosis

Which ONE of the following statements about the management of diabetic ketoacidosis (DKA) is true? Select ONE option only.

○ A   Emergency treatment involves an immediate insulin injection and fluid rehydration

○ B   DKA usually has no prodromal phase

○ C   The respiratory rate is often reduced

○ D   Polydipsia often causes fluid overload and hyponatraemia

○ E   Initial treatment should include stat injection of intramuscular glucagon

P2.131 Shin lesions

A 21-year-old student presents with a 1-week history of tender lumps on her shins. She is otherwise fit and well and takes no regular medication. A photograph of her shins is shown below.

Which ONE of the following statements about this condition is NOT true? Select ONE option only.

○ A   It may be caused by cat scratch disease

○ B   Patients should have a throat swab and chest X-ray as routine investigations

○ C   It may be caused by the oral contraceptive pill

○ D   Non-steroidal anti-inflammatory drugs (NSAIDs) may provide symptomatic relief

○ E   It is usually a sign of underlying malignancy

P2.132 Weaning

With regard to weaning of healthy infants, MATCH each type of food to the appropriate age of the child. All four must be correctly matched to score one mark.

A   Adult food
B   Meat
C   Milk
D   Rice

Age	Food
<4 months	
4-6 months	
6-9 months	
9-12 months	

P2.133 Breathing problems

A 79-year-old man who is having chemotherapy for lung cancer complains of difficulty breathing. On examination he has dilated veins over his neck and shoulders, oedema in both arms and stridor at rest. Which ONE of the following is the SINGLE MOST LIKELY diagnosis? Select ONE option only.

O   A   Angioedema

O   B   Asthma

O   C   Foreign body aspiration

O   D   Pulmonary embolus

O   E   Superior vena caval obstruction

Psychological therapies for alcohol abuse

P2.134–P2.136

Options

A   12-step facilitation
B   Aversion therapy
C   Behavioural couples therapy
D   Cognitive–behavioural therapy
E   Self-help-based treatments
F   Social skills training
G   Structured brief advice

For each description below, select the SINGLE most appropriate option from the list above.

P2.134   Identifies high-risk situations, alters expectancies and increases self-efficacy

P2.135   Utilises the concept that alcohol misuse is a spiritual and medical disease

P2.136   Suitable for use in primary care

P2.137   Type 2 diabetes
A 49-year-old patient with type 2 diabetes arthritis and obstructive sleep apnoea has a BMI of 37 and is taking maximally tolerated doses of metformin, gliclazide and pioglitazone. His most recent HbA1c is 103 mmol/mol. You suggest that he start insulin treatment, but due to his occupation he cannot risk hypoglycaemia. According to NICE guidance, what would be the most appropriate class of drug to use at this stage?

Write your answer in the box below.

P2.138   Epidemiology
The prevalence of a disease is 8.3 per 100 000 of the population.
Which ONE of the following is CORRECT with regard to this information?
Select ONE option only.

○   A   On the date that the data were collected, 8.3 per 100 000 people had the disease

○   B   Over their lifetime, 8.3 per 100 000 patients will have the disease

○   C   There are 8.3 new cases per 100 000 patients diagnosed per year

○   D   These data suggest that the disease has a poor prognosis

○   E   These data suggest that the disease is chronic

P2.139 Rheumatological treatments

With regard to drug treatments for rheumatological conditions, which ONE of the following statements is true? Select ONE option only.

- ○ A Infliximab is licensed for the prevention of recurrence in rheumatoid arthritis
- ○ B Hydroxychloroquine will reduce pain, swelling and stiffness in systemic lupus erythematosus (SLE)
- ○ C Penicillamine is given by intramuscular injection
- ○ D Methotrexate produces immediate benefit in rheumatoid arthritis
- ○ E Sulfasalazine has no effect on fertility, so it can be safely used in younger patients

P2.140 Hand pain

A 53-year-old woman presents with 6 weeks of malaise and fatigue associated with swelling and erythema affecting her metacarpophalangeal joints in both hands. These are particularly stiff first thing in the morning. Which ONE of the following is a likely diagnosis? Select ONE option only.

- ○ A Primary nodal osteoarthritis
- ○ B Rheumatoid arthritis
- ○ C Reiter syndrome
- ○ D Gout
- ○ E Rheumatic fever

P2.141 Audit

Which ONE of the following statements is true with regard to audit in primary care? Select ONE option only.

- ○ A Audit involves researching the effects of new treatment protocols
- ○ B Standards must be defined and agreed before an audit is carried out
- ○ C The 'audit cycle' refers to the continual need to refine our audit criteria
- ○ D The implementation of change is implicit in the audit cycle
- ○ E Audits should be doctor led

P2.142 Ear discharge
A 46-year-old man with no previous history complains of recurrent otitis externa and deafness. You look in his ear and note thick yellow debris. This is removed with a probe and is shown below.

Which ONE of the following is the SINGLE MOST LIKELY underlying diagnosis? Select ONE option only.

○　A　Acute otitis externa

○　B　Chronic otitis externa

○　C　Cholesteatoma

○　D　Foreign body

○　E　Fungal otitis externa

Shoulder problems

P2.143–P2.147

Options

A   Cervical spondylosis
B   Frozen shoulder
C   Osteoarthritis
D   Referred pain
E   Ruptured supraspinatus
F   Shoulder dystocia
G   Shoulder–hand syndrome
H   Subluxation of the glenohumeral joint
I   Supraspinatus tendonitis

For each of the cases described below select the SINGLE MOST appropriate choice from the list of options. Each option may be used once, more than once or not at all.

P2.143   A 19-year-old girl who is 5 weeks pregnant presents with vaginal bleeding and pain in the tip of her left shoulder. On examination she has a full range of movement in the shoulder.

P2.144   A 56-year-old man presents with several years of pain and reduced range of movement in his right shoulder. On examination there is limited range of movement and extensive crepitus.

P2.145   A 67-year-old woman with a history of chronic neck pain complains of pain in her right shoulder with weakness in abduction. She also reports paraesthesiae in her arm at times.

P2.146   A 45-year-old man is seen with a 12-week history of reduced range of movement in his left shoulder. This started without obvious cause and on examination you note that external rotation is particularly affected.

P2.147   A 23-year-old man presents with pain and reduced range of movement in his left shoulder. He thinks that he may have fallen on to his shoulder the previous night after drinking, but cannot remember. On examination his shoulder looks flattened and, in addition to inability to abduct his shoulder, he has a numb patch on the side of his humerus.

P2.148 Itching in pregnancy
A 27-year-old woman in week 36 of pregnancy complains of severe itching of her hands and feet, particularly at night. She has no rash or signs of jaundice, but there are signs of scratching. She has been feeling regular fetal movements. Bilirubin and ALT are both normal, and alkaline phosphatase is slightly elevated. What is the SINGLE MOST appropriate management option?

- O A Prescribe a sedating antihistamine to use at night
- O B Prescribe topical emollients only
- O C Prescribe ursodeoxycholic acid
- O D Send blood for bile acid levels, and if these are normal no further action is needed
- O E Send bloods for bile acid levels, and if these are normal repeat if itching persists

Medical records legislation

P2.149–P2.154

Options

A Access to Health Records Act
B Access to Medical Reports Act
C Children's Act
D Community Care Act
E Data Protection Act
F Freedom of Information Act
G Mental Health Act 1983
H Public Records Act

For each of the scenarios below, select the ONE SINGLE MOST appropriate option from the list above. Each option may be used once, more than once, or not at all.

P2.149   It allows patients to see entries in their medical records made since 1991.
P2.150   It allows patients to access and request alterations to be made to computer records.
P2.151   It allows a charge of up to £10 to be made for access to records, plus copying expenses.
P2.152   It assumes that a mother automatically has responsibility for a child.
P2.153   It allows patients to attach a codicil to the record in question if he or she disagrees with it.
P2.154   It allows doctors to withhold information from a patient's record that would be damaging to his or her mental health.

Red eye

P2.155–P2.160

Options

A   Acute glaucoma
B   Anterior uveitis
C   Conjunctivitis
D   Episcleritis
E   Keratitis
F   Scleritis

Complete the table opposite from the list of options above. Each option may be used once, more than once, or not at all.

Suspected condition	P2.155	P2.156	P2.157	P2.158	P2.159	P2.160
Common symptoms	Severe pain, photophobia, haloes, no discharge	Photophobia, foreign body sensation, purulent discharge	Photophobia, pain, blurred vision	Severe pain without discharge, insidious onset, history of connective tissue disease	Minimal pain, no discharge, no photophobia. Foreign body sensation	Foreign body sensation, discharge
Common signs	Hazy cornea, fixed pupil, reduced acuity	Corneal defect visible with fluorescein, pus in anterior chamber	Circumcorneal erythema, irregular pupil, reduced acuity	Acuity maybe normal	Localised erythema, normal acuity	Conjunctival injection and mucopurulent discharge, normal visual acuity

P2.161 Colic

A new mum comes to see you at the end of her tether. Her 4-week-old son has had awful colic every night for the last 2 weeks. He is otherwise well but she demands that something be done. On examination no abnormalities are found. Which ONE of the following statements about colic is true? Select ONE option only.

○ A It is usually associated with vomiting at the end of an attack

○ B It occurs in 1% of infants

○ C It usually resolves over 1–2 weeks

○ D It may be helped with dicyclomine

○ E It may be helped with lactase added to feeds

Female urinary problems

P2.162–P2.164

Options

A   Cystocele
B   Genuine stress incontinence
C   Mixed urinary incontinence
D   Overflow urinary incontinence
E   True urinary incontinence
F   Urethrocele

For each patient described below, select the SINGLE MOST likely diagnosis from the list of options. Each option may be used once, more than once, or not at all.

P2.162   A 39-year-old woman with a history of spinal cord injury complains of continuous dribbling of urine, with a feeling of inability to empty her bladder.

P2.163   A 78-year-old woman with a previous history of bladder cancer complains of continuous dribbling of urine from her vagina.

P2.164   A 63-year-old woman complains of urinary leakage with coughing and sneezing, often immediately preceded by a sense of urgency.

P2.165 Management of thyroid disease in pregnancy

A 32-year-old woman with a previous history of hypothyroidism has just found out that she is pregnant. She is currently taking 100 μg of levothyroxine every day. Which ONE of the following statements is correct with regard to management of hypothyroidism in pregnancy?

- O   A   In most cases levothyroxine requirement falls during pregnancy

- O   B   Levothyroxine dose should be increased by 30% at the booking appointment

- O   C   Levothyroxine dose should be increased only when blood tests show an elevated TSH level

- O   D   Treatment of subclinical hypothyroidism in pregnancy is associated with adverse outcomes for the fetus

- O   E   TSH assays are unreliable in pregnancy due to interference from hCG

P2.166 Notifiable diseases

A   *Chlamydia trachomatis* infection
B   Chickenpox
C   Influenza
D   Leptospirosis
E   Lyme disease
F   Measles
G   Mumps
H   Ophthalmia neonatorum
I   Rubella
J   Scarlet fever
K   Tuberculosis
L   Whooping cough

Place the name of EACH disease listed into ONE of the columns below to indicate whether it is a notifiable disease or not. All options must be correctly matched to score one mark.

Notifiable disease	Not notifiable disease

P2.167 Haemoptysis

A 67-year-old man who has been a lifelong smoker presents with haemoptysis, progressive shortness of breath and weight loss. His hands have the appearance shown below.

What is the probable underlying diagnosis? Select ONE option only.

○ A   Inflammatory bowel disease

○ B   Congenital heart disease

○ C   Pneumonia

○ D   Cystic fibrosis

○ E   Lung cancer

P2.168 Urinary problems in babies

You are referred a 3-month-old baby boy by the health visitor after his mother noticed that he is leaking urine from the middle of his penis. On examination there seems to be a small pit on the underside of the penis. Which ONE of the following statements about this condition is true? Select ONE option only.

○ A   The condition is rare, with an incidence of 1:5000

○ B   It always presents in infancy

○ C   Surgery is always indicated

○ D   It is usually associated with other abnormalities of the urogenital tract

○ E   It may be a sign of female virilisation

Hirsutism

P2.169–P2.173

Options

A   Combined oral contraceptive
B   Cyproterone acetate
C   Dianette
D   Electrolysis
E   Finasteride
F   Metformin
G   Minoxidil
H   Referral
I   Spironolactone
J   Weight loss

For each of the patients described below, select the SINGLE MOST appropriate therapy from the list of options. Each option may be used once, more than once or not at all.

P2.169   A 22-year-old woman with excessive facial hair and irregular periods. Blood tests are normal.

P2.170   A 47-year-old woman with hirsutism who has a history of DVT on the contraceptive pill and who has not found electrolysis or camouflage effective.

P2.171   A 27-year-old woman of Mediterranean origin with normal periods who has a prominent hair on her upper lip only and is unable to take the pill.

P2.172   An 18-year-old girl with hirsutism and acne, not responding to the combined oral contraceptive pill (COCP).

P2.173   A 23-year-old woman who is hirsute with irregular periods and primary infertility.

Dizziness and vertigo

P2.174–P2.178

Options

A   Acoustic neuroma
B   Benign paroxysmal positional vertigo
C   Cardiogenic syncope
D   Cervical vertigo
E   Hyperventilation
F   Ménière's disease
G   Ramsay Hunt syndrome
H   Round window rupture
I   Migraine
J   Vestibular neuronitis

For each scenario described below, select the SINGLE MOST likely diagnosis from the list of options. Each option may be used once, more than once or not at all.

P2.174   Recurrent attacks of pressure in the ear are associated with tinnitus, deafness and vertigo.

P2.175   There is an acute onset of severe vertigo with vomiting, which usually settles over several days.

P2.176   It is associated with a sensation of light-headedness and palpitations before fainting.

P2.177   It is associated with vertigo only on moving the head in certain planes.

P2.178   Vertigo is accompanied by facial palsy and deafness.

P2.179 Prostate tests
A 63-year-old man requests a PSA (prostate-specific antigen) test to see if he has prostate cancer. Before testing you spend some time counselling him about the test and its use. Which ONE of the following statements about PSA testing is true? Select ONE option only.

O   A   The test is highly sensitive

O   B   The test is highly specific

O   C   A raised PSA may be caused by urinary infection

O   D   PSA testing is a proven diagnostic test

O   E   Anyone with a PSA >4.0 mmol/l should be referred

P2.180 Drug abuse

A 29-year-old man registers at the practice, having just moved to the area. At his first consultation he admits that he has been injecting heroin for the last 8 months and would like help in stopping. Which ONE of the following statements about this area of practice is NOT true?

- ○ A He should be converted to a twice-daily maintenance dose of methadone and this should be gradually reduced

- ○ B He should be advised about the importance of safe sex

- ○ C GPs are not obliged under the terms of the GMS contract to provide substitution treatment for opiate dependency

- ○ D A treatment contract should be agreed with the patient that covers the responsibilities of each party

- ○ E A hierarchy of goals is recommended that will initially minimise harm and aim for eventual abstinence

P2.181 Breathlessness

A 19-year-old man presents complaining of an acute onset of breathlessness and pain in his left chest. He has no previous history of note. On examination he is tall and lean, and seems to be in good health. He has reduced air entry on the left side of his chest and is tachypnoeic. Which ONE of the following is the SINGLE MOST likely diagnosis? Select ONE option only

- ○ A Pleurisy

- ○ B Pulmonary embolus

- ○ C Panic attack

- ○ D Pneumothorax

- ○ E Bronchopneumonia

P2.182 Travel advice

A 24-year-old girl who is about to go travelling for a year consults you for advice on antimalarials. Which ONE of the following statements about prevention of malaria is true? Select ONE option only.

- ○ A Malarone is taken weekly starting 1 week before travel until 4 weeks after return from a malaria region

- ○ B Patients who are entitled to free prescriptions can get antimalarials on an FP10

- ○ C As long as patients take antimalarials as prescribed they are at very low risk of catching malaria

- ○ D Mefloquine is associated with neuropsychiatric side effects in up to 10% of patients

- ○ E Doxycycline is associated with photosensitivity

P2.183 Patient complaints
You receive a letter of complaint from a patient. Which ONE of the following is a requirement relating to the practice response? Select ONE option only.

○ A A written response must be received by the patient within 10 working days

○ B The complaint must be acknowledged within 5 working days

○ C The complaint needs to be considered only if it is received on paper

○ D If the patient's concerns are not satisfied by the practice response, the patient can take the complaint to the Healthcare Commission

○ E There is a time limit of 12 months for practice complaints

P2.184 Mumps
You are telephoned by the mother of a 15-year-old boy who is away on school camp. One of his classmates has just been diagnosed with mumps and his mother is concerned that he is at risk. Which ONE of the following statements about mumps is true? Select ONE option only.

○ A The incubation period is 7–10 days

○ B Salivary gland swelling is pathognomonic and seen in all cases

○ C Ten per cent of patients with mumps develop symptomatic meningeal involvement

○ D Of postpubertal males 80% develop bilateral orchitis

○ E Of those with orchitis 70% become infertile

P2.185 Data interpretation

A trial comparing a new intervention for acute stroke with standard care is carried out, with disability score at 12 months as the primary outcome. The disability score was ranked from 1 to 3, with 1 being the least disabled and 3 the most disabled. The results of the trial are shown below.

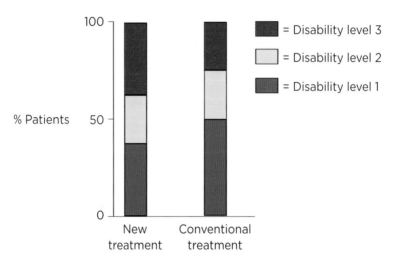

Which ONE of the following statements is correct about these data? Select ONE option only.

○ A The new treatment increases severe disability compared with standard treatment

○ B The new treatment reduces disability at all levels compared with standard treatment

○ C The new treatment reduces severe disability but has no effect on minor disability, compared with conventional treatment

○ D The results are not statistically significant

○ E The results are prone to bias

P2.186 Cholesterol

A 42-year-old man attends having read an article in a newspaper suggesting that people with arcus cornea are at high risk of heart disease and should have statins. He is concerned because he has this condition. His blood pressure is 124/70 mmHg and he does not smoke, is of normal weight and has recently been tested for diabetes as part of a private insurance well man check. Which ONE of the following statements is true about this condition? Select ONE option only.

- ○ A Arcus cornea is a sign of high triglycerides rather than high cholesterol and he should be prescribed a fibrate
- ○ B He is at high risk of cardiovascular disease and should be prescribed aspirin and a statin regardless of his cholesterol level
- ○ C He should be referred to an endocrine clinic due to the association of this condition with the metabolic syndrome
- ○ D He should have his cholesterol measured and be treated according to his calculated cardiovascular risk score, using QRISK or a similar method
- ○ E He should start simvastatin 40 mg once daily

P2.187 Nappy rash

Parents of a formula-fed 4-month-old girl bring her in to see you for a second opinion regarding her nappy rash. Examining her you note a florid rash on the perineum, including the skin creases. They have tried zinc oxide barrier cream and medicated wipes to no avail. Which ONE of the following would be the SINGLE MOST appropriate next step in her management? Select ONE option only.

- ○ A Advise the parents to increase the frequency of nappy changes
- ○ B Change her milk to a hypoallergenic preparation
- ○ C Clotrimazole
- ○ D Hydrocortisone
- ○ E Tacrolimus

P2.188 Breast cancer
You see a 62-year-old woman after she has been diagnosed with ductal carcinoma *in situ* (DCIS) on routine mammography. She asks you to tell her what the diagnosis means for her. Which ONE of the following statements is true regarding DCIS? Select ONE option only.

O   A   It is associated with Paget's disease of the nipple

O   B   It is not usually sensitive to tamoxifen

O   C   It is not associated with invasive disease

O   D   It is rare

O   E   Patients with confirmed DCIS can be treated with watchful waiting

P2.189 Earache
A 9-month-old boy has had earache for the last 2 days. In spite of regular analgesia he is inconsolable and febrile. Examining him his right tympanic membrane is bulging. You decide to prescribe amoxicillin. Write the correct dose in milligrams based on his age in the box below.

P2.190 and P2.191   Diarrhoea and vomiting in children
Which TWO of the following are correct with regard to the management of gastroenteritis in children? Select TWO options only.

O   A   Antidiarrhoeal medications should not be used in children

O   B   Breastfeeding children with gastroenteritis should continue to breastfeed

O   C   Children with gastroenteritis but without clinical dehydration should be advised to drink fruit juice

O   D   Children with gastroenteritis with clinical dehydration should have rehydration via a nasogastric tube

O   E   Milk should be avoided for 7 days after the onset of diarrhoea, to avoid lactose intolerance

P2.192 **Fever**

A 3-year-old child has a 72-hour history of fever of 38–39°C. He has no other symptoms apart from not wanting to walk anywhere. On examination you find no signs of focal infection, and apart from being a little miserable the child seems fine. Urine dipstick is negative. Which ONE of the following must be excluded at this point? Select ONE option only.

○ A Influenza

○ B Irritable hip

○ C Kawasaki's disease

○ D Meningococcal disease

○ E Septic arthritis

P2.193 **Eye problems**

A 77-year-old man complains of difficulty reading over the last few months. His peripheral vision seems normal but he struggles to read print. He has no previous medical history of note apart from having recently stopped smoking. You find his visual acuity to be 6/18 in each eye but visual fields are normal to confrontation. What is the SINGLE MOST likely diagnosis? Select ONE option only.

○ A Acute glaucoma

○ B Age-related macular degeneration

○ C Cataract

○ D Chronic simple glaucoma

○ E Diabetic retinopathy

P2.194 Spasticity

A 9-year-old boy comes to see you with his parents. He has cerebral palsy and attends a specialist school where he has regular physical therapy. In spite of this he gets frequent episodes of pain throughout the day due to muscle spasm. He asks if there is anything that can be done to help. Which ONE of the following would be the SINGLE MOST appropriate management option at this stage?

○ A Baclofen

○ B Botox

○ C Clonazepam

○ D Diazepam

○ E Dorsal rhizotomy

P2.195 Haematuria

A 34-year-old man with no previous medical history of note attends for a new patient check. He brings in a urine sample as instructed, but on dipstick testing is strongly positive for blood. He is asymptomatic and there are no nitrites or leukocytes detected on urinalysis. Which ONE of the following would be the SINGLE MOST appropriate action at this point in his management?

○ A Check blood pressure

○ B Digital rectal examination

○ C Refer for renal ultrasound

○ D Refer to 2-week wait clinic

○ E Send urine for microscopy to confirm haematuria

P2.196 Shortness of breath

A 73-year-old man who is an ex-smoker complains of several months of increasing shortness of breath. On examination he has a few fine crepitations in both lung bases. ECG and blood tests including BNP are normal. You arrange for spirometry at your local hospital, the results of which are shown below.

	FEV_1	FVC	FEV_1/FVC	Transfer factor
Patient reading	2.48	3.26	76	2.91
Percentage predicted	77	78		35

What is the most likely diagnosis? Write your answer in the box below.

P2.197 Dementia

Mr Smith has just been diagnosed with vascular dementia. He comes to see you with his wife to discuss the diagnosis and treatments that may help. Which ONE of the following interventions has been shown to have a significant impact on the rate of decline in cognitive function in patients with vascular dementia? Select ONE option only.

○ A   Acetylcholinesterase inhibitors

○ B   Aggressive control of blood pressure

○ C   Antiplatelet treatment

○ D   Memantine

○ E   Statins

P2.198 Hearing problems

A 76-year-old woman complains of difficulty hearing and bilateral tinnitus. Her audiogram is shown below. What is the SINGLE MOST likely diagnosis? Select ONE option only.

- O A Sudden-onset sensorineural hearing loss
- O B Presbyacusis
- O C Acoustic neuroma
- O D Noise-induced hearing loss
- O E Otosclerosis

P2.199 Data interpretation

Your local commissioning group is looking at the variation in emergency admission rates across the area in an attempt to reduce referrals. They present the following data:

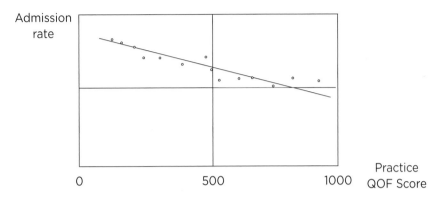

Which ONE of the following statements is true with regard to possible explanations for these results? Select ONE option only.

- ○ A Practices with high QOF scores are more likely to be located in areas with high deprivation scores

- ○ B Practices with high QOF scores might be making more earlier diagnoses, resulting in higher admission rates for elective treatment

- ○ C Practices with high QOF scores might be exception reporting the most sick patients to inflate their QOF scores artificially

- ○ D It is easier to obtain high QOF scores in areas of high morbidity where there are naturally high admission rates

- ○ E Practices with high QOF scores have devolved much of their routine work to non-medical staff, who are better able to manage complex medical problems

P2.200 Fainting

A 74-year-old woman complains of recurrent episodes where she feels dizzy and has fallen on two occasions, once while queuing in the bank and once while waiting for a bus. She denies palpitations. She is being treated for hypertension but is otherwise well. On examination her pulse is 84 and regular, and her heart sounds are normal. Her blood pressure is 124/62 mmHg. What would be the SINGLE MOST appropriate examination to carry out at this stage? Select ONE option only.

- ○ A 24-hour blood pressure

- ○ B 24-hour tape

- ○ C Electrocardiogram

- ○ D Full blood count

- ○ E Standing blood pressure

Paper 2 Answers

P2.1   **D:**   **Push the hook through and out of the skin before cutting off the barb**

The best technique to remove barbed fishing hooks is to inject local anaesthetic around the likely exit point of the barb (or use a ring block for digits) before pushing the hook out through the skin. Once the barb is clear of the skin it can be cut off and the hook then pulled back out through the entry wound. This gives two small scars rather than a much larger scar with incision along the hook or pulling it back out of the wound without removing the barb first. Tetanus status should be checked and wound toilet carried out afterwards.

P2.2   **C:**   **Check his FBC**

This child has symptoms of leukaemia, which is the most common malignant disease in children and often presents with muscle and joint pain. Signs of marrow failure include anaemia, frequent infections and thrombocytopenia, although blast activity may also cause headache, fits and gum hypertrophy.

Lower urinary tract symptoms in men

P2.3   **B:**   α Blocker

P2.4   **D:**   Anticholinergic

P2.5   **A:**   5α-Reductase inhibitor

P2.6   **C:**   α Blocker plus 5α-reductase inhibitor

P2.7   **F:**   Desmopressin

NICE recommend the following as drug treatment for patients bothered by LUTS. An alternative to desmopressin for nocturnal polyuria is a loop diuretic in the late afternoon.

Symptoms	Moderate-to-severe LUTS	Detrusor instability	LUTS with enlarged prostate	LUTS with enlarged prostate despite treatment with 3	Nocturnal polyuria
Treatment	α Blocker	Anticholinergic	5α-Reductase inhibitor	α Blocker + 5α-reductase inhibitor	Desmopressin

P2.8   D: Topical tacrolimus

Vitamin D analogues and coal tar are not suitable for facial psoriasis. If lesions fail to respond to short courses of topical steroids or continuous treatment is needed, topical tacrolimus is more suitable due to a lower risk of side effects. Emollients are unlikely to be effective in this situation.

P2.9   E: Breech presentation is a risk factor

Breech presentation and positive family history are risk factors. Ortolani testing involves attempting to relocate a dislocated hip whereas Barlow testing attempts to dislocate a hip. Ultrasound screening has a high pickup rate but is associated with a high false-positive rate. Most children require splinting only.

P2.10   E: Topical glyceryl trinitrate (GTN)

This patient has symptoms suggestive of an anal fissure; where this is not settling with dietary changes or topical treatment, GTN or diltiazem application may be of benefit.

P2.11   20 mg

In a patient with normal renal and liver function no dose adjustment is required. The total daily morphine dose is 60 mg × 2 = 120 mg.

The bolus dose is therefore 120/6 = 20 mg.

P2.12   A: Asbestosis

Asbestosis is a progressive lung fibrosis caused by inhalation of blue asbestos. It increases the risk of lung cancer 5-fold and in smokers by 55-fold. Industrial compensation is available. The prognosis is poor. Spirometry shows a restrictive defect; however, a chest X-ray may miss fibrosis and CT (computed tomography) may be more appropriate.

P2.13   1 mg

Hypoglycaemia should be treated if possible with oral glucose. If they are unconscious they should be given glucagon. The dose for glucagon is 1 mg for patients over 8 years and 500 mcg for those under 8 kg (or <25 kg). Both oral glucose and glucagon produce a short-lived rise in blood glucose levels and close monitoring is necessary to spot relapse. If not responding 50 ml of 20% intravenous glucose may be given.

Common infections

P2.14   C: 1 week

P2.15   E: 3 weeks

P2.16   D: 2½ weeks

P2.17   B: 4 days

Explaining to patients the natural history of self-limiting infections encourages appropriate use of antibiotics and may potentially improve the utilisation of health resources, through reduced use of appointments for self-limiting illness.

P2.18   D: Refer for lithotripsy

Plantar fasciitis usually responds to orthotics and taping. Where there is no response a steroid injection may provide short-term relief. Where a heel spur is shown on X-ray, lithotripsy is often helpful. Botox is indicated for patients with pes cavus, but is not suitable for athletes. Further injection is unlikely to help.

P2.19   E: She should be treated with a permanent pacemaker

The diagnosis is complete heart block. She should be referred immediately for a pacemaker. The most common cause is ischaemic heart disease. If compromised, atropine 1 mg can be used.

P2.20   E: Vasectomy is reversible in only 50% of cases

The lifetime failure rate is <1:1000. Bruising is very common and the most common long-term complication is pain. It is usually performed under local anaesthetic and sterility should not be assumed until 3 months and two negative sperm counts have passed.

P2.21   E: Silver nitrate cautery may cause septal perforation

Most bleeds are anterior and unilateral with bleeding from Little's area, the plexus of capillaries derived ultimately from the internal and external carotid. The most common cause is idiopathic followed by iatrogenic, with aspirin and warfarin therapy being particular culprits. Bleeding points may be cauterised with silver nitrate but over-zealous or too frequent use of this may result in perforation of the nasal septum. Where pressure fails to settle the bleeding, Merocel packs are easily inserted by nurses or doctors and are extremely effective. BIPP packing is seldom used.

P2.22   A: Dendritic ulcer

This is a typical history of a dendritic ulcer. The appearance could also be seen in corneal abrasion or corneal ulcer in a contact lens wearer, but not with this history. Treatment is with aciclovir five times a day.

P2.23   B: Clarithromycin

This ECG shows a long corrected Q–T interval (>440 ms in men, >460 ms in women). Long Q–T syndrome may be inherited or acquired, usually due to medication or in malnutrition, eg anorexia nervosa where there is low potassium or magnesium. It is associated with syncope and sudden death due to ventricular fibrillation. Iatrogenic long Q–T syndrome is seen with antiarrhythmics (sotalol, amiodarone), macrolide and quinolone antibiotics, antifungals (ketoconazole, fluconazole), diuretics that cause hypokalaemia, eg furosemide, antipsychotics (haloperidol, olanzapine, risperidone quetiapine), methadone and tamoxifen.

P2.24   A: Dementia is usually associated with altered cognition and consciousness

Dementia does not affect consciousness. Where consciousness is affected, consider causes of delirium. Young patients may have metabolic defects, eg Wilson's disease or HIV.

Liver function tests

P2.25   B: Gilbert syndrome

Isolated hyperbilirubinaemia is almost never of pathological significance. This can be demonstrated by taking a fasting bilirubin after an overnight fast.

P2.26   F: Iatrogenic

Enzyme-inducing drugs and alcohol can elevate GGT levels.

P2.27   H: Physiological

ALP may be elevated in adolescence, bone tumours and Paget's disease.

P2.28   E: Hepatitis

Acute hepatitis usually presents with a greatly elevated ALT.

P2.29   A: Gallstones

LFTs usually return to normal after the obstruction has been removed.

P2.30   C: Postural instability is a key symptom in Parkinson's disease

Parkinson's disease is characterized by bradykinesia with muscular rigidity, resting tremor and postural instability. It is usually unilateral initially, progressive and responds well at first to a trial of levodopa. Asymmetry usually persists, and affects the side of onset most. Early dementia, a history of cerebrovascular disease, head injury or encephalitis suggest alternative diagnoses, and use of antipsychotic and dopamine-depleting drugs should be considered in the initial diagnosis.

P2.31   E: This could be a presentation of a renal tumour

Renal colic can be due to direct obstruction by tumour or bleeding from the tumour. Calcium levels can be raised and should be measured. Signs of infection should prompt admission. Stones are not usually visible on a plain film. An NSAID should be used unless contraindicated.

Erectile dysfunction

P2.32   E: Sildenafil

Sildenafil may cause chromatopsia, usually green.

P2.33   A: All of them

Patients who are prone to priapism, such as those with sickle cell disease, should not take treatments for erectile dysfunction.

P2.34   C: MUSE

MUSE is a transurethral system and should not be used in urethral stricture.

P2.35   F: Tadalafil

Tadalafil should be taken at least 30 minutes before sexual activity and the effect may persist for up to 36 hours.

P2.36   A: All of them

Patients with neurological disease, renal failure, diabetes or prostate cancer, or who have had radical pelvic surgery qualify for impotence drugs on the NHS.

P2.37   D: The results should be treated with caution because of inclusion bias

Qualitative studies are notoriously prone to bias. This study has no standardised measure of depression scores at either the outset or the end, consists of self-reporting by patients who self-refer and pay for a treatment in which they presumably have faith, has no control group and relies on the use of only one therapist. It is therefore prone to inclusion bias, reporting bias and a strong placebo effect. The economic analysis is not valid because most patients with mild depression would not need drug treatment. The number needed to treat (NNT) cannot be calculated because there is no comparison group.

P2.38   A: Refer for colonoscopy

This patient has symptoms of a right-sided colonic cancer. Sigmoidoscopy will not visualise the area and barium enema can miss up to 20% of lesions. Raised ESR is consistent with cancer.

P2.39   A: Approximately 4000 people a year commit suicide in England and Wales

There is a bimodal social-class distribution, with middle classes being at lowest risk. Older divorced men who have just lost their jobs and live in towns are most likely to commit suicide. Overdose is the most common method, and violent attempts, such as hanging, are the most likely to succeed. There is a 1–2% risk of deliberate self-harmers committing suicide within 12 months.

Child development

P2.40   A: 6 weeks

P2.41   H: 36 months

P2.42   C: 9 months

At 6 weeks a baby will smile at its mother and watch faces. At 6 months he or she will drink from a cup held up to his or her mouth and smile at his or her image in a mirror and show excitement. At 9 months a baby will respond to his or her name, feed him- or herself with a biscuit and reach for toys. By 12 months there is some understanding of simple instructions and by 15 months the baby will start to feed him- or herself with a spoon, scribble and take shoes off. By 18 months babies may be dry by day and will drink unaided from a cup. By 36 months a child will be able to dress him- or herself with help.

P2.43 and P2.44   Malaise

Part A   Glandular fever

Part B   E: None of the above

This patient has signs, symptoms and blood tests indicative of glandular fever, caused by the Epstein–Barr virus. Treatment is symptomatic and patients should avoid contact sports for at least 6 weeks afterwards, due to the risk of splenic rupture. Ampicillin and amoxicillin should be avoided because they invariably cause a rash. Treatment should be supportive, with fluids, analgesia and antipyretics. Admission is usually required only if there is airway obstruction and most patients recover within 2–3 weeks, although some suffer a prolonged period of malaise.

P2.45   A: Private fees can be set at whatever level the practice wishes

Private fees can be set on a free-market basis but practices should beware exploiting patients where they have no option to go elsewhere, eg for occupational medicals where their registered GP is required to complete a report. The Monopolies Commission banned the BMA from setting recommended fees some years ago. Private work is not covered by the GMS Contract. Private fees should be displayed prominently and patients made aware of these before services are provided.

P2.46   A: Ninety per cent of hip replacements last for more than 10 years

The infection rate is approximately 1%. Crossing the surgical leg over the nonsurgical leg is associated with dislocation. The incidence of deep vein thrombosis (DVT) is 1.5% and of pulmonary embolus (PE) 1.1%. Hip resurfacing is superior to conventional arthroplasty for survival of the prosthesis and preservation of bone mineral density, but is usually indicated only in early disease.

Headache

P2.47   D: Migraine

P2.48   E: Tension headache

P2.49   A: Cluster headache

P2.50   B: Cervicogenic headache

P2.51   C: Medication overuse headache

P2.52   A: Kawasaki's disease

This child has Kawasaki's disease, a febrile vasculitis affecting children. It may cause coronary artery aneurysms in a third of patients and has a mortality rate of around 3%. ECG changes are seen including arrhythmias and long QT interval. Treatment is with aspirin or intravenous immunoglobulin.

P2.53   E: Biventricular failure

This patient has signs of right- and left-sided heart failure. Cor pulmonale is right-sided heart failure secondary to pulmonary disease. The presence of a regular pulse precludes new-onset AF as a diagnosis.

P2.54   D: It may cause phimosis

Balanitis is usually caused by *Candida* sp. or coliforms. Topical antifungals and sometimes fusidic acid are often helpful. Recurrent attacks may cause phimosis and need circumcision. Fifty per cent of 6-year-olds cannot fully retract their foreskin.

P2.55   E: She can start taking the combined oral contraceptive pill immediately but should use condoms or avoid sex for 14 days

Patients who start hormonal contraception immediately after progesterone-only contraception should use condoms or avoid sex for 2 days if using the progesterone-only pill, 7 days for the combined oral contraceptive pill and 9 days for Qlaira. Patients who start hormonal contraception immediately after using ulipristal should use barrier methods for 9 days if starting the progesterone-only pill, 14 days for the combined oral contraceptive and 16 days for Qlaira.

P2.56   D: The condition may be associated with corneal thinning

Keratoconus may be unilateral or bilateral and is characterised by progressive irregularity of the cornea, resulting in astigmatism. In some patients it progresses to corneal thinning and eventually corneal transplantation is required. It can be inherited as either an autosomal recessive or dominant trait, and may be associated with syndromes such as Down, Marfan or Ehlers–Danlos. Milder cases can be treated with contact lenses or glasses, or corneal implants to modify the corneal distortion.

P2.57   E: Scoliosis may be associated with deformity of the skull and ribcage

Of infants with scoliosis 50% will resolve spontaneously. Primary scoliosis often presents in adolescence where it is more common in girls. It is usually midthoracic and the curve is usually concave to the right. It may be associated with plagiocephaly in infants and prominence of the posterior rib cage in teenagers. Treatment where indicated usually involves insertion of rods.

Bleeding in early pregnancy

P2.58   F: Septic abortion

She should be admitted for intravenous antibiotics and ERPC (evacuation of retained products of conception).

P2.59   D: Ectopic pregnancy

An empty uterus and a climbing or static quantitative bhCG suggests a nonuterine pregnancy.

P2.60   B: Cervical incompetence

Cervical incompetence typically causes mid-trimester loss with few contractions.

P2.61   G: Threatened abortion

Of threatened abortions 75% settle spontaneously.

P2.62   D: Ectopic pregnancy

All women with abdominal pain should have a pregnancy test because there may be few gynaecological signs.

P2.63   B: Bronchiolitis

Bronchiolitis occurs in epidemics in winter, caused by respiratory syncytial virus. It is particularly severe in those under 6 months old and can be fatal. High-risk patients (eg congenital heart disease), those with apnoeas or tachypnoeas, and those with failure to feed should be admitted to hospital. Well children can often be managed at home.

P2.64   C: Employers must write to employees in advance of their retirement date and advise them of their rights to apply to work beyond this date

Age discrimination protects elderly and young people. Mandatory retirement cannot be lower than 65 years for men and women. The maximum qualifying length of service for benefits is 5 years. Dismissal on the basis of age is legal from 65 onwards, as long as it can be justified.

P2.65   24 hours

This child has scarlet fever, caused by group B streptococci. It is highly infectious and can be spread by droplets. The Health Protection Agency (2010) 'Guidance on infection control in schools and other childcare settings' suggests school exclusion until 24 hours after commencing antibiotics.

P2.66   E: If *Staphylococcus* sp. is suspected flucloxacillin should be added.

The first-line treatment for community-acquired pneumonia is amoxicillin at a dose of 500–1000 mg three times daily (BTS guidelines), which should cover intermediate resistant strains of *Streptococcus pneumoniae*. In allergic individuals or where atypical pneumonia is suspected, a macrolide is appropriate. During flu outbreaks staphylococcal pneumonia has a high mortality and should be treated with flucloxacillin.

P2.67   C: Paroxetine can increase the period before ejaculation up to eight times longer than placebo

Up to 31% of male respondents to surveys reported premature ejaculation. Clomipramine is useful when taken before intercourse or as a once-daily treatment, but has an adverse side-effect profile in many patients. Paroxetine once daily is the most effective treatment.

Management of epididymitis

P2.68   E: Doxycyline

P2.69   D: Contact tracing

P2.70   C: Ciprofloxacin

Epididymo-orchitis in men <35 is usually caused by sexually transmitted infection such as chlamydial infection, although, in men >35 without risk factors for STIs, it is usually caused by enteric Gram-negative organisms. All patients presenting with symptoms of epidymo-orchitis should have a sexual history taken and antibiotic choice should be guided by this history.

P2.71   C: Lithium is associated with an increase in risk of hypothyroidism

Lithium toxicity is still seen frequently, particularly in the elderly, despite the QOF targets on monitoring and frequent safety advice. Patients should have renal and thyroid function monitored before and regularly after starting treatment, and patients should be warned of common side effects such as tremor, dry mouth, thirst and urinary frequency. Lithium has a narrow therapeutic window and toxicity may develop rapidly with dehydration, pregnancy or renal impairment. There is also a reported association with hyperparathyroidism so calcium levels should also be monitored.

P2.72 and P2.73   Speech problems
A: Language delay has a worse prognosis than speech delay;
E: There is often a family history of speech and language delay

Speech and language delay is seen in 6% of 3- to 4-year-old children, and is more common in boys and those with a family history of the condition. Speech delay is less serious than language delay, but prognosis depends on the underlying cause. First-line investigation should be a hearing test because undiagnosed hearing problems such as glue ear are common reversible causes. It should be noted that there is a wide range of variation within the normal range, particularly with regard to vocabulary.

P2.74   C: The ramipril should be stopped and specialist advice sought

NICE guidance suggests that an increase of 50% in creatinine or a rise to >200 mg/ml should prompt referral. Most cases are caused by occult renal artery stenosis which may cause secondary hypertension. Angiotensin receptor antagonists (ARBs) have the same effect and NICE recommend that both be started under specialist supervision if baseline creatinine >150 mg/ml.

P2.75   B: All prescriptions for controlled drugs must specify the quantity in words and numbers

Controlled drug prescriptions do not need to be hand written but must be written in indelible ink, must be signed in the prescriber's own handwriting, specify the prescriber's address, state the name, strength and form of the medication, and in the case of under-12s the patient's age must be specified in addition to the date of birth. They cannot be sent by Electronic Prescription Service (EPS).

P2.76   C: It is typically triggered by particular head movements

BPPV is rotatory vertigo brought on by head movements in a certain plane, eg lying back in a dentist's chair. It is not associated with any other neuro-otological symptoms and can be demonstrated with Hallpike testing, whereby torsional nystagmus is provoked after a latent period of 15–30 seconds. This fatigues with repeat testing. The presence of other neuro-otological symptoms should prompt further investigations to exclude alternative diagnoses, eg Ménière's disease or cholesteatoma. Acoustic neuromas rarely cause vertigo without other otoneurological symptoms.

P2.77   D: Malignant melanoma

This lesion has the following features of melanoma: asymmetry, size >6 mm, irregular edges or surface and non-uniform pigmentation.

P2.78   A: Patients can be screened for this condition using the SCOFF questionnaire

Anorexia requires a BMI <17.5 kg/m^2 and an inability to eat. Prevalence is 1–2% in women, much lower in men. Over a 4- to 8-year follow-up 2% of patients died and 65% achieved normal weight. The SCOFF questionnaire includes the following questions:

Do you make yourself **S**ick because you feel uncomfortably full?
Do you worry that you have lost **C**ontrol over how much you eat?
Have you recently lost more than **O**ne stone in a 3-month period?
Do you believe yourself to be **F**at when others say that you are too thin?
Would you say that **F**ood dominates your life?

A score of ≥2 indicates a likely case of anorexia nervosa or bulimia.

Cardiovascular drugs

P2.79   B: Atorvastatin

Atorvastatin and rosuvastatin have a triglyceride reducing action, in addition to their effects on cholesterol.

P2.80   L: Sotalol

Sotalol is effective in prophylaxis of AF and may be used while awaiting DC cardioversion to try to cardiovert patients chemically. Flecainide is sometimes used in a 'pill in the pocket' fashion for treating acute attacks of PAF, but is not routinely used for prophylaxis.

P2.81   N: Valsartan

Angiotensin II receptor antagonists are licensed in heart failure and after myocardial infarction.

P2.82   O: Verapamil

Verapamil should not be used in patients with bradycardias or heart block, or those who take β blockers.

P2.83   H: Isosorbide mononitrate

P2.84   M: Spironolactone

P2.85   A: Amiodarone

Amiodarone has a long half-life and is associated with ophthalmic, dermatological and thyroid dysfunction.

P2.86   G: Indapamide

ACE inhibitors and angiotensin II receptor antagonists are first-line treatment in young hypertensive patients, but where renal artery stenosis is present a thiazide is a better choice.

P2.87   B: **Aspirin use in primary prevention reduces risk of non-fatal myocardial infarction**

Aspirin in primary prevention studies has been shown to reduce the risk of myocardial infarction, but the gains are offset by an increase in risk of gastrointestinal bleeding. The risk of bleeding seems highest in the first 1–2 years and falls off with duration of use. There is a large body of evidence that aspirin will reduce the risk of cancer, particularly colorectal, and also reduce the risk of metastases. There is also a transient increase in risk of MI on stopping aspirin. At present, the consensus is that there is insufficient evidence to recommend aspirin or other antiplatelets for primary prevention in patients who are otherwise well.

P2.88   B: **Cryotherapy**

Cryotherapy given at 3-weekly intervals will cure 75% of warts after four treatments. Side effects such as pain and blistering are common, and patients should be warned of the risk of hypopigmentation and tendon damage. Excision should be avoided due to risk of scarring, and all patients should be advised that two-thirds of cases of warts spontaneously resolve within 2 years, and a third within 6 months. Podophyllin and bleomycin are not usually used for simple warts due to their side-effect profile.

P2.89   E: **Patients with recurrent symptoms can use flecainide as a 'pill-in-the-pocket' treatment**

AF affects 0.4% of the general population, but incidence increases sharply with age, with a lifetime risk of 1:4 shown in the Framingham study. Patients should be anticoagulated if they have persistent prolonged attacks and are at high risk, eg coexisting hypertension, smoking. Reductions in alcohol, caffeine, stress and smoking help to reduce the incidence of the condition. In patients with a structurally normal heart flecainide is effective as treatment.

P2.90   E: Raised ALP suggests that the diagnosis is gallstones

Gallstones cause either a flatulent dyspepsia or biliary colic. Colic tends to be severe and can require treatment with pethidine injection. Pain usually comes 60–120 minutes after fatty meals and can last several hours. It is usually associated with raised ALP and stones can cause pancreatitis or obstructive jaundice. Where associated with weight loss, cancer should be considered in the differential diagnosis.

P2.91   C: Earache, trismus and dysphagia are typical symptoms

Most cases are caused by streptococcal infections, and the abscess is outside the tonsillar capsule close to the upper pole of the tonsil. The patient is usually unwell and unable to swallow fluids or solids. Intravenous fluids and intravenous broad-spectrum antibiotics, with interval tonsillectomy, are the usual management options.

P2.92   B: Excision biopsy

The main differentials for this lesion are squamous cell carcinoma and keratoacanthoma. The rapid growth merits urgent excision biopsy and this patient should be referred under the 2-week rule. Cryotherapy does not provide tissue for histological diagnosis and is therefore unsuitable. 5-Fluorouracil and ingenol mebutate are treatments for solar keratosis. Although keratoacanthomas spontaneously regress in most cases, watchful waiting is not suitable, without histological diagnosis, for confirmation that this is not a squamous cell carcinoma.

Traveller's diarrhoea

P2.93   E: *Giardia lamblia*

This is a protozoal diarrhoea and accounts for between 1% and 6% of cases of traveller's diarrhoea. It is common in travellers to south and south-east Asia and may cause chronic diarrhoea with steatorrhoea; it is often associated with upper GI side effects such as bloating and belching.

P2.94   D: ETEC

This causes a profuse watery diarrhoea often preceded by cramps and nausea, and usually settles within 48–72 hours. It is more commonly reported in sub-Saharan Africa and Latin America.

P2.95   G: Cholera

This is asymptomatic in 75% of infections but, of those patients with symptoms, 20% develop profound watery diarrhoea and hypovolaemia. Without treatment death can occur, but with adequate fluid rehydration most patients recover within 24–72 hours.

ETEC is the most common reported cause of traveller's diarrhoea, accounting for up to 34% of reported cases, followed by *Campylobacter* spp. (up to 32% cases). Rotavirus and norovirus account for between 20% and 25% of cases combined. *Campylobacter* and *Shigella* spp. tend to cause lower GI symptoms such as tenesmus, blood diarrhoea and urgency, whereas *Giardia* sp. tends to cause upper

GI symptoms such as bloating and belching. Of cases of traveller's diarrhoea 90% last for ≤7 days and only 1% last ≥30 days. *Giardia*, *Cryptosporidium* and *Shigella* spp. tend to cause more prolonged infection.

P2.96 and P2.97   Chest infection

Part A   2

Part B   A: Admit to hospital

This patient's CRB-65 score is 2 (age, tachypnoea) so he should be admitted to hospital. The CRB-65 score awards one point for each of confusion, respiratory rate >30, blood pressure with systolic <90 mmHg or diastolic <60 mmHg and age ≥65 years.

Patients with a score of 0 can safely be managed at home, whereas those with a score of 1 or 2 should be admitted to hospital. Patients with a score of ≥3 are at high risk of death and should be admitted immediately. Oxygen saturation <92% suggests admission is likely to be necessary.

P2.98   D: It often gets worse during pregnancy

Otosclerosis is an autosomal dominant disease with incomplete penetrance that affects 0.5–2% of the population, has a sex ratio of 2 females:1 male, and is more common in white people. It tends to worsen during pregnancy, menstruation and the menopause. Most patients present before the age of 30. It causes a conductive hearing loss, slightly worse at lower frequencies, often with a dip in the bone-conduction thresholds at 2 kHz. Stapedectomy is an effective treatment but there is a risk of hearing loss, so many patients choose to wear hearing aids instead. There is some evidence that the incidence is falling, thought to be a result of the use of fluoride in drinking water.

P2.99   D: Long-term oral tetracycline is effective in reducing frequency of attacks

Hidradenitis suppurativa is not a disease of apocrine glands, but rather an acne-like condition. Treatment options include short courses of antibiotics and oral steroids or local steroid injections. Long-term antibiotics may be useful and as a last resort some patients may require surgery. Dianette may be helpful in women because of the cyproterone acetate component.

P2.100   E: None

This patient has ruptured the long head of biceps, which produces a characteristic Popeye appearance. No treatment is needed.

P2.101   E: It is exclusively seen in children

Epiglottitis is usually seen in young children, but may be seen in adults, where the principal complaint is of severe pain on swallowing. The most common differential is croup, but children with epiglottitis are much sicker and should be admitted as an emergency before attempting to examine the child.

P2.102   C: Reassurance with safety netting advice

This lesion is a lipoma. Typically lipomas have a soft, fluctuant feeling, and are non-tender, lobulated and free of overlying skin. There is no punctum, and no associated lymphadenopathy. Suspected lipomas that are >5 cm in diameter or slowly growing should be referred under the 2-week rule to exclude liposarcoma. The contents of the lipoma cannot be aspirated, but they can usually be removed easily under local anaesthetic. Removal may be indicated for cosmetic reasons or when it causes functional impairment. If there is diagnostic uncertainty as to whether this is a lymph node an ultrasound may be helpful.

P2.103   D: Prucalopride

Prucalopride, a $5\text{-}HT_4$ agonist, is licensed for the treatment of chronic idiopathic constipation in women in whom treatment with two different classes of laxative at the highest tolerated dose has failed. Co-danthrusate is no longer recommended due to risk of carcinogenicity, whereas methylnaltrexone is an acute treatment for opioid-related constipation. Sodium picosulfate is used in preparation for surgery or colonoscopy. The trial data used to license prucalopride included only women, so it is licensed only for use in women.

P2.104   B: The wounds should be cleaned with saline, and closed

The human mouth is full of anaerobes and aerobes that can rapidly cause severe illness. All patients in whom the skin is punctured should receive antibiotics and a tetanus booster, and those with any signs of spread should be admitted to either orthopaedics or plastic surgery according to the site of the bite. Always consider a foreign body as a cause of infection in traumatic wounds.

P2.105   B: Graduated loading with eccentric exercises should be used as first-line treatment

Steroid injections provide good short-term relief of symptoms, but there is evidence that they increase the risk of recurrence and may delay healing. Avoidance of the irritating action together with eccentric muscle loading is the first-line treatment. There is some evidence for the short-term use of topical NSAIDs and GTN patches in resistant cases. Where these treatments fail, referral for surgery or Botox should be considered.

Drug management of Parkinson's disease

P2.106   G: Pramipexole

Pramipexole and ropinirole are associated with impulse control disorders, with a 14% lifetime risk. Common symptoms are hypersexuality and pathological gambling.

P2.107   C: Citalopram

SSRIs are the first-line choice for depression, which affects up to 50% of patients. Tricyclics should be avoided due to sedation and risk of falls.

P2.108   I: Selegiline

MAO-B inhibitors such as selegiline are useful on their own or in combination with dopamine.

P2.109   D: Clozapine

Psychotic symptoms such as hallucinations are very common in Parkinson's disease in advanced stages. Clozapine is an effective treatment.

P2.110   E: Vertebrobasilar stroke

The presence of brain-stem symptoms with dizziness is suggestive of a brainstem ischaemic event, rather than a labyrinthine process. Labyrinthitis would normally cause rotatory vertigo, with nystagmus but not dysarthria or upper limb symptoms. Ménière's disease causes vertigo, fluctuating hearing and tinnitus, which recur, with asymptomatic periods in between. Vestibular neuronitis causes acute severe rotatory vertigo with unilateral tinnitus and nausea, without associated neurological symptoms. Migraine may cause labyrinthine or isolated neurological symptoms but this pattern is much more suggestive of a brain-stem event.

P2.111   E: Chickenpox

Chickenpox typically presents with a non-specific febrile illness followed by the development of a vesicular rash. Measles usually starts on the back of the neck and is also associated with conjunctival symptoms. Parvovirus B19 causes a slapped cheek appearance.

Prescription charges

P2.112   H: Not entitled to free prescriptions

Patients with diabetes treated with drugs are entitled to free prescriptions.

P2.113   C: Entitled to free NHS dental treatment

Women who are pregnant and up to 12 months postpartum are entitled to free dental treatment and NHS prescriptions.

P2.114   G: Not entitled to free NHS sight test

Myxoedema gives exemption from prescription charges not eye tests.

P2.115   B: Automatically entitled to free prescriptions

People aged 16, 17 or 18 and in full-time education are exempt from charges.

P2.116   E: Entitled to free prescriptions on applying for an exemption certificate

Those patients who need replacement therapy, or have medically treated diabetes, epilepsy or a fistula, are entitled to free prescriptions on applying and receiving an exemption certificate.

P2.117   B: Varicose eczema

Asteatotic eczema results from loss of lubricating fluid from the skin; it presents as a crazy paving pattern on the lower legs. Psoriasis causes thickened plaques of skin over flexor aspects, eg elbows. Pompholyx affects the soles of the feet and the palms of the hands.

Examination of the eye

P2.118   H: Retinoblastoma

Retinoblastoma is often diagnosed by loss of red reflex and has been picked up from family photos when one person has no red eye.

P2.119   F: Optic atrophy

Optic neuritis causes disc pallor; in the acute phase the disc may also be swollen.

P2.120   A: Acute angle-closure glaucoma

Unlike uveitis, the pupil is fixed but round.

P2.121   G: Recurrent uveitis

Recurrent uveitis causes adhesions around the periphery of the iris.

P2.122   C: Chronic glaucoma

The cup:disc ratio is used to monitor the progression of glaucoma.

P2.123   E: None of the above

Café-au-lait patches are brown macules, usually present from birth. They affect up to 10% of people and, when there are fewer than four patches <0.5 cm and no patches >1.5 cm, they are of no significance. Multiple patches are suggestive of neurofibromatosis or Albright syndrome, characterised by cystic bone lesions and precocious puberty. Tuberous sclerosis is characterised by shagreen patches that fluoresce under UV light. Patients with Bloom syndrome have short stature, telangiectasia and facial erythema.

P2.124   D: Chalazion

Chalazions are retention cysts in meibomian glands. They are similar in appearance to styes but lack signs of acute inflammation. Often settling spontaneously, where this does not happen and patients are symptomatic, incision and curettage may be indicated. Infected chalazions are treated in the same way as styes.

Antibiotic prescribing

P2.125   L: Nitrofurantoin

Nitrofurantoin is the most appropriate choice in this case. Co-trimoxazole (Septrin) is a combination of trimethoprim and sulfamethoxazole.

P2.126   F: Ciprofloxacin

Ciprofloxacin is a useful alternative to rifampicin as prophylaxis.

P2.127   M: Phenoxymethylpenicillin

Phenoxymethylpenicillin is the first-line treatment for tonsillitis in patients who do not have penicillin allergy.

P2.128   H: Erythromycin

Erythromycin has a similar spectrum of activity to amoxicillin and also covers atypical pneumonia.

P2.129   C: Co-amoxiclav

All dog and cat bites or scratches should be treated with co-amoxiclav or doxycycline and metronidazole if penicillin allergic.

P2.130   A: Emergency treatment involves an immediate insulin injection and fluid rehydration

DKA may follow a prodromal illness or present acutely as a consequence of an intercurrent illness. There is often abdominal pain and vomiting, and polydipsia with polyuria. Patients are often significantly dehydrated, although frequently they have an apparent hyperkalaemia on blood testing. Examination findings include tachypnoea and ketotic breath.

P2.131   E: It is usually a sign of underlying malignancy

Common causes of erythema nodosum include streptococcal infections, sarcoidosis, infections and drugs. Treatment is conservative and aimed at the underlying cause.

P2.132

Age	Food
<4 months	Milk
4–6 months	Rice
6–9 months	Meat
9–12 months	Adult food

Ideal starting foods for weaning are fruit or vegetable purées and non-wheat cereal such as rice. Eggs, fish and meat are usually introduced at 6–9 months and most babies should be able to manage mashed family meals at 9–12 months.

P2.133   E: Superior vena caval obstruction

Superior vena caval obstruction may develop rapidly and may be thrombotic. Stridor suggests obstruction of the main bronchus or trachea. The oedema and venous engorgement are seen in the watershed area of the SVC, and in some cases collateral circulation may cause dilated veins on the abdomen. The most common cause is primary bronchial carcinoma, followed by lymphoma, thymoma, retrosternal goitre and thoracic aortic aneurysm. Initial treatment is usually with dexamethasone followed by treatment of the cause.

Psychological therapies for alcohol abuse

P2.134   D: Cognitive–behavioural therapy

P2.135   A: 12-step facilitation

P2.136   G: Structured brief advice

The 12-step facilitation is based on the Alcoholics Anonymous approach and seeks to combine abstinence with active participation in group meetings. Structured brief advice can be carried out by non-specialists in 5–15 minutes and is based on the FRAMES principles (feedback, responsibility, advice, menu, empathy and self-efficacy) and uses structured advice tools. Aversion therapy uses noxious stimuli to reinforce abstinence, whereas social skills training seeks to deal with the underlying stressors that stimulate alcohol abuse. Couples therapy focuses on the harm caused to relationships.

P2.137   GLP-1 mimetic

NICE (NG 28, 2015) suggests addition of a glucagon-like peptide 1 (GLP-1) mimetic at this stage in patients who are overweight and will not take insulin. Exenatide and liraglutide are available in the UK for this purpose. They stimulate endogenous insulin production in a glucose-dependent fashion and delay gastric emptying, encouraging weight loss. They do not cause hypoglycaemia unless used with sulfonylureas, and can cause pancreatitis.

P2.138   A: On the date that the data were collected, 8.3 per 100 000 people had the disease

Prevalence gives a snapshot of the number of people with a specified disease on the sampling date. It does not matter whether the disease is acute and self-limiting, eg influenza, or chronic, eg hypertension; it is simply the number of people suffering on that day. Incidence of a disease is the number of people diagnosed with a disease within a specified time frame, usually annually. For an acute self-limiting disease that is seen annually, eg influenza, the prevalence will be much lower than the incidence, because most people are acutely affected and recover within a short period, so only appear in prevalence figures for 2–3 weeks. They will, however, appear in incidence figures until the next sampling time frame.

P2.139   B: Hydroxychloroquine will reduce pain, swelling and stiffness in SLE

Hydroxychloroquine is effective in SLE and RA. Infliximab is for use in active RA only. Sulfasalazine causes reversible effects on fertility. Methotrexate may take some weeks to become effective.

P2.140   B: Rheumatoid arthritis

Primary nodal osteoarthritis affects the distal interphalangeal joints of the fingers. Reiter syndrome usually involves iritis or conjunctivitis. Gout would be unlikely to affect both sides simultaneously.

P2.141   D: The implementation of change is implicit in the audit cycle

The audit cycle is the process of setting standards, measuring performance, diagnosing the problem, implementing change and then re-measuring. Standards can be 'soft', such as the number of complaints, or 'hard', such as the number of patients treated to a blood pressure target.

P2.142   D: Foreign body

These are the tips of cotton buds. They frequently dislodge during ear cleaning to leave the cotton wool in the ear canal. This then causes a recurrent otitis externa and is often associated with an offensive smell. It is good practice when atypical or recurrent otitis externa presents in a patient to arrange review after treatment to ensure no underlying causes such as perforation, foreign body or cholesteatoma. Fungal otitis externa is usually identifiable by hyphae and spores, but does not usually cause large lumps of material. Cholesteatoma usually causes scant debris deep in the canal, rather than large lumps of debris.

Shoulder problems

P2.143   D: Referred pain

Pain in the shoulder may be a sign of diaphragmatic irritation, eg cholecystitis or ruptured ectopic.

P2.144   C: Osteoarthritis

Long-standing pain and reduced range of movement suggest osteoarthritis rather than rotator cuff and the history is too long for frozen shoulder. There is often prominent lipping of the joint.

P2.145   A: Cervical spondylosis

Cervical spondylosis may be present with or without neurological symptoms.

P2.146   B: Frozen shoulder

Frozen shoulder affects all movements but external rotation is particularly affected.

P2.147   H: Subluxation of the glenohumeral joint

This is a typical description of a dislocated shoulder.

P2.148   E: Send bloods for bile acid levels, and if these are normal repeat if itching persists

Intrahepatic cholestasis of pregnancy, characterised by intense itching in the absence of a rash, should be considered in all women complaining of itching, especially during the third trimester. Liver function tests using trimester-specific ranges, including bile acids, should be checked. Alkaline phosphatase is usually elevated in pregnancy and bile acids must be checked, together with fetal monitoring. If these are normal, and itching persists, the blood test should be repeated weekly. Delayed diagnosis is associated with an increased risk of stillbirth and perinatal morbidity. Although 23% of women experience pruritus during pregnancy <1.5% develop intrahepatic cholestasis.

Medical records legislation

P2.149   A: Access to Health Records Act

P2.150   E: Data Protection Act

P2.151   A: Access to Health Records Act

P2.152   C: Children's Act

P2.153   B: Access to Medical Reports Act

P2.154   A: Access to Health Records Act

Red eye

P2.155   A: Acute glaucoma

P2.156   E: Keratitis

P2.157   B: Anterior uveitis

P2.158   F: Scleritis

P2.159   D: Episcleritis

P2.160   C: Conjunctivitis

P2.161   E: It may be helped with lactase added to feeds

Colic is a disease of unknown origin but some evidence suggests that it may be caused by temporary lactose intolerance. It occurs in 20% of infants and usually lasts up to 3 months of age. Dicyclomine is contraindicated in those aged under 6 months. Vomiting suggests alternative diagnoses, eg constipation, Hirschsprung's disease.

Female Urinary Problems

P2.162   D: Overflow urinary incontinence

This results from a lack of detrusor contraction and the bladder accommodates excessive urine without an increase in intravesical pressure. It is most commonly due to hypotonic bladder or chronic retention caused by bladder outflow obstruction. It may also follow radical pelvic surgery. Treatment is by intermittent self-catheterisation.

P2.163   E: True urinary incontinence

This is the result of a fistula between the ureter or bladder and the uterus or vagina. Most cases are the result of pelvic surgery or irradiation, and 50% are caused by simple hysterectomy. In developing countries, obstructed labour or forceps delivery is a common cause. Surgical repair is the treatment of choice.

P2.164   C: Mixed urinary incontinence

Patients may complain of pure urge incontinence, pure stress incontinence or mixed urinary incontinence. Where urgency is associated with nocturia and frequency, this suggests overactive bladder syndrome. This can be confirmed on urodynamics where detrusor overactivity is evident.

Accurate classification of incontinence is crucial in management. NICE guidelines (2013) recommend, where urgency or overactive bladder syndrome, is suspected a trial of weight loss, reducing caffeine and modification of fluid intake, together with pelvic floor exercises for a minimum of 3 months in stress or mixed incontinence. Anticholinergic drugs should be used where there is no response, but with caution in frail elderly women.

P2.165 B: Levothyroxine dose should be increased by 30% at the booking appointment.

The required dose in pregnancy always increases, and dose should be increased by 30–50% at booking to avoid maternal hypothyroidism. Regular monitoring every 6 weeks is recommended to maintain a low normal TSH in the first trimester, unless trimester-specific TSH rages are available. The aim is to maintain a euthyroid state, and levothyroxine treatment of women with subclinical hypothyroidism is associated with better maternal obstetric outcomes.

P2.166 Notifiable diseases

Notifiable disease	Not notifiable disease
Measles	*Chlamydia trachomatis* infection
Mumps	Chickenpox
Rubella	Leptospirosis
Scarlet fever	Ophthalmia neonatorum
Tuberculosis	Lyme disease
Whooping cough	Influenza

The Health Protection (notification) Regulations (2010) require doctors to notify the local health protection team of any cases of the following diseases: encephalitis, meningitis, poliomyelitis, acute hepatitis, anthrax, botulism, brucellosis, cholera, diphtheria, enteric fever, food poisoning, HUS, group A streptococci (including scarlet fever), Legionnaires' disease, leprosy, malaria, measles, mumps, rubella, plague, rabies, severe acute respiratory syndrome (SARS), smallpox, tetanus, TB, typhus, whooping cough and yellow fever. Since 2010 it has no longer been a requirement to notify dysentery, ophthalmia neonatorum, leptospirosis or relapsing fever.

P2.167 E: Lung cancer

With a smoking history, clubbing and weight loss, cancer is the most likely diagnosis. Cystic fibrosis and congenital heart disease cause shortness of breath and clubbing but present earlier. Pneumonia would not normally cause clubbing; however, bronchiectasis may cause shortness of breath and clubbing.

P2.168   E: It may be a sign of female virilisation

Crypto-orchidism and hypospadias raise the possibility of female virilisation. The condition is seen in 1:300 male births. Epispadias, where the opening is on the upper, dorsal side of the penis, may be associated with bladder abnormalities. Mild cases of hypospadias may present in adulthood.

Hirsutism

P2.169   A: Combined oral contraceptive

In women with no biochemical evidence of hormonal imbalance a combined oral contraceptive is the best initial treatment.

P2.170   E: Finasteride

In women who are unable to take the COCP, or in whom it is not effective, finasteride may be effective. Adequate contraception is essential.

P2.171   D: Electrolysis

Cosmetic techniques should be considered for all women, particularly where hair is localised.

P2.172   C: Dianette

Dianette is licensed for the treatment of hirsutism and acne. It is preferable to cyproterone alone because adequate contraception is needed to prevent feminisation of a male fetus in the event of unplanned pregnancy.

P2.173   H: Referral

This woman probably has polycystic ovary syndrome. Referral is indicated to optimise chances of conception and control symptoms.

Dizziness and vertigo

P2.174   F: Ménière's disease

This is a classic description of Ménière's disease.

P2.175   J: Vestibular neuronitis

Vestibular neuronitis tends to produce severe vertigo, which often causes people to take to their beds for several days. It is thought to be viral.

P2.176   C: Cardiogenic syncope

Vestibular disease causes rotatory vertigo. Light-headedness without vertigo is seldom caused by otological disease.

P2.177   B: Benign paroxysmal positional vertigo

Benign paroxysmal positional vertigo causes maximal symptoms when the affected semicircular canal is stimulated more than the others.

P2.178   G: Ramsay Hunt syndrome

Herpes zoster affecting the geniculate ganglion may cause facial nerve paralysis, vertigo and sensorineural deafness. It should be treated with aciclovir and steroids.

P2.179   C: A raised PSA may be caused by urinary infection

PSA is neither highly specific nor sensitive. A significant number of people with prostate cancer are missed by PSA testing and many undergo prostate biopsy without having cancer confirmed. Old age, prostatic hyperplasia, infection and instrumentation can all elevate the PSA. There are age-specific cut-offs for elevated PSA.

P2.180   A: He should be converted to a twice-daily maintenance dose of methadone and this should be gradually reduced

Methadone is given once daily and has a long half-life. Buprenorphine is safer in overdose and less addictive than methadone. Management of opiate abuse includes a holistic approach to lifestyle risk factors.

P2.181   D: Pneumothorax

Spontaneous pneumothorax is often idiopathic but, where recurrent, CT may demonstrate bullae. In this instance surgical pleurodesis may be indicated. In spontaneous pneumothorax cyanosis is rare. Spontaneous pneumothorax can often be treated with needle aspiration.

P2.182   E: Doxycycline is associated with photosensitivity

Malarone needs to be taken only from 2 days before entering a malaria zone until 1 week after leaving. It is taken daily. Antimalarials are available only on private prescription. Mefloquine causes serious neuropsychiatric side effects in less than 1% of patients, but patients often report milder symptoms such as vivid dreams. It should be avoided in patients with a history of psychiatric illness. All patients should use insect repellents, long trousers and sleeves, and consider insect nets.

P2.183   A: A written response must be received by the patient within 10 working days

There is a time limit of 6 months for practice complaints. The complaint must be acknowledged within 2 working days. Complaints may be verbal, written or emailed to the practice. The Healthcare Commission deals with the process of the complaint, not the substance. There is a time limit of 6 months from the incident, but this can be extended, eg if a patient was too ill to complain. Out-of-hours complaints should be made to the relevant PCO (primary care organisation).

P2.184   C: Ten per cent of patients with mumps develop symptomatic meningeal involvement

The incubation period is usually around 18 days. Of patients 70% develop salivary gland involvement, and infection is by droplets or fomites. Although 25% of postpubertal males develop orchitis, it is unilateral in 80% and hence the risk of infertility is low.

P2.185   A: The new treatment increases severe disability compared with standard treatment

The graph suggests that more patients in the new treatment group will experience severe disability than in the usual treatment group. This type of study is prone to recording and inclusion bias but without information on study design and confidence intervals it is not possible to comment on statistical significance or possible bias.

P2.186.   D: He should have his cholesterol measured and be treated according to his calculated cardiovascular risk score, using QRISK or a similar method

The Copenhagen Heart Study found that xanthelasmas are a predictor of ischaemic heart disease, myocardial infarction, atherosclerosis and death independent of other risk factors, including lipid levels. Arcus cornea, on the other hand, was not associated with increased risk. This patient is not therefore at increased risk due to his arcus but he should have his cholesterol measured so that he can be reassured about his 10-year risk scores. It is unlikely, however, that he would reach the threshold for intervention given his normal blood pressure, lack of smoking and diabetes.

P2.187   C: Clotrimazole

Nappy rash that affects the skin creases is usually caused by *Candida* sp. Less commonly it can be caused by bacterial infection or dermatitis. Treatment with clotrimazole and more regular nappy changes/leaving the nappy off help. Where nappy rash spares creases, it is usually caused by irritant dermatitis. Barrier creams, regular nappy changes and use of baby wipes all help in this situation.

P2.188   A: It is associated with Paget's disease of the nipple

Eczematous lesions on the nipple, often associated with discharge, are frequently associated with DCIS. The rate of progression to invasive cancer is 30–50% and the tumours are usually estrogen receptor positive. DCIS is frequently picked up at an early stage on mammography due to the presence of microcalcification.

P2.189   62.5 mg three times daily

The dose for amoxicillin based on age is 62.5 mg three times daily up to 1 year, from 1 year to 8 years 125 mg three times daily, and >8 years 250 mg three times daily.

P2.190 and 2.191   Diarrhoea and vomiting in children
A: Antidiarrheal medications should not be used in children;
B: Breastfeeding children with gastroenteritis should continue to breastfeed

Most cases of gastroenteritis in the UK are viral and usually self-limiting. Breastfeeding mothers should continue to breastfeed, but if there is concern over dehydration supplemental fluids should be given. Fruit juice should be avoided in the presence of dehydration because these are hyperosmolar and may worsen dehydration. Where there is evidence of clinical dehydration, oral rehydration solutions (ORSs) should be used. If an ORS is not tolerated, admission for nasogastric fluids may be indicated. Neither antibiotics nor antispasmodics should be used routinely and, once rehydrated, full-strength milk should be reinstituted.

P2.192   E: Septic arthritis

A child with a fever and joint or limb swelling, failure to use a limb or inability/reluctance to weight bear should have septic arthritis or osteomyelitis excluded. Irritable hip has a subacute presentation and affects older children, usually around age 6 years. Kawasaki's disease causes fever and all of: bilateral conjunctival injection, change in mucous membranes, polymorphous rash and cervical lymphadenopathy. Children with meningococcal disease are usually very ill, often with a non-blanching rash.

P2.193   B: Age-related macular degeneration

Age-related macular degeneration (ARMD) typically causes painless loss of central vision, often with visual distortion, and relative sparing of peripheral vision. It typically affects the over-50 age group and is the most common cause of blindness in the over-65s. The risk of developing ARMD is 3.6 times higher in smokers. Chronic simple glaucoma causes loss of peripheral vision with central preservation until late in the disease, and acute glaucoma causes severe pain at onset. It would be unusual to develop symptomatic diabetic retinopathy without overt features of diabetes, and vision is usually relatively normal, unless macular oedema or haemorrhages occur.

P2.194   A: Baclofen

NICE guidance for management of spasticity in patients with cerebral palsy advises that all patients should have physical therapy as part of a multidisciplinary team approach, with consideration of orthoses. Where these fail to control symptoms, oral baclofen is the most appropriate medication for day-time use. Benzodiazepines are helpful at night where sedation is less of a problem. Focal spasticity affecting motor function, eg in the hand, can be treated with Botox, whereas intrathecal baclofen or dorsal rhizotomy may help if medication fails.

P2.195   A: Check blood pressure

Persistent microscopic haematuria is common, and usually benign, but may be a sign of renal disease. The most common cause is infection, so this should be excluded with urinary culture. A blood pressure check as part of the initial assessment is mandatory to pick up renal disease and, if elevated, should prompt a routine referral. All patients with persistent haematuria should have baseline renal function and urine protein assessment. Urine microscopy, unless on very fresh urine, has low sensitivity and prostate cancer is an unlikely cause for microscopic haematuria in asymptomatic men. Renal ultrasound is indicated if there are symptoms suggestive of renal colic.

P2.196   Pulmonary fibrosis

Pulmonary fibrosis causes a restrictive lung defect so the FEV_1 and FVC will both be reduced, hence the normal FEV_1/FVC. The transfer factor is markedly reduced, however, confirming the probable diagnosis of pulmonary fibrosis.

P2.197   B: Aggressive control of blood pressure

Unlike Alzheimer's disease, vascular dementia is usually unresponsive to acetylcholinesterase inhibitors or memantine. Slight benefits in cognition have been reported in some trials, but these are thought to be due to presumed coexistent Alzheimer's disease-type neuropathology. Aggressive treatment of blood pressure has been shown to reduce the risk of the disease and also slow its rate of decline if used early in the disease. This has not been shown to be true for antiplatelet or statin use.

P2.198   B: Presbyacusis

A symmetrical, high-frequency, sensorineural loss is characteristic of presbyacusis. Bilateral tinnitus is not a sign of acoustic neuroma.

P2.199   B: Practices with high QOF scores might be making more earlier diagnoses, resulting in greater admission rates for elective treatment

Practices with high QOF scores are more likely to be in areas of low deprivation. Exception reporting will inflate the QOF score but not affect the admission rate. Non-medical staff tend to be very good at rigid, protocol-led work, such as collecting data, but are less capable of managing complex problems.

P2.200   E: Standing blood pressure

This woman has symptoms of postural hypotension and this can be confirmed by checking blood pressure supine and standing. A drop of 20 mmHg is considered significant. Common causes include antihypertensives, L-dopa and anxiolytics. Other common causes include venous pooling after prolonged standing, poor muscle tone, eg bed-bound patients or hypovolaemia (blood loss, diarrhoea). A 24-hour tape is useful for the diagnosis of intermittent arrhythmia whereas a 24-hour blood pressure can differentiate white coat hypertension from sustained hypertension. An ECG is also indicated in this situation but a standing blood pressure should be carried out as part of her baseline observations.

Index

Question numbers beginning with 'P' refer to the practice papers at the end of the book.